CBT TREATMENT PLANS AND INTERVENTIONS FOR DEPRESSION AND ANXIETY DISORDERS IN YOUTH

TREATMENT PLANS AND INTERVENTIONS
FOR EVIDENCE-BASED PSYCHOTHERAPY
Robert L. Leahy, Series Editor

Each volume in this practical series synthesizes current information on a particular disorder or clinical population; shows practitioners how to develop specific, tailored treatment plans; and describes interventions proven to promote behavior change, reduce distress, and alleviate symptoms. Step-by-step guidelines for planning and implementing treatment are illustrated with rich case examples. User-friendly features include reproducible self-report forms, handouts, and symptom checklists, all in a convenient large-size format. Specific strategies for handling treatment roadblocks are also detailed. Emphasizing a collaborative approach to treatment, books in this series enable practitioners to offer their clients the very best in evidence-based practice.

TREATMENT PLANS AND INTERVENTIONS FOR DEPRESSION
AND ANXIETY DISORDERS, SECOND EDITION
Robert L. Leahy, Stephen J. F. Holland, and Lata K. McGinn

TREATMENT PLANS AND INTERVENTIONS FOR BULIMIA
AND BINGE-EATING DISORDER
Rene D. Zweig and Robert L. Leahy

TREATMENT PLANS AND INTERVENTIONS FOR INSOMNIA:
A CASE FORMULATION APPROACH
Rachel Manber and Colleen E. Carney

TREATMENT PLANS AND INTERVENTIONS
FOR OBSESSIVE–COMPULSIVE DISORDER
Simon A. Rego

CBT WITH JUSTICE-INVOLVED CLIENTS:
INTERVENTIONS FOR ANTISOCIAL AND SELF-DESTRUCTIVE BEHAVIORS
Raymond Chip Tafrate, Damon Mitchell, and David J. Simourd

CBT TREATMENT PLANS AND INTERVENTIONS
FOR DEPRESSION AND ANXIETY DISORDERS IN YOUTH
Brian C. Chu and Sandra S. Pimentel

CBT Treatment Plans and Interventions for Depression and Anxiety Disorders in Youth

Brian C. Chu
Sandra S. Pimentel

Series Editor's Note by Robert L. Leahy

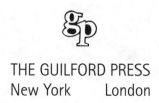

THE GUILFORD PRESS
New York   London

Copyright © 2023 The Guilford Press
A Division of Guilford Publications, Inc.
370 Seventh Avenue, Suite 1200, New York, NY 10001
www.guilford.com

Printed in the United States of America

Last digit is print number: 9   8   7   6   5   4   3   2

The authors have checked with sources believed to be reliable in their efforts to provide information that is complete
and generally in accord with the standards of practice that are accepted at the time of publication. However, in view
of the possibility of human error or changes in behavioral, mental health, or medical sciences, neither the authors, nor
the editors and publisher, nor any other party who has been involved in the preparation or publication of this work
warrants that the information contained herein is in every respect accurate or complete, and they are not responsible
for any errors or omissions or the results obtained from the use of such information. Readers are encouraged to confirm
the information contained in this book with other sources.

Library of Congress Cataloging-in-Publication data

Names: Chu, Brian C., author. | Pimentel, Sandra S., author.
Title: CBT treatment plans and interventions for depression and anxiety
  disorders in youth / Brian C. Chu, Sandra S. Pimentel.
Other titles: Cognitive-behavioral therapy treatment plans and
  interventions for depression and anxiety disorders in youth
Description: First edition. | New York, NY : The Guilford Press, a Division
  of Guilford Publications, Inc., 2023. | Series: Treatment plans and
  interventions for evidence-based psychotherapy | Includes
  bibliographical references and index. |
Identifiers: LCCN 2022055855 | ISBN 9781462551149 (paperback ; acid-free paper) |
  ISBN 9781462551156 (hardcover ; acid-free paper)
Subjects: LCSH: Depression in adolescence—Treatment. | Anxiety in
  adolescence—Treatment. | Cognitive therapy for teenagers. | BISAC:
  PSYCHOLOGY / Psychotherapy / Child & Adolescent | PSYCHOLOGY / Movements
  / Cognitive Behavioral Therapy (CBT)
Classification: LCC RJ506.D4 C39 2023 | DDC
616.85/2700835—dc23/eng/20230210
LC record available at https://lccn.loc.gov/2022055855

About the Authors

Brian C. Chu, PhD, is Professor and Department Chair of Clinical Psychology at the Graduate School of Applied and Professional Psychology, Rutgers, The State University of New Jersey, where he is Founder and Director of the Youth Anxiety and Depression Clinic. Dr. Chu is a recipient of the Klingenstein Third Generation Foundation Young Investigator Award. He is a Fellow of the Association for Behavioral and Cognitive Therapies and past editor of *Cognitive and Behavioral Practice*. Dr. Chu's work focuses on anxiety and mood problems in children and adolescents, with a special emphasis on therapy processes, mechanisms of change, and dissemination of evidence-based practices. He collaborates with community organizations to optimize access to care for underserved and marginalized communities.

Sandra S. Pimentel, PhD, is Chief of Child and Adolescent Psychology, Associate Director of Psychology Training, and Associate Professor of Clinical Psychology in the Department of Psychiatry and Behavioral Sciences at Montefiore Medical Center and the Albert Einstein College of Medicine. She is Founder and Director of the Anxiety and Mood Program, a specialty training program in the Child Outpatient Psychiatry Division. Dr. Pimentel serves on the editorial board of *Evidence-Based Practice in Child and Adolescent Mental Health* and is President (2023–2024) of the Association for Behavioral and Cognitive Therapies. As a scientist-practitioner, Dr. Pimentel specializes in cognitive-behavioral treatments for youth and young adults. She is a health advocate dedicated to creatively engaging communities to optimize care for children and families.

Series Editor's Note

CBT Treatment Plans and Interventions for Depression and Anxiety Disorders in Youth, by Brian C. Chu and Sandra S. Pimentel, provides an excellent balance of serious scholarship with accessible, readable, clinical application. Whether you are a seasoned clinician or just getting started, the authors of this valuable resource provide the reader with the necessary research reviews, conceptualizations, and clinical tools that can make your work as a clinician more effective, while drawing on the latest research and advances in cognitive-behavioral therapy (CBT) with children and adolescents. The book is not simply a list of techniques—although the techniques are there; it also helps you make sense of what you are doing. Each chapter provides a clear and concise overview of the important topics that the clinician should address. What is certain to me in reading this book is that it combines the immense strengths of the authors' scholarly knowledge with their sensitivity and wisdom as clinicians.

The first chapter is an excellent primer on CBT in general. It also alerts the reader—who is a practicing clinician—on the important subjects to cover in the initial assessment as well as providing additional online resources. The authors make the point that case conceptualization is an important part of CBT and that CBT is not simply the application of techniques. You have to know why you are using techniques and interventions before you implement your treatment. The second chapter continues the introduction of some common processes or issues across anxiety and depressive disorders and outlines for the clinician the main points that should be addressed in conducting a functional analysis, exposure, activity scheduling, and skill acquisition. The third chapter moves to the third phase of therapy as one begins to consider termination in preparation for avoiding relapse. As clinicians learn, many problems run the risk of relapse, so planning ahead to identify when things begin to slip back and having a plan to address recurring problems can assure that the short-term positive effects of therapy become long-term clinical gains. These three introductory chapters are quite important in preparing the clinician for structuring therapy in phases and pulling it all together, not only with the common processes, but also with the case conceptualization (that should be continually updated).

Child and adolescent therapy is often a collaborative process with medical professionals who bring their set of tools to the work with clients. Keep in mind that we, as clinicians, have one shared value—the welfare of the client. Chapter 4 (coauthored with Dr. Uri Meller) is a much needed addition to a cognitive-behavioral treatment planner, illustrating the importance of biological treatments to help clients. The authors indicate where this sort of referral is an important part of the treatment and how to socialize the family members to the relevance of medication. No one clinician has all the answers. There are helpful suggestions on how to contact and share information with a prescribing psychiatrist that will make collaboration more seamless.

As anyone who has worked with children understands, it is essential to include caregivers in their treatment. Chapter 5 does exactly this. Drs. Chu and Pimentel address the importance of normalizing anxiety, avoiding avoidance, and learning coping skills. They also identify certain spirals of interaction between parents and children that may either precipitate or maintain the problems that are the focus of treatment.

From there, the authors turn with excellent practical focus to the most common presenting problems clinicians will treat in children and adolescents: depression, suicide and self-injury, separation anxiety, social anxiety disorder, generalized anxiety disorder, and school refusal. Across these chapters, they retain the collaborative, compassionate mindset that makes evidence-based techniques effective.

Proudly welcoming *CBT Treatment Plans and Interventions for Depression and Anxiety Disorders in Youth* into this series, I strongly recommend it as an important, scholarly, and useful resource for clinicians at all levels. It will be the go-to guide for clinicians working with children and adolescents. The sign of a good treatment planner is when clinicians tell you, "This is a core part of my practice." Chu and Pimentel's book will become that core for many clinicians.

ROBERT L. LEAHY, PhD
Director, American Institute for Cognitive Therapy;
Clinical Professor of Psychology, Department of Psychiatry,
Weill Cornell Medical College, New York, New York

Preface

Recently, one of us began a class by asking the students, "What makes CBT hard to deliver in everyday settings?" The responses varied by setting and client population, but common themes emerged. Many had concerns about what they understood as CBT's "simple" approach and its "limitations" in addressing complex diagnostic problems or complicated clinical profiles. Associated with this were concerns that CBT produced efficacious outcomes only under highly controlled conditions. Or, that the "rigid structure" of CBT made it a poor fit for community settings that suffered from limited resources and served disadvantaged communities. Others voiced concerns that CBT did not permit the flexibility needed to respond to the frequent shifts in clinical focus or crises of the week that plague typical therapy, or that it did not focus on the therapeutic relationship. Some noted the advantages of modular and principles-based approaches and wished that CBT could be delivered in these ways.

In other words, to these students, CBT offered the promise of a "simple," "straightforward" treatment that might work for relatively concrete problems, like a specific phobia, but had little relevance to addressing the complex and nuanced problems that face everyday clients and are confronted in daily practice. Furthermore, they assumed the only way to conduct CBT was to deliver it in some predetermined set of rigid steps, as in a tightly controlled research project in the form of a treatment manual. The notion that CBT could be delivered in a principles-based manner, in which clinical judgment served as a guide for delivering flexible, personalized therapy, was foreign to these students.

Thus began our mission to demonstrate that CBT is a rich and flexible theoretical approach that requires active assessment, case conceptualization, flexible delivery of strategies, and active reassessment. At each stage, the competent CBT clinician actively incorporates data from the client's subjective experience, accounts for the client's individual strengths and weaknesses, and accommodates environmental resources and disadvantages. CBT clinicians evaluate their effectiveness by observing the impact of their intervention choices on the client's functioning. CBT as a theory is indeed designed to simplify and clarify complex psychological experiences, but employing that theory as a set of principles requires active hypothesis testing by engaging the client in a dynamic trial-and-error approach (also known as "collaborative empiricism"). Conducted as it is intended, CBT offers a relatively straightforward set of principles that can address a wide diversity of client problems and concerns.

This mission motivates our book. As lifelong practitioners of CBT across a number of settings and client populations, we have tried to accomplish three goals with this book:

- Distill CBT to its core components so readers can see its simplicity.
- Show how CBT principles and practices can *flexibly* be applied to meet the needs of diverse clients with complex problems who are experiencing challenging life circumstances. Numerous case illustrations permeate each chapter to help bring this work to life. (All identifying details have been obscured and all dialogues are fictionalized.)
- Make CBT easier for the busy clinician. To that end, we have provided a lavish library of clinical FAQ sheets, worksheets, handouts, and other therapist tools that the reader can print and use whenever the need calls for it.

The focus of this book is anxiety and depression disorders in youth, highlighting middle childhood through adolescence. This is a critical group of clients, as internalizing problems represent the most common forms of impairment in young people. Over 8% of youth will report major depression, and over 30% will report a major anxiety disorder at some time during adolescence (Merikangas et al., 2010). These problems often co-occur and almost always present clinicians with a diverse profile of mixed anxiety and depressive symptoms (Garber & Weersing, 2010). Youth presenting with a mix of anxiety and mood problems are associated with higher clinical severity and impairment, and so deserve special attention (Garber & Weersing, 2010; Ollendick, Jarrett, Grills-Taquechel, Hovey, & Wolff, 2008). This book provides a common set of principles and strategies that can be flexibly applied across these related target problems.

CBTs have received strong support for reducing distress in youth, especially compared with other psychological therapies (Higa-McMillan, Francis, Rith-Najarian, & Chorpita, 2016; Weersing, Jeffreys, Do, Schwartz, & Bolano, 2017). CBT's effectiveness seems to extend to traditional practice settings across diverse communities (Chorpita et al., 2011). For both anxiety and depression, the efficacy of CBT can be enhanced when it is provided in combination with medication treatment, particularly selective serotonin reuptake inhibitors (SSRIs; March et al., 2004; Walkup et al., 2008). In total, the evidence is strong for CBT, and it ought to serve as a first line of treatment for most young people with anxiety, depression, or their combination.

Although CBT proceeds in an iterative fashion in which assessment, conceptualization, and intervention inform each other, we present elements of CBT in early, middle, and later phases of treatment to help orient the clinician. Chapter 1 presents CBT theory and case conceptualization, introducing functional assessment and integrative cognitive-behavioral frameworks. It then discusses evidence-based assessment and how to translate conceptualization into a workable treatment plan. The treatment plan is designed to give clinicians a working roadmap that keeps therapist and client working toward common goals while also leaving room for adjustments when new problems emerge. Chapter 2 describes core treatment strategies, including rapport building, psychoeducation, self-talk and cognitive restructuring, mindfulness, and problem solving. We then provide a comprehensive tutorial on designing and implementing exposure exercises and behavioral experiments to help youth challenge expectations in difficult situations. Chapter 3 describes termination processes, including progress review, termination itself, and relapse prevention.

Medication therapy, especially in combination with CBT, has garnered increasing support as an important component of efficacious treatment for youth with anxiety and depression (Birmaher, Brent, & AACAP Work Group, 2007; Connolly & Bernstein, 2007). Yet, making psychiatric referrals and coordinating care across disciplines can seem like daunting tasks. Chapter 4 was co-authored by child and adolescent psychiatrist Uri Meller, MD, who offers pragmatic recommendations for therapists in seeking psychiatric evaluation and in fostering productive collaboration with psychiatry. The chapter walks readers through initial considerations when making a referral, how to discuss psychiatric referrals with families, and how to optimize continuity of care. Additional information on common antidepressant and anti-anxiety medications makes the reader better prepared to facilitate medication referrals.

Any work with youth populations will require clinicians to enlist the help of caregivers (parents or otherwise) and foster active, respectful collaborations. Chapter 5 highlights the various roles that caregivers can play in youth-based CBT, including as therapeutic partners or as agents of change. The chapter offers psychoeducation that can set the right tone and expectations for treatment and describes caregiver–youth interaction patterns that are common to youth with anxiety and depression. We present tips for fostering healthy communication styles for families and describe reward and contingency management strategies to shape youth behaviors.

Chapters 6–11 are designed to provide detailed case illustrations of conducting CBT with common anxiety and depression problems, including depression, separation anxiety disorder (SEP), social anxiety disorder (SAD), and generalized anxiety disorder (GAD). These chapters present case illustrations on problems commonly associated with anxiety and mood disorders, including a chapter on suicide and self-harm (Chapter 7) and a chapter on school refusal (SR) behaviors (Chapter 11). Each chapter demonstrates how a clinician would conduct assessment, conceptualize a youth's target problems, plan treatment, and monitor progress for an illustrative case. Detailed descriptions are provided for delivering CBT in a principles-based manner that follows the therapist's initial conceptualization and adapts to the unpredictable vicissitudes of clinical work. Clinical vignettes representing composites of real-life cases help bring the casework to life; in them, we have attempted to capture a variety of key scenarios and targets. Each chapter ends with a summary and key points to help readers identify the commonalities and distinguish differences in working with diverse client problems. The reader will notice that pronoun usage may change between she/he and they/them when referring to singular subjects throughout the volume. We are following the *APA Publication Manual*'s latest guidance to use gender-neutral language whenever the gender of the subject is unknown for singular verb tenses, but to use the appropriate pronoun (she/he/they) when the gender of the subject is known (e.g., when presenting a case study).

Throughout all chapters, we refer to multiple tools that can facilitate implementation of CBT strategies in session. Many handouts and worksheets are available as reproducibles in Appendix A at the end of the book and also online (see the box at the end of the table of contents). We hope these handouts and worksheets will serve as "go-to" resources for all your work with youth and families.

Appendix B presents curated lists of resources that clinicians can access for their own learning or to provide to families to facilitate therapy. The first is a list of recommended organization websites that provide useful information for professionals and consumers alike. Each website provides education on common youth psychological concerns in lay language. Some offer FAQ sheets that can be shared with families; others offer professional training opportunities. Furthermore, caregivers often request recommendations for parent-oriented books to get a better understanding of what their child is experiencing. The second list includes books for both youth and caregivers to facilitate your work.

As practicing clinicians, we aim to provide therapists with a straightforward, comprehensive resource for conducting CBT with anxious and depressed children and teens. We hope it will work for you on multiple levels. For the novice therapist (e.g., first-year graduate student), we hope this book will provide an outline and structure for approaching one's initial cases. For the seasoned clinician, we hope the case vignettes will illustrate the nuanced ways in which CBT principles can be used to address complex needs. The worksheets should ease the burden of reinventing the wheel. Together, we hope to dispel some of the long-held myths and make the work you do with young clients rich, engaging, fun, and effective!

Acknowledgments

We would like to thank the countless family, friends, and colleagues who have supported us. In particular, we acknowledge Philip Kendall, without whom our partnership would not have occurred, and who laid the foundation for the clinical, research, and training wisdom underpinning this book. Other vital and inspiring mentors on our professional and personal journeys include Anne Marie Albano, John Weisz, Ellen Flannery-Schroeder, Michael Southam-Gerow, Elizabeth Gosch, Simon Rego, John Piacentini, Terry Wilson, Bob and Toni Zeiss, Stephen Shirk, and our peers, from whom we have learned equally.

Brian Chu could never have fulfilled his promise without the light and lightness that Laura, Carter, and Cayleigh bring every day. He thanks his mother and father for giving the tools, heart, and humor needed for this life-long path and his extended family for the lessons and stories that craft this work.

Sandra S. Pimentel is grateful for her parents, Maria and Manuel, for the enduring gift and promise of education, and the love of her large Portuguese family—avós, brothers, godparents, tios and tias, in-laws, niece, godchildren, and cousins—all of them! She is a lucky Muh, too. From Ponta Garça, Açores, to Newark, New Jersey, she is proud of the roots and communities that shaped her.

This book would not have come to fruition without the tireless persistence of Jim Nageotte, Jane Keislar, and the entire Guilford Press team—we are forever grateful.

Undoubtedly, the greatest teachers have been the youth, families, and students over the years, who have entrusted their care and education to us. This book is for them.

Contents

Contents

List of Figures, Tables, Handouts, and Worksheets

FIGURES

TABLES

HANDOUTS

WORKSHEETS

CHAPTER 1

The CBT Model and Early Treatment Phase

This chapter reviews the overall CBT model and the components that the early phase of treatment usually comprises. Collecting comprehensive multimodal, multireporter assessment is critical to developing a holistic picture of your client. Assessment data are then used to develop a case formulation that highlights the cognitive, behavioral, and interpersonal processes maintaining the youth's anxiety and depression. The therapist subsequently plans the course of treatment and selects specific interventions based on this understanding of the youth's strengths and needs. Collecting and reviewing progress data help inform the clinician's treatment planning and improves therapy outcomes. Progress monitoring can include symptom reports or achievement of goals. Each of these activities is soundly grounded in the overarching CBT model. Over the next three chapters, we discuss CBT in the early, middle, and later phases of treatment to help orient the clinician. However, CBT proceeds in an iterative fashion, implementing interventions based on initial and then ongoing assessment, formulation, and treatment goals. Rarely is treatment linear, but there are common elements across CBT cases that tend to occur in phases.

THE COGNITIVE-BEHAVIORAL THERAPY MODEL

The cognitive-behavioral therapy (CBT) model attempts to clarify emotional states (e.g., sadness, anxiety, shame, happiness, anger) that can often feel diffuse and uncontrollable into more observable and describable components: cognitions, physical feelings, and behaviors (Badin, Alvarez, & Chu, 2020). This CBT triangle, or thoughts–physical feelings–action cycle, has abundant utility. The clinician can use the framework to interpret objective and subjective (client or parent impression) data presented by the client to build a case conceptualization of how the client responds to stressors in the environment. It can also be used to provide psychoeducation to the client by describing the unique and interrelated roles of thoughts, feelings, and actions. The triangle construct holds whether considering clinical or more commonplace content. The triangle graphic (see Figure 1.1; a reproducible version is available as Handout 1 in Appendix A) often helps kids of diverse ages to understand their own emotional cycles. Finally, it helps set up treatment planning. As you analyze a client's idiographic responses to a trigger, you can note particular strengths and weaknesses. As you recognize where the client is getting stuck (e.g., pervasive negative thoughts,

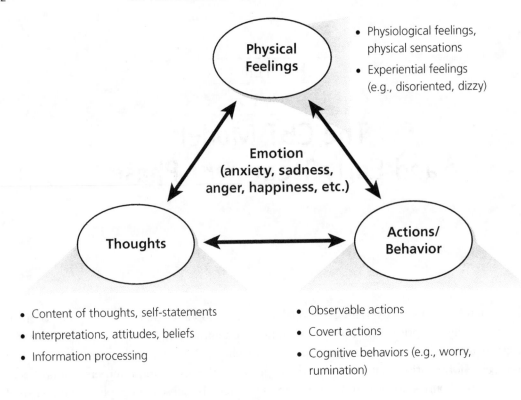

FIGURE 1.1. General cognitive-behavioral model.

severe physiological symptoms, freezing or escape behavior), you can then prioritize CBT interventions that target the client's weak spots.

Cognitive Components

The cognitive components of the model can be viewed at any level in the hierarchy of cognitive processes, from basic executive functioning (e.g., attention, memory), to information processing (e.g., conscious automatic thoughts, interpretations, distortions), to abstract meta-thinking (e.g., intermediate and core beliefs). The information processing and abstract thinking levels tend to focus on the *content* of thought. For example, when a youth is depressed, cognitive content tends to be unrealistically negative ("Soccer is for losers!" "My teacher has it out for me"), pessimistic ("Why bother trying when things never work out?"), and self-critical ("I mess up everything"). For a socially anxious youth, cognitive content tends to overfocus on a lack of control or self-efficacy ("I'll never be prepared for that talk!" "I can't handle the pressure") and an exaggerated estimation of risk ("I know I'll flub in front of everyone") and magnitude of negative consequences ("Everyone will laugh at me!" "I'll be known as the loser of the school").

In addition to understanding the content of thoughts, evaluating cognitive *processes*, like worry, rumination, and distraction, can be helpful (Aldao & Nolen-Hoeksema, 2010; Chu, Chen, Mele, Temkin, & Xue, 2017). The benefit of treating cognitions as a process is that they can be viewed in terms of their behavioral functions. As a brief example, when a depressed teen is ruminating, it is critical to identify the triggers and consequences that surround that rumination. If a teen reports substantial rumination while doing homework after school, it is critical to examine the initial triggers (opening a math book) and reactions (negative thoughts and feelings about the day) that lead to a cascade of rumination. This ruminative process helps the teen avoid their homework and helps us understand the *avoidant functions* of rumination. Being clear about the distinction between cognitive content and cognitive processes will help clients distinguish the distinct roles and consequences of behaviors, physical feelings, and emotions in their daily lives.

Behavioral Components

Behavioral components can also be viewed at multiple levels. Observable actions are most associated with the term "behavior" (Chu, Skriner, & Staples, 2014). They consist of controllable, overt behaviors such as, talking, walking, socializing, exercising, sleeping, arguing, freezing, escaping, smiling, and laughing. But intentional behaviors can include discrete, covert behaviors that are not obvious to outside observers, such as muscle tensing, staring blankly, and the like. Sometimes it is difficult to identify the behaviors associated with emotional states because the intensity of emotions attracts our attention. For example, feeling love generally includes acting in a loving way even when the emotional sensations of love feel most salient. Acting lovingly could include attending to one's partner when they are talking, holding hands, or thinking about the person during the day. You can select from a cornucopia of behaviors. Every emotional state offers the same diversity of options. Being "wakeful and alert" includes sitting up straight, breathing evenly, making eye contact with a conversation partner, exchanging thoughts and reciprocating attention. Feeling "lonely" might include withdrawal, isolation, self-pity, cascading rumination, pushing away available social resources and invitations. How any client acts happy, sad, mad, or anxious provides an idiographic behavioral conceptualization of that person. The more specifically and accurately one can identify the client's unique behavioral response with various emotions, the more accurate one's case conceptualization will be.

Physical Components

The physical components of the model tend to refer to automatic physiological responses and other physical sensations that the body has in reaction to stressors. Physiological indices include heart rate, breathing rate and depth, galvanic skin response (leading to sweaty palms), dilated or constricted pupils, and blurry vision. Physical feelings that imply physiological reactions include: headaches, dry mouth, lump in the throat, tightness in the chest, stomachaches, muscle tension, coldness, feeling flush, muscle cramping, sweating. Such components can also include experiential feelings, such as disorientation, derealization, and depersonalization. The client will describe these feelings as automatic and out of their control (though we know that many of these responses can be put under the client's control; Badin et al., 2020).

How the Components Interact

There are several key aspects to the CBT model that bear emphasizing. First, no one component takes priority over the others in terms of understanding a client's concerns. Second, the relations among thoughts, feelings, and actions are mutually reciprocal and bidirectional. Third, emotional cycles do not stop naturally after one cycle of thoughts, actions, and behaviors. Emotional cycles are frequently self-perpetuating unless intervention is used.

All Components Are Equally Important

A common misperception when applying a CBT framework is that thoughts, particularly the negative content of thoughts, are the key element to understand and to intervene with. However, as shown in Figure 1.1, the triangular shape of the model gives the same weight to each component, implying that each component contributes equally to the overall emotional experience for the individual. The particular salience of one component over the others will be completely individual. One depressed youth may be particularly aware of their negative thoughts and embrace cognitive restructuring as a way to challenge negative thoughts. Another depressed youth might be especially sensitive to the fatigue and somatic symptoms that come with their sadness. In this case, relaxation exercises may help alleviate the tension and increased physical activity may help address the fatigue. Yet another teen may not be aware of their pessimistic thinking or of any particular physical symptoms. Instead, they note that they are most depressed when they retreat to their room after school and crash on their bed, avoiding family and friends for the rest of the day. The CBT model encourages the therapist to identify the individual profile that reflects each youth's emotional experience. It also encourages affective education to teach youth to be able to differentiate among the components and to label thoughts, feelings, and actions. In this way, the general CBT model can be individualized, creating an idiographic understanding of how the youth expresses their particular depression. When designing a treatment plan, this individualized case formulation lends itself directly to choosing the most appropriate intervention strategies.

Thoughts, Feelings, and Actions Are Bidirectionally Influential

The second key aspect to this model is the bidirectional nature of the thoughts–feelings–action components. When an individual encounters a trigger, any component can be activated "first." In reality, each component works in simultaneous, rapid sequencing that escapes human observation. For clinical purposes, the clinician or client will often (but not necessarily) notice one component responding first. From there, each of the other components become activated and can reciprocally affect the first component as well. The bidirectional arrows reflect these reciprocal, mutually causative relations among all three components. This is best illustrated by tracing a person's reaction to a trigger around the thoughts–feelings–actions triangle. For example (see Figure 1.2; a reproducible version of a general CBT model is available in Handout 12 in Appendix A), the first thought a depressed teen who has received a bad grade on a test might have is "I really messed that up," upon which they notice feeling a little flushed in their face and some pressure in their forehead (physical feeling). They then put their head against the school bus window on the ride home (action). This triggers a second thought, "I'll never be able to catch up now," leading to increased pressure in the youth's temples and a slight queasiness in their stomach. They look down at their lap and begin to tear. "My parents are going to be so angry with me" is their next thought before feeling a lump in their throat and clasping their head in their hands. The teen is thinking, "Everyone else has it so much easier than me," and feels heat build in their face right before they snap at a friend who has asked if everything is all right. The result of this downward spiral is the experience of sadness or depressed mood.

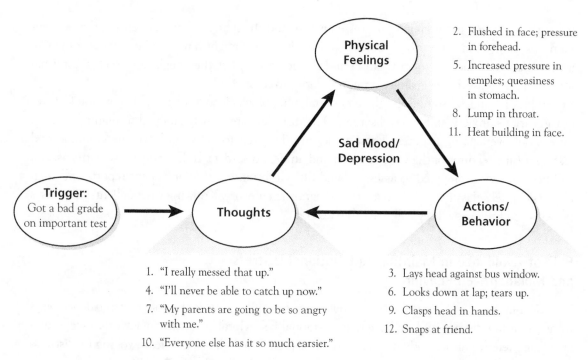

FIGURE 1.2. Individualized CBT conceptualization for depressed youth.

Emotional Cycles Can Be Self-Perpetuating

The above example highlights the reciprocal and self-perpetuating nature of emotional cycles. Such sequences are often called the "distress spiral," "depression cycle," or "feelings tornado" (Badin et al., 2020). These terms highlight the cycling, seemingly unstoppable nature of thoughts, feelings, and actions after one is activated in high emotional situations. These feelings snowball from seemingly innocuous starting points to become seemingly uncontrollable emotional catastrophes. It would not have mattered whether the cycle "started" with feelings, actions, or thoughts; once it starts, it self-perpetuates until stopped. Thus, all components carry equal weight with regard to impacting emotions, and most emotional cycles do not stop naturally after one trip around the cycle.

Different emotional experiences, and hence different psychological disorders, are characterized by different expressions of thoughts, feelings, and actions. Disorders that are more experientially similar will also have more similar thoughts, feelings, and actions. For example, depression and persistent depressive disorder (formerly called "dysthymia") have a number of common expressions of each component, with slight variations in feelings and actions that reflect the more persistent but less acute nature of persistent depressive disorder. If one compares the CBT model for depression to the model for social anxiety disorder (see Chapters 6 and 9), one will notice greater differences. Social anxiety is characterized by acute fear or panic-like symptoms when exposed to social situations. Thoughts are characterized by fears of embarrassment or evaluation and of catastrophic consequences of failure. Socially anxious individuals have less difficulty getting moving (anhedonia) like a depressed individual, but are prone to freezing and escaping frightening situations. If one were to look at the CBT model for generalized anxiety disorder (GAD), one sees commonalities in both depression and social anxiety disorder. One recognizes the diffuse negative affect that is common to depressed youth, and the increased muscle tension that is common to socially anxious youth. A worried youth with GAD might have trouble getting going like a depressed teen due to procrastination and perfectionism, but they might also seek substantial attention and reassurance that is common in most anxious youth.

Tables 1.1 and 1.2 summarize the emotional, physiological, cognitive, and behavioral features of the various anxiety and mood disorders. The disorders are loosely grouped to highlight which have more overlapping features. These tables are designed to help you learn the common and distinguishing features of the various mood and anxiety disorders. In learning these patterns, you will become better prepared to assess for and filter information that any client reports and then more accurately classify them into a useful diagnostic category. Knowing where clients' responses fit helps you know how they will react to stressors.

Role of Avoidance in Maintaining Emotional Distress and Maladaptive Behavior

A critical mechanism that the CBT triangle does not fully cover is the role that *avoidance* plays in maintaining distress and maladaptive emotional-behavioral patterns. Behavioral escape and avoidance refer to an individual not entering, or prematurely leaving, a fear-evoking or distressing situation. These are types of "action." Cognitive forms of avoidance can include maladaptive coping attempts, such as distraction and thought suppression. Automatic emotional processes can also serve the function of avoidance, such as when an individual experiences numbing, dissociation, or freezing. The individual engages in these activities either with or without control as attempts to cope with distress.

Avoidance can present a number of problems in adequately processing emotions and learning (Chu, Skriner, & Staples, 2014; Harvey, Watkins, Mansell, & Shafran, 2004). According to the emotion-processing model of anxiety (Foa, Huppert, & Cahill, 2006), pathological fear structures contain associations among a stimulus, response, and meaning representations that distort reality. Repeated avoidance prevents sufficient activation of the fear network, precluding new, anti-anxiety information from being learned. Likewise, according to the habituation model, prolonged exposure to a feared stimulus is required to decrease anxiety (brief exposure periods may "sensitize" patients to feared stimuli). In both the habituation and emotion-processing models, avoidance prevents prolonged exposure (Figure 1.3).

In terms of learning theory, avoidance has a number of impairing functions. First, avoidance behavior is often negatively reinforced because it provides immediate relief through escape. Second, avoidance denies the person opportunities for positive reinforcement and contributes to a deprived environment (Hoffman & Chu, 2019; Ferster, 1973; Jacobson, Martel, & Dimidjian, 2001). Third, it may exacerbate self-focused attention and ruminative thinking because avoidance narrows the person's interests and reduces their exposure to external stimuli. From a cognitive perspective, avoidance removes the opportunity to disconfirm negative beliefs (Salkovskis, 1991). Finally, avoidance behavior is intrinsically functionally problematic because it can result in increased absence from school, work, and social opportunities. By contrast, preventing avoidance can increase a sense of self-control and self-efficacy that promotes approach behavior. Working with youth often requires working with caregivers to catch how their actions may promote youth escape or avoidance of distressing situations. No matter the theory, behavioral, emotional, and cognitive processes are impacted when avoidance is used as a solution to a stressful trigger.

TABLE 1.1. Distinguishing Features of Youth Anxiety Disorders

Disorder	Emotional experience	Physiological experience	Cognitive experience	Behaviors
Generalized anxiety disorder	• Apprehension and anxiety about friends, family, future, physical health, etc. • Diffuse negative affect	• Muscle tension, fatigue, restlessness, agitation when worried • Difficulty relaxing, particularly during sleep	• Persistent "What if's" • Self-imposed perfectionism; rigid rule sets; worries about self, family, school, health, etc.	• Worry, rumination • Avoidance/procrastination • Reassurance seeking, neediness • Perfectionism, rigidity • Excessive planning
Separation anxiety disorder	• Fear/panic at separation and apprehension in advance	• Panic-like symptoms upon separation (increased heart rate, rapid breathing, crying) • Complaints of stomachaches, sickness, nausea	• Worry about harm to self or parent upon separation, inability to handle self during separation	• Clinging behavior, reassurance seeking • Protests, arguments, complaints, oppositionality • Refusal to separate at home, school, or elsewhere
Social anxiety disorder	• Fear and anxiety of social situations and social evaluation	• Tension, sickness when anticipating social setting • Panic-like symptoms in social situations	• Fear of evaluation, embarrassment, and the consequences of poor performance	• Avoidance/refusal/escape of social activities or demands • Disruption in performance and social presentation
Specific phobia	• Fear/panic of specific objects: animal, heights, darkness, blood, etc.	• Panic-like symptoms in presence of specific trigger	• Fear of catastrophic outcomes (e.g., bodily injury) or inability to control oneself	• Avoidance, escape of feared object • Endure under great duress
Panic disorder	• Acute panic attacks plus worry of future attacks	• Persistent anxious arousal worrying about next attack • Panic symptoms and fear of death or losing control	• Persistent/acute fears of catastrophic outcomes of having attack and being trapped	• Avoidance, escape of contexts where panic occurred • Withdrawal, isolation
Obsessive–compulsive disorder	• Distress-inducing obsessions that compel repetitive/idiosyncratic compulsions	• Intense distress, discomfort triggered by intrusive thoughts • Relief at completion of compulsive act	• Idiosyncratic fears of catastrophic consequences if compulsions aren't completed	• Behavioral and mental rituals (e.g., washing, checking, ordering, repetitive behaviors)

TABLE 1.2. Distinguishing Features of Youth Unipolar Depression Disorders

Disorder	Emotional experience	Physiological experience	Cognitive experience	Actions
Depression	• Depressed mood • Sad, down, blue • Persistent enduring sadness • Heavy, "weight of the world" feeling or pit in the stomach pain. • Irritability, anger • Hopelessness, helplessness	• Pit in the stomach, pressure in chest, feeling like crying (teary), weight on shoulders • Feeling heavy, fatigued, like a dead weight • Cloudy head, unfocused • Eating/appetite problems • Restlessness/sleeping disturbances • Psychomotor retardation • Anxiety, tenseness	• Difficulty thinking, concentrating, focusing • Negativity • Self-criticism • Hopelessness, helplessness • Negative automatic thoughts/cognitive distortions (e.g., all or nothing; blaming self; catastrophizing; discounting positives)	• Rumination, worry • Social withdrawal, isolation, pushing others away, poor assertiveness • Avoidance of stressors, hassles, poor problem solving • Passivity, poor self-direction, inability to get going • Limited self-reward, limited seeking of pleasant activities and rewards • Repetition of passive and unrewarding behavior • Diffident, unengaging social skills • Negative behavior toward others (rejecting, neediness, complaining) • Peer and family conflict
Persistent depressive disorder (dysthymia)	• "Down in the dumps," lazy, heavy, dragging • Bored, apathetic • Drowsy • Poor connectedness to experience and others	• Lazy, heavy, dragging • Cloudy, hazy, unfocused • Poor appetite/eating • Restlessness/sleeping disturbances • Tired, fatigued	• Low self-esteem • Difficulty thinking, making decisions • Negativity • Hopelessness, pessimistic about future	• Rumination, worry • "Lazing" around, anhedonia, inability to get going • Withdrawal, isolation • Avoidance of challenges/hassles, low motivation to strive, pursues low-effort activities

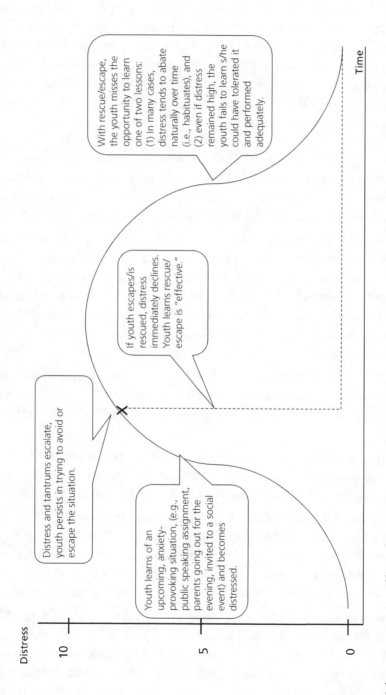

FIGURE 1.3. Habituation curve: effect of rescue/escape on learning. Rescue or escape is negatively reinforced by its immediate impact on distress reduction. The youth fails both to experience natural habituation of distress and to learn distress tolerance.

CONDUCTING AN INITIAL ASSESSMENT

The first step in applying the CBT model to an individual client is conducting an initial assessment. Take an evidence-based approach that consists of diagnostic, symptom, and functional assessment of the individual youth within their full interpersonal (family, community) context. This approach is consistent with the recommendations of the American Psychological Association (APA) for evidence-based psychological practice in that it starts with a comprehensive understanding of the identified client and then prioritizes available research in selecting potential interventions (APA Presidential Task Force on Evidence-Based Practice, 2006). An evidence-based assessment (EBA) approach for children and adolescents includes the following characteristics:

1. Ground your assessment in the child's or adolescent's presenting problem and target problems. The goal of any therapy is to help youth achieve the goals that are most meaningful for them. Choosing assessment tools focused on the domains that bring the youth to therapy are most likely to engage them, their caregivers, and enhance their motivation to participate.

2. Assess multiple domains, the different aspects of a youth's functioning to obtain a holistic sense of their strengths, limits, and impairment. This can include diagnosis of psychological disorders, measurement of symptoms (e.g., anxiety, depression), and evaluation of functional impairment (performance at school, in extracurriculars, with friends). Within each of these levels, assessing multiple domains (e.g., social anxiety, fear of evaluation) can be more informative than assessing one global dimension (e.g., anxiety). Choose measures and measure subscales that match the child's primary problems.

3. Obtain data from multiple reporters. Youth exist within multiple social systems. Obtain input from the individual youth, caregivers, and when possible other collaterals who may have pertinent information about the youth's functioning (e.g., teachers, coaches, other adults living with the youth).

4. Take social context into account. As youth are embedded in multiple social systems, collect data about the adults, siblings, and peers with whom the youth lives or interacts; understanding the youth's community and school provides valuable data for case conceptualization.

5. Use developmentally and culturally appropriate measures. They should assess constructs that are relevant and should be written at the appropriate reading level for the youth. For example, having a teen complete a questionnaire that asks about bedwetting may immediately reduce a clinician's credibility in the youth's eyes. If youth or caregivers are non-English-speaking, therapists should find measures that have been translated to the preferred language when possible.

6. Make use of psychometrically sound measures when comparisons count. When assessing broad symptoms or constructs that benefit from national or international comparisons, it is essential to use psychometrically sound measures. For example, evaluating a youth's anxiety, depressive symptoms, academic competence, or social skills may benefit from normative comparisons. This allows you to compare the youth's functioning against other individuals who are the same age, sex, or other important trait.

7. Use idiographic measures to assess and monitor individual goals. Idiographic tools (e.g., fear hierarchies, top problems lists) are sometimes best to capture specific functional impairment that might be lost by broad symptom measures. These are particularly useful to measure weekly changes that are tied to the client's treatment goals.

Several resources exist to help clinicians obtain and use EBA tools. For those with access to scholarly journals, there are several excellent issues and articles that span a wide range of domains. These include Mash and Hunsley's (2005) special issue on EBA, key resource articles (Beidas et al., 2015; Becker-Haimes et al., 2020) that list publicly available assessment tools, and the article by Youngstrom and colleagues (2015) that provides case examples of how clinicians can use EBA in everyday clinical practice. Publicly available online resources also exist to aid clinicians. Some professional organizations curate freely available assessment tools that are published in the public domain. Helping Give Away Psychological Science (HGAPS) has created an online assessment center where caregivers, adolescents, and adults can complete mental health screeners and get immediate feedback (*www.hgaps.org/ac.html*). The APA's Society of Clinical Psychology has created a repository for EBA instruments (*www.div12.org/assessment-repository*). Here, the practicing clinician can find a broad range of downloadable EBA tools that assess various problems across age groups. The Society of Clinical Child and Adolescent Psychology (SCCAP, Division 53 of APA) has developed a website (*www.EffectiveChildTherapy.com*) that has freely available resources, including informational fact sheets, brief informational videos for families, didactic seminars for professionals, and full-length workshops for professionals. The Association for Behavioral and Cognitive Therapies (ABCT) website also includes a special page on self-help resources that have received the organization's stamp of approval (*www.abct.org/SHBooks*).

Collaborative learning projects, like Wikiversity, additionally provide a public resource where therapists can obtain and share knowledge. For example, SCCAP has developed tutorials to guide therapist planning around EBA (e.g., planning, selection of measures, interpreting data, and emphasis on incremental assessment). See, for example, *https://en.wikiversity.org/wiki/Evidence_based_assessment* and *https://en.wikiversity.org/wiki/Category:Vignettes*. Online collaboratives allow content to be updated continuously to reflect growing knowledge, a common barrier to dissemination by more traditional means.

CASE CONCEPTUALIZATION

Once a set of assessment tools has been selected and administered, you can use the information to inform a case conceptualization, also called "case formulation." Case conceptualizations represent the therapist's working explanation of the factors contributing to and maintaining the youth's presenting problems (Christon, McLeod, & Jensen-Doss, 2015; Persons, 2006). It is grounded in the CBT model and incorporates knowledge about triggers (e.g., events, interpersonal interactions) and consequences (functional outcomes) for the individual youth. Case formulation begins the moment clinicians meet their clients, and they revise their formulations continuously as new data present themselves. For example, cognitive-behavioral theory attributes significant maintenance roles for unrealistic negative thinking, inactivity, behavioral avoidance, skills deficits, and physiological reactivity in youth pathology. When operating within a principles-based CBT approach, it is up to the therapist to tailor strategies to the individual youth by: (1) identifying the unique triggers that precede depressed moods, (2) assessing which specific mechanisms (e.g., thoughts, avoidance, problem solving) are most critical, and (3) observing what consequences maintain the maladaptive behavior. Based on this individualized conceptualization (i.e., functional assessment), the therapist emphasizes some strategies over others. If the youth responds to perceived failures (e.g., getting into a fight with a friend at school) with withdrawal and isolation (i.e., avoidance), the therapist might choose to focus on behavioral activation and behavioral experiments to foster problem-solving and approach behaviors. Even when the crisis of the week shifts from session to session, the formulation keeps the therapist focused on the core mechanisms (avoidance, unrealistic thinking). In the presence of complicating comorbidities (e.g., drug use), the therapist might choose supplemental interventions that complement the ongoing formulation, such as motivational interviewing (MI), which has a focus on encouraging personalized goal-oriented behaviors. In this way, a therapist can view daily challenges from a consolidated lens that narrows the number of choices that need to be made.

Data should be collected continuously throughout treatment to test out the therapist's thinking about maintaining mechanisms. It is critical to view this thinking as a working hypothesis, not a fixed theory. The therapist must then revise the case conceptualization as new information becomes available and treatment progresses. This process has been described as the assessment–treatment dialectic (Weisz et al., 2011). In other words, clinicians continuously integrate new information in an ongoing feedback loop of Assessment → Case formulation → Treatment planning → Strategy implementation → and Outcome monitoring and Assessment. Successful interventions can be used with greater intensity or dose. Unsuccessful interventions can be discontinued.

Certain commonalities emerge within a diagnostic classification. Youth diagnosed with social anxiety disorder will express much of their fears around performance evaluation and social comparison. Social settings (e.g., parties, meeting novel people, answering questions in class) reflect a common context that evokes fear, and within these contexts, similar specific triggers will precede fear (e.g., making eye contact with a stranger; the teacher calling on them). Youth with social anxiety will then respond with common internal and behavioral responses (e.g., upset stomach, avoidance of social settings, escape from uncomfortable situations) and have similar thinking patterns (e.g., unrealistic predictions and evaluations of their performance). At the same time, any two individuals who meet criteria for the same diagnosis can look fairly different. For example, one teen with social anxiety disorder may have a very critical parent, while another might have a parent who is overly accommodating (*context*). One teen's fear may be triggered by the parent claiming they will never amount to anything, while a second teen may be triggered by a party invitation that comes via text (*triggers, antecedents*). The *maintaining mechanism* for one teen may be catastrophic negative thoughts ("I'll never amount to anything") and it may be an overwhelming physiological reaction for another teen. The immediate consequence for each might be the relief they feel when escaping the stressful scene. However, the long-term consequences may differ in that the first teen may compensate for their fears by studying really hard and acing their exams. The second teen might become intensely isolated.

The two examples illustrate the centrality of case conceptualization. Each story is plausible (indeed, highly common) among youth with social anxiety. Knowing that each youth qualifies for a diagnosis of social anxiety helps narrow the field. Individualized case conceptualization helps develop a specific, working model to pick interventions tailored to each child. The layout of the current book aims to facilitate both. Treatment plans are grouped by diagnostic category, but individualized case formulation is highlighted in each chapter to emphasize the diversity of cases that appear within each disorder.

Building an Individualized Case Conceptualization

How does a clinician make use of the CBT and avoidance models to form a conceptualization? The first step is to create a target problems list from the youth's major areas of impairment. Goals are then developed for these areas of impairment, and the impairments are subsequently broken down into smaller problems. The functional assessment of each problem can then identify its maintaining mechanisms. Thoughts are next integrated into the conceptualization along with interpersonal contexts. Each of these steps is described in greater detail below.

Goals and the Target Problems List

To set treatment goals, the therapist, youth, and caregivers collaboratively develop a target problems list based on the youth's major areas of functional impairment. The therapist summarizes information from the multidomain, multireporter assessment to provide feedback to the family about possible areas of concern (e.g., intense symptomatology, skills deficits). The youth and caregivers identify concrete areas where change would improve the youth's functioning. Together, a joint target problems list provides a clear sense of the outcomes the youth, family, and therapist care most about. The therapist can use the following common prompt: "If you had the power to change three things, what would they be?" Above all, treatment goals should focus on real-life changes the client and family want to see in the child's life.

If the targets on the list appear too broad (e.g., "too anxious," "feeling better about myself"), the therapist encourages the family to break the goals into smaller, specific goals. The therapist helps the family concretize broad emotional states and take the first steps toward achievable goals. You can help the family visualize the kind of day-to-day change they would like to see in meaningful life domains (school, peers, family, health). How would the parents know if the youth was feeling less "anxious" or "sad"? How would the youth be acting if they "felt better about themself"? What would be different on a daily basis? After devising this list, the therapist can use functional assessment to identify triggers, mechanisms, and consequences of problematic behaviors.

As an example, the lists of parent and youth goals below show a mixture of diffuse emotional goals ("decrease anxiety," "not be afraid or overwhelmed"), as well as more concrete, achievable goals ("Go to a party and talk to people—don't hide in a corner"). The broader goals offer a general domain to work on, but we also need to identify concrete, observable goals that give more direction to the work.

Parents' Goals for Their Child

- Decrease anxiety [too broad].
- Stop worrying so much [too broad].
- Spend more time with friends; get out of the house more [moderately specific].
- Improve sleep [moderately specific].
- Make schoolwork a priority by completing homework before dinner [mostly specific].

Child's Goals for Themself

- Not be afraid or overwhelmed so much [too broad].
- Make friends and accept more invitations to go out [moderately specific].
- Spend less time in my room and more time hanging out with the family [moderately specific].
- Have my parents stop nagging me to talk to other kids [moderately specific; also common].
- Be able to ask my teachers for help when I need to [mostly specific].
- Go to a party and talk to people—don't hide in a corner [mostly specific].

After devising a reasonably specific target problems list, the therapist can use functional assessment to identify the mechanisms maintaining the problematic behaviors.

Identifying Maintenance Mechanisms through Functional Assessment

The purpose of forming a case conceptualization is to understand the origin and maintenance of a client's problems. A CBT conceptualization connects the dots between problematic situations (contexts) and the individual's distress response (thought–feeling–action) to give the clinician direction on where to intervene. In CBT conceptualizations, the *maintaining mechanisms* serve as targets for treatment. They are the client's cognitive, physiological, or behavioral patterns that perpetuate maladaptive cycles.

How does one identify maintaining mechanisms? By conducting functional assessment! This is one of the most flexible and robust CBT techniques. "Functional assessment" means assessing *antecedent–behavior–consequence* (ABC) sequences, also called "behavioral chains" (Kazdin, 2001; Rizvi & Ritschel, 2014). An "antecedent" is any trigger or circumstance (e.g., person, place, object, event, thought, feeling, action) that has some kind of meaning to the individual. "Behavior" refers to any client response (action, cognition, emotion, physiological response) that follows the antecedent. The "consequence" refers to any outcomes that follow the client's response. Figure 1.4 (a blank version is available as Worksheet 1 in Appendix A) illustrates the ABC functional assessment model. In the dialogue below, the clinician conducts a series of assessments to determine the triggers, behavioral responses, and environmental responses that characterize a client's problematic behavior.

THERAPIST: I'd like to get to know you better and learn what situations seem to get you stuck. Can you think of a situation where you've felt sad or anxious this past week?

CLIENT: Well, I had to give a speech in class, and I was freaked out.

THERAPIST: Oh, yes, that can be a scary challenge for any of us. Was this a spontaneous speech or a talk you had been planning for a while?

CLIENT: Well, it was assigned a while ago, but I could never push myself to really prepare.

THERAPIST: And so, on the day of the talk, you felt really unprepared?

CLIENT: Yeah.

THERAPIST: And what feeling did you feel in class that day?

CLIENT: Pure panic! I was for sure certain the teacher would yell at me in class and embarrass me.

THERAPIST: What did you do?

CLIENT: Well, we didn't know who the teacher was going to call on. You know, there were more people who had to go than could fit in the class. So, I kept trying to keep my head low, so the teacher wouldn't see me. . . .

THERAPIST: How'd that work?

CLIENT: I don't know—but I just kept freaking out and couldn't think of anything other than how I was going to fail.

THERAPIST: How did you end up getting through?

WORKSHEET 1. Trigger and Response

Tell us about your triggers and how you reacted. Describe your feelings, what you did (action), what happened right away (immediate outcome), and then what happened later (long-term outcome).

Antecedent → Behavioral and Emotional Response → Consequences

Trigger	Feeling (emotional response)	Action (behavioral response)	Immediate Results (What keeps it going?)	Long-Term Results (What gets you in trouble?)
I had to give a speech in class.	Fear, panic	Asked my teacher if I could go to nurse's office—feeling sick.	Teacher said "yes." Huge relief!	Now I have to do the speech another time. Teacher seemed annoyed at me.
My parents are fighting.	Sadness	Go to my room, put in my earbuds.	Phased out. Numbed.	Feeling lonely, isolated. Avoid my parents.
My coach told me I'll be benched if I don't get it together.	Nervous, scared	Skip practice, because I know the coach already hates me.	Feel better because don't have to face coach.	I'm not getting any better and probably will be benched.

FIGURE 1.4. Functional assessment of multiple moods and actions.

15

CLIENT: I finally just asked if I could go to the nurse. Like, I had a bad stomachache or something.

THERAPIST: And?

CLIENT: The teacher kind of looked at me weird—like kind of annoyed. But then they said, "OK." I was so excited!

THERAPIST: So, you were pretty relieved.

CLIENT: Yeah, I got out of there as soon as I could.

THERAPIST: (*laughing*) OK, so it seemed to get you out of giving your speech that day. I guess that solution worked for the moment. . . .

CLIENT: Uh, yeah.

THERAPIST: I wonder, has anything happened since? Have you noticed any positive or negative outcomes coming from this? I mean, did it work totally?

CLIENT: Well, I've kind of been avoiding my teacher since, and she's always looking at me kind of annoyed. And I'll have to give the speech eventually. And I'm still not prepared!

This dialogue illustrates how a therapist could conduct an ABC assessment in a very conversational manner, yet can accrue the information necessary to understand how the client responds to the trigger of speech giving and what outcomes typically result in the client's natural environment. Figure 1.5 (a blank version is available as Worksheet 1 in Appendix A) demonstrates the flexibility of an ABC assessment to cover a variety of triggers and emotional responses. Eventually, a clinician might want to group behavioral sequences into "themes," sorted by either common emotional responses or behavioral patterns (see below). At first, it is suitable to simply collect data and learn more about the client's natural response patterns.

ANTECEDENTS SHOULD BE SPECIFIC

There are several challenges in conducting useful functional assessments. First, when identifying antecedents, the clinician should try to identify as specific a trigger as possible. "When my parents fight" is OK to the extent that the youth responds in similar ways whenever their parents argue. However, we recommend identifying a specific event ("My parents fought about my poor grades [on Wednesday]"). It is true that there are rarely "right" or "wrong" answers to pinpointing the one single event prompting a response (Rizvi & Ritschel, 2014). Nevertheless, identifying a specific trigger on which the client and family can focus helps give a starting point for intervention.

ORGANIZE ASSESSMENTS BY EMOTION

A second challenge is that clients can experience multiple emotions in response to a single distressing trigger. We recommend creating a separate ABC row for each distinctive emotion, because each usually indicates distinctive reactions that lead to distinctive behavioral responses. The youth may not be aware of how each emotion triggers unique responses, but explicitly separating these emotions helps clarify the complexity of the response and stimulates varying solutions to address maladaptive patterns. Figure 1.5 helps demonstrate the value of clarifying separate ABC sequences for distinct emotions. In the first row, there are too many emotions to understand, and

WORKSHEET 1. Trigger and Response

Tell us about your triggers and how you reacted. Describe your feelings, what you did (action), what happened right away (immediate outcome), and then what happened later (long-term outcome).

```
Antecedent  →  Behavioral and Emotional Response  →  Consequences
```

Trigger	Feeling (emotional response)	Action (behavioral response)	Immediate Results (What keeps it going?)	Long-Term Results (What gets you in trouble?)
My parents fought about my bad grades.	Sadness, fear, nervousness, anger	Didn't do my homework, didn't talk to friends. Fought with parents.	Everyone's angry at me.	Still failing.
Separate the first row into three separate ABC sequences based on distinct feelings!				
My parents fought about my bad grades.	Sadness	Went to my room, put in my earbuds.	Phased out. Numbed.	Feeling lonely, isolated. Avoid my parents.
My parents fought about my bad grades.	Fear, nervousness	Nothing . . . can't think of what to do. Didn't do my homework.	Didn't do homework.	Fail the class.
My parents fought about my bad grades.	Anger	Yell at my parents—tell them I'm not studying any more.	Parents stop fighting.	Get punished for yelling. Fall further behind in class.

FIGURE 1.5. Functional assessment by emotion. Focus on just one emotion per row to keep the functional analysis clear. In the first row, there are too many emotions to understand; in the second, you can gain insight by analyzing each set of emotions.

17

this does not provide the therapist or the client with clear next steps for intervention. The second and third rows are separated into two sets of more specific feelings (sadness and fear/nervousness). Sadness is characterized by the youth avoiding other people and phasing out, which leads to growing isolation from family members. Nervousness is characterized by avoiding homework, which leads to incomplete homework and poor grades. The more specific ABC sequences give the clinician specific leads of what behaviors to target (avoiding people and homework) and what outcomes to pursue (social isolation, poor grades).

DEFINE SHORT- AND LONG-TERM CONSEQUENCES

Third, you can expect multiple outcomes (consequences) to result from the youth's behavioral response to any distressing challenge. Consequences comprise any specific events, thoughts, and emotions that occur after the behavior of concern (Rizvi & Ritschel, 2014). The therapist seeks to identify factors that might influence the recurrence of the behavior or that might be helpful in preventing future occurrences. These consequences fall into the categories of positive and negative reinforcers and punishers [for a full review of reinforcers and punishers, see Kazdin (2001) or Yoman (2008)]. Briefly, a "reinforcer" is any consequence that increases the likelihood of the behavior occurring again in the future, and a "punisher" is any consequence that decreases the likelihood of the behavior occurring again (Rizvi & Ritschel, 2014). Clinically, you can assess the reinforcing and punishing effects of outcomes by inquiring about both the positive and negative consequences that follow any antecedent–behavior sequence.

Some outcomes are apparent in the short term, and others only become apparent in the long term, after some time has passed. Returning to our example above, sadness may lead to the youth self-isolating, contributing to the short-term outcomes of isolation and failure to receive necessary social support. In the long term, the parent–youth relationship may deteriorate (the youth learns they cannot count on their parents) and the youth's grades may suffer. When a youth reacts angrily, they get their parents to stop fighting but also are punished for yelling. In this case, the short- and long-term outcomes diverge depending on the youth's immediate reaction in the moment. Specifying the short-and long-term consequences of the youth's choices help make clear the costs of choosing each behavioral path. The information can be used for goal setting and motivational interviewing as treatment planning begins.

TRIGGERS AND RESPONSES CAN BE BOTH INTERNAL AND EXTERNAL

Be mindful that triggers *and* responses can include both internal and external events (Kazdin, 2001; Rizvi & Ritschel, 2014). Most people commonly associate triggers with external events, such as learning bad news, having a difficult discussion with a friend or family member, receiving criticism or a bad performance review. However, internal stimuli, like thoughts, memories, and physiological feelings, can trigger further emotional response as well. The behavioral link in the ABC chain also refers to any individual response to the trigger; it is not limited to overt behaviors. Instead, be interested in knowing what youth thoughts, behaviors, and physiological feelings occur following the trigger. It may be unusual to view feelings and thoughts as behaviors at first, but from a learning theory point of view, these various responses are indistinguishable in terms of their potential role in a functional assessment. You should only be concerned about the *function* that the response plays in either maintaining or minimizing distress. Does the response serve to minimize distress, gain attention or support, garner some instrumental gain, avoid stressors, or punish aversive stimuli? The overt form (thought, feeling, behavior) of the behavior is less significant for the purposes of knowing the client better. To understand the function of the response better, it is critical to detail the short- and long-term consequences that follow. Is the youth's response reinforced (increased) or punished (decreased)? Knowing the immediate and secondary consequences will help reveal what factors are maintaining maladaptive behavior in the face of apparent impairment.

Conducting functional assessments accomplishes several clinical goals (Rizvi & Ritschel, 2014). It gives the youth (and family members) an opportunity to disclose intimate details of problematic behavior and gain insight into the triggers and emotional reactions that precede problematic behavior. A functional assessment acts as an essential assessment tool, as it helps the client, family, and therapist identify which behavioral chains lead to the most concerning problem behaviors and most impairing consequences. These will begin to illuminate details and patterns that lay the groundwork for case formulation and opportunities for intervention.

Integrating Thoughts into the Conceptualization

So far, our discussion of functional assessment has focused on emotions and behaviors. But thoughts play a key role in the CBT model. Assessing thoughts using one of the functional assessment tools (see also Worksheets 1 and 2 in Appendix A) can be easy. Figure 1.6 integrates thoughts with the functional analysis that we conducted previously with the youth whose parents were fighting over the youth's poor grades. In this example, when the youth feels sad, the primary thought that surfaces is "I'm causing my parents to fight with each other," leading the youth to isolate in their bedroom, feel guilty, and avoid their parents. When the youth feels frustration or anger, persecutory automatic thoughts surface: "They don't care how much I studied," which might lead the youth to act out against their parents. Knowing that the youth has two distinct response patterns helps the youth and therapist develop specific game plans for each occurrence. When the youth feels nervous, anxious thoughts are triggered: "I'm going to fail this class," leading to freezing and failing to complete their homework. In each ABC sequence, exploring the automatic thoughts that underlie the youth's emotions provides information about the specific fear or barrier that is keeping the youth from responding healthfully.

Integrating Interpersonal Contexts into the Conceptualization

A substantial evidence base highlights the role of interpersonal context and social interactions in triggering and maintaining anxiety and mood disorders in youth. In depression, interpersonal conflict and rejection are some of the most salient negative events to trigger depressive episodes and self-harming behaviors (Hammen, 2009; King & Merchant, 2008). Other research shows that depressed people both reject and end up being rejected by others in their lives (Joiner, 2000). The increased isolation and withdrawal also contribute to a decreasingly narrow social network from which to garner support when needed. Family members are frequently found to be facilitating anxious behaviors in youth by transmitting anxious information, by reinforcing anxious responding via rescue and escape, and by accommodating the fears of anxious youth.

Thus, assessing how the youth interacts with others is critical to understanding how the problematic behavior is being maintained. You will want to keep interpersonal contexts in mind when

WORKSHEET 2. Thoughts, Feelings, and Actions Tracker

What kind of thoughts do you have when feeling sad, anxious, or distressed? How do you act when thinking that way? What happens (outcome) from thinking that way?

Trigger	Feeling	Thought	Action	Outcome?
My parents fought about my bad grades.	Sadness	"I'm causing my parents to fight with each other."	Go to my room, put in my earbuds.	Feeling lonely, isolated. Avoid my parents.
My parents fought about my bad grades.	Frustration	"They don't care how much I studied."	Yell at my parents—tell them I'm not studying any more.	Get punished for yelling. Fall further behind in class.
My parents fought about my bad grades.	Fear, nervousness	"I'm going to fail this class."	Nothing . . . can't think of what to do.	Fail the class.

FIGURE 1.6. The same event can trigger multiple unique thought–feeling–action sequences.

generating problems lists, understanding the maintaining mechanisms (case formulation), and planning out the intervention. We provide examples of doing this in each of the disorder-specific chapters.

TREATMENT PLANNING

Armed with a multidimensional assessment, case conceptualization, and list of target problems, the therapist can then plan interventions to address the youth's concerns. Each disorder-specific chapter (Chapters 6–11) provides a treatment plan that contains common interventions for each problem area. Research suggests significant overlap in the interventions used across evidence-based programs for anxiety and depression in youth (Chorpita & Daleiden, 2009). There remains limited research to suggest the order or dose of specific treatment elements. Some research suggests that social skills and problem solving are among the most potent interventions for depressed adolescents (Kennard et al., 2009) even as behavioral activation and cognitive restructuring remain key elements (Oud et al., 2019). Other research supports programs that contain exposure-based interventions as the most efficacious treatments for anxiety in youth (Higa-McMillan, Francis, Rith-Najarian, & Chorpita, 2016). When such evidence is available, it makes sense to present social and problem-solving skills early in treatment, and we will highlight these decisions in upcoming disorder-specific chapters when relevant.

At the same time, match interventions to the client's particular profile (Chu, 2019). Youth who are primarily presenting with anhedonia, isolation, and limited activation would likely benefit from behavioral activation and exposure. For youth whose negative assumptions lead to protracted rumination or for those who report more diffuse self-esteem issues, cognitive restructuring may be helpful. Youth who experience significant conflict with family members require parent intervention.

Based on selected strategies, the therapist can then provide an overview of the treatment plan to the family, including a general sequence and time frame. Research suggests that involving youth and caregivers in this process improves attendance, treatment engagement, and ultimate outcomes (Langer & Jensen-Doss, 2018). Thus, making treatment selection a collaborative decision process can start off the therapy from a good place.

PROGRESS MONITORING

Cognitive-behavioral therapists ensure they are moving toward their clients' goals by monitoring progress routinely through therapy. Growing evidence suggests that the process of obtaining and reviewing regular outcome data can be an effective intervention in itself (Bickman, 2008; Bickman, Kelley, Breda, de Andrade, & Riemer, 2011; Lambert et al., 2003; Lambert Harmon, Slade, Whipple, & Hawkins, 2005). In these studies, clinicians who received feedback routinely (e.g., alerts related to current symptoms) have clients who demonstrate improved outcomes (Bickman et al., 2011), less deterioration (Lambert et al., 2005), and greater therapy engagement (Jensen-Doss & Weisz, 2008) compared to the clients of clinicians who did not receive feedback. Furthermore, visual feedback that graphically depicts provider or student behaviors has been associated with promising intervention outcomes (Hawkins & Heflin, 2011; Nadeem, Cappella, Holland, Coccaro, & Crisonino, 2016; Reinke, Lewis-Palmer, & Martin, 2007). Similar systems have been implemented in schools (e.g., Deno et al., 2009) as requirements for greater accountability call for active progress monitoring (U.S. Department of Education, 2001). Thus, monitoring and feedback systems may be useful and acceptable across youth intervention settings.

Monitoring systems can include tracking of standardized outcome measures (e.g., RCADS, SCARED, CES-DC), idiographic behavioral goals, or individualized "top problems" (Weisz et al., 2011). Feedback can consist of scale scores, graphs of outcomes over time, or simple indicators that the treatment is not progressing. For example, in a series of studies examining monitoring and feedback systems in adults, therapists simply needed to receive a colored dot (e.g., red = client not progressing as expected; green = client making expected progress) to self-correct and engender better outcomes (Lambert et al., 2003). There are commercial systems available for this (e.g., *www.practicewise.com*), but simple Excel graphs can also suffice. Smartphone apps are also quickly proliferating that help keep track of individual client data as part of treatment (see *https://psyberguide.org* for a guide of relevant smartphone apps).

SUMMARY AND KEY POINTS

The initial stages of CBT include the initial assessment and case formulation that help the clinician choose appropriate interventions and plan the course and sequence of therapy. Critical elements include:

- A firm grounding in the CBT model, with an understanding of the reciprocal relations among thoughts, physical feelings, emotions, and actions
- A holistic but focused initial assessment that evaluates multiple domains of functioning and obtains the perspective of multiple participants in the youth's life
- A case conceptualization that integrates the theoretical model with assessment data
- A treatment plan that takes into account the youth's individual target goals and data from their functional assessment that identifies specific antecedents and maintaining mechanisms
- A plan for monitoring progress over time, including standardized and idiographic assessments

CHAPTER 2

Middle Treatment Phase

Intervention Strategies

Cognitive-behavioral therapy (CBT) comprises a core set of intervention skills designed to help youth identify and change unrealistically negative assumptions and beliefs, manage their emotions, and approach problems rather than avoid them. In this chapter, we provide an overview of the most common CBT techniques and strategies. Each disorder chapter then provides examples of relevant strategies and discusses how to implement them with a specific case. Table 2.1 summarizes the intervention strategies described in this chapter.

BUILDING A STRONG RAPPORT AND WORKING ALLIANCE

Building a trusting rapport and collaborative relationship with youth and parents is critical to the success of treatment. The CBT therapist is often likened to a coach or tutor. The therapist is not there to authoritatively tell the client how to respond or how to act, nor would it be appropriate for the therapist to be passively introspective in the midst of active behavioral practice. Instead, the therapist is there to play the role of diagnostician, consultant, and cheerleader. For example, if a teen were looking to improve their backhand in tennis, they might enlist the help of a tennis coach. Ideally, that coach might bring the teen out to a tennis court and watch as they took some serves and attempted their backhand. As a diagnostician, the coach would look for strengths and flaws in how the teen was approaching or executing their swing. As a consultant, the coach would provide feedback to the teen, testing out hypotheses about the teen's mechanics. The coach might note that the teen is opening up their stance as they finished their follow-through or that they were taking their eyes off the ball. After giving this feedback, the coach would ask the teen to take new swings and help the teen execute the recommended fixes. The suggestions that produce better results stay, while the less effective suggestions are abandoned. All the while, the teen's feedback and experience are solicited so that the coach can personalize each suggestion.

Similarly, the therapist serves as an empathic and encouraging cheerleader. The teen has come explicitly to the therapist because they are *struggling*. If the therapist were to employ criti-

TABLE 2.1. Summary of CBT Intervention Strategies

Tone Setting

- Rapport and alliance building
- Client engagement and motivational interviewing
- Goal setting

Psychoeducation

- About the disorder or problem
- About the CBT model: emotions, thoughts, actions
- Emotions education
- Self-monitoring

Cognitive Interventions

- Thought–feeling–action tracking
- Cognitive restructuring
- Identifying self-talk
- Labeling thinking traps
- Coping thoughts
- Mindfulness training: creating distance from thoughts

Behavioral Interventions

- Problem solving
- Behavior activation
- Activity monitoring
- Functional assessment
- Activity scheduling
- Behavioral experiments (imaginal, *in vivo*)
- Fear and challenge hierarchies
- Exposures and behavioral experiments
- Homework
- Social skills training
- Reward charts and self-rewards

Physical

- Relaxation
- Breathing retraining
- Sleep, dietary, and exercise hygiene

Parenting

- Identifying parent–child interaction patterns
- Communication skills and labeled praise
- Empathize and encourage
- Contingency management

cal or punishing comments, or act frustrated with each failed attempt, the teen would inevitably become demotivated and discouraged. Instead, the therapist can maintain high motivation by reinforcing the teen's willingness to attempt new suggestions and their efforts to cope with their own frustration as they learned novel skills. A CBT therapist embodies this role of active and responsive coach—using their expertise to make personalized suggestions and to shepherd the youth through tough challenges. All the while the therapist treats the youth's experiences as critical data. In this way, the CBT relationship is characterized by active collaboration between therapist and client, reflecting a mixture of education, assessment, encouraging feedback, concrete interventions, and trial and error (hypothesis testing).

Some therapists have told us that they feel they have to "establish trust" and a good relationship before they start the work of therapy. Specific relationship-building exercises (e.g., icebreakers, get-to-know-you games) are always welcome at the beginning of treatment. However, we want to emphasize that relationship building is an active and *continuous* part of CBT. There is also a bidirectional relationship between relationship building and targeted techniques. Early interventions (e.g., goal setting, motivational interviewing, psychoeducation) help demonstrate understanding and build trust. Greater collaboration sets the context for greater interest in skills and active participation in behavioral exercises. For these reasons, the therapist's commitment to learning (*and remembering*) the youth's interests and needs is critical. What are the youth's likes and dislikes? What are the child's strengths and vulnerabilities? Is there a particular role model they admire? The more that interventions can be tailored to the youth's and family's specific needs, interests, and abilities, the greater the chance for connection as well as treatment uptake and benefit.

MOTIVATIONAL INTERVIEWING AND ENGAGEMENT TECHNIQUES

Motivational interviewing (MI; Miller & Rollnick, 2012) is a systematic approach that encourages behavior change by helping clients explore and resolve the ambivalence that impedes forward movement. It makes use of a directive, but client-centered approach that entrusts the client to make the change they seek. Briefer engagement strategies (e.g., Nock & Kazdin, 2005) have been developed for use in early phases of CBT to help therapist and client in clarifying therapy goals, identify potential barriers to progress, and problem-solve solutions to these impediments. Using this approach, the therapist elicits the kinds of changes the youth and caregivers want to make, the reasons they have made such choices, and the steps they plan to take. This approach conveys that youth and caregivers are responsible for active engagement in treatment. In the Change Plan worksheet (see Figure 2.1; a blank version is available as Worksheet 3 in Appendix A), a therapist helps clients anticipate common impediments to therapy participation and to practicing lessons at home. It is impossible to anticipate all upcoming barriers. It is also unlikely that the youth and therapist will be able to develop solutions to overcome all the anticipated barriers. However, this approach puts the topic explicitly on the table for future conversations. In the example below, a teen identifies attending basketball practice as a core goal, but they assume the basketball coach will be unforgiving and absolute about attendance. The youth has identified a future barrier that will require active intervention, but the Change Plan worksheet highlights for both youth and therapist where the key barriers reside. Easier challenges can be problem-solved at this point, including soliciting the mother's help in prompting the youth's attendance at therapy sessions.

The therapist can use a decision matrix to help clarify conflicting motivations and barriers that have stymied efforts to change in the past (see Figure 2.2). The therapist draws a four-box square and elicits from the teen the pros and cons of both doing the behavior and not doing it. The example in Figure 2.2 is about deciding to go back to basketball after a long layoff or to not go back. It is important for the therapist to stay fairly neutral through this process as the youth spells out their reasons, even if the therapist is required to provide examples of what they have heard the youth say before. Once all cells within the matrix are completed, the therapist reviews the pros of engaging the behavior and the cons of not engaging it, as well as the pros of not engaging the behavior and the cons of engaging it. It is in these last two cells where one can identify the barriers that have kept the youth stuck to date. Reviewing these cells highlights the role that negative evaluation (e.g., "Everyone will see how bad I am") and lack of physical activation (e.g., "I'm so tired in the afternoons") have served in maintaining this youth's depressive behavior. As the therapist reviews these pieces of information, they need to stay agnostic with regard to the outcome; it is not up to the therapist to advocate for a particular goal. It is not up to the therapist to "push" the youth to attend basketball practices again. Rather, the point of this exercise is to make clear the choices before the teen and to help them weigh the pros and cons of their choices. Will attending basketball, or not attending, bring more value to the youth's life? The therapist helps guide the youth in realistically seeing the choice before them, but it is then up to the youth to make those choices.

WORKSHEET 3. Change Plan

> The therapist and youth can fill this out together (use help from parents as needed) to discuss what they would like to get out of their collaborative work. Using this worksheet, try to identify the youth's goals, and the challenges and supports that are needed to reach those goals.

1) The changes I want to make are:

(e.g., decrease anxiety/sad mood, improve grades, make more friends, do more fun activities)

Get to basketball practice regularly. Spend more time with friends.

2) The most important reasons I want to make these changes are:

(e.g., my happiness, my family, my social life, my grades)

I used to love basketball. It makes me feel good about myself. I have fun when I'm with friends.

3) The steps I plan to take in changing are:

(e.g., come to sessions, try skills at home, practice)

Try out things my therapist says. Try to push myself to get back to basketball.

Things that could interfere with the change plan:

4) How much trouble do you think you'll have getting to session each week (e.g., scheduling)?

0   1   ②   3   4

Not at all   Very Much

To overcome this, I will: (e.g., talk to my teacher)

Schedule it in my phone. Have my mom remind me.

(continued)

FIGURE 2.1. Completed Change Plan worksheet on basis of a case example. Adapted with permission from Nock, M. K. (2005). *Participation Enhancement Intervention: A brief manual for a brief intervention.* Unpublished manuscript. Harvard University, Cambridge, MA.

WORKSHEET 3. Change Plan (p. 2 of 3)

5) How much do you think things will get in the way of you practicing the skills we go over here at home? 0   1   2   3   ④

Not at all   Very Much

> To overcome this, I will: (e.g., use reminders to self to practice each day)
>
> *Not being in the mood. Being worried what my coach and friends will think when I come back. What if I stink?*

6) How much do you feel as if coming to session each week might be too much work? 0   1   ②   3   4

Not at all   Very Much

> To overcome this, I will: (e.g., talk to my group leaders, make a deal with myself to work hard now for a better future)
>
> *I might feel embarrassed about coming if I haven't done the homework. I'll make sure to do the homework. If that doesn't work, we'll problem-solve in session.*

7) How much do you feel as if using these skills at home will be too much work? 0   1   2   3   ④

Not at all   Very Much

> To overcome this, I will: (e.g., ask parents for help, make a deal with myself to work hard now for a better future)
>
> *Ask my mom to help schedule it in. Tell friends that I'll be at practice—put pressure on myself. Or ask them to hang out early in the week.*

8) How much do you feel that a lack of support from others will be a problem for you in using the skills we practice here at home? 0   1   2   ③   4

Not at all   Very Much

> Person: (e.g., parents, friends, group leaders)
>
> *Mom will be helpful. Not sure coach and friends would understand. What if I bail out on them, and then they're mad?*
>
> Possible ways to help: (e.g., share work, ask group leaders, parents, or friends for more support)
>
> *Ask mom to make me accountable. Ask my one friend who knows I'm struggling—Tia. She can help figure out the best way to set up low-key hang-outs.*

(continued)

FIGURE 2.1. *(continued)*

WORKSHEET 3. Change Plan (p. 3 of 3)

9) How much do you feel as if these skills will work at home?   0   1   ②   3   4

Not at all   Very Much

> To overcome this, I will: (e.g., remember it takes time and practice, talk to my group leaders)
>
> *I think practicing b-ball at home or having friends over would be OK. Going to practice or hanging out outside might be tougher. My friend Tia will help set up low-key hang-outs. I'll have to speak to the coach eventually.*

10) Overall, how comfortable do you think you'll feel practicing these skills with us in session?   0   1   2   ③   4

Not at all   Very Much

> To overcome this, I will: (e.g., practice until I feel more comfortable)
>
> *In session should be OK. At home will be harder. The therapist tells me we can do phone coaching or Web-coaching to practice together at home.*

11) How comfortable do you think you'll feel practicing these skills at home?   0   ①   2   3   4

Not at all   Very Much

> To overcome this, I will: (e.g., practice until I feel more comfortable)
>
> *This is the hard part. And I'll ask my therapist to do phone coaching.*

12) How likely do you think it is that you will continue for the entire treatment?   0   1   2   ③   4

Not at all   Very Much

> To overcome this, I will: (e.g., remember initial treatment goal and make sure I meet it)
>
> *I think I'll be fine with that.*

FIGURE 2.1. *(continued)*

Decision to Make: Whether to go back to basketball practice after a long layoff

	Pros	Cons
Going Back	• I see my teammates again. • I get to practice; I get better. • I'm part of a team. • I could get scouted by colleges.	• It's too much effort. I'm so tired in the afternoons. • Everyone will see how bad I am. • I might have to come off the bench. • I need to pull up my grades to stay eligible.
Not Going Back	• People won't see me as being all rusty. • I don't have to explain why I've been gone. • It's easier.	• I'll only get worse. • I'll lose more playing time. • My friends all hang out afterward. • I won't have a chance to get a scholarship.

FIGURE 2.2. Using a decision matrix to clarify the pros and cons of two choices.

PSYCHOEDUCATION

About the Disorder or Problem

CBT provides two forms of psychoeducation over the course of treatment. One form focuses on providing specific information about the youth's diagnosis (e.g., social anxiety) or problem area (e.g., school avoidance, self-harming behaviors) to educate the family on the nature and course of the problem, associated impairments and skills deficits, and effective treatments for the problem. The therapist generally provides this information at the start of treatment, after a comprehensive assessment has been completed. This allows the family to make educated choices about treatment options and to set expectations for realistic goals. Chapter 5 refers to handouts on depression and anxiety disorders. Fact sheets are also provided when specific phenomena are clinically relevant to specific disorders (e.g., establishing sleep hygiene in depression). Use these to guide discussion about each of the covered disorders.

About the CBT Model

The second form of psychoeducation centers on information about the CBT model. This includes a description of the CBT triangle (thoughts, actions, physical feelings), the role of thinking traps and behavioral avoidance, functional assessments, and a review of common parent–child interaction patterns that interfere with functioning. Explicitly describing the CBT model helps the youth and family understand the therapist's approach and become equal partners in generating target goals and forming a treatment plan. Chapter 1 describes the CBT model in more depth, but we recommend that therapists emphasize the following key points:

1. **Emotions are natural.** The goal of CBT is to help youth learn how they react in challenging situations and to utilize strategies to cope. CBT does not aim to neutralize or eliminate emotions. Feelings are natural and helpful experiences that contribute to a full life when the cli-

ent feels they are in proper balance. Some youth may require more remedial affective education, including help in labeling and defining emotions. We provide examples of affective education below.

2. **CBT depends on the active participation of clients.** This does not mean we should expect a youth client to bound into therapy excited to execute change. Indeed, most youth do not self-refer for therapy. They arrive at the direction of parents, teachers, or other adults. It is vital to acknowledge this fact to the youth, and also emphasize that any benefit will only come from their contributing to the process. CBT does not work by taking some passive agent (e.g., medication); it requires kids to be open, to self-disclose, and to participate. You can express this by saying, "I may be an expert or coach in CBT and helping kids deal with anxiety and depression, but you're the expert on you." Working with youth also requires some level of active participation from caregivers; that level may be dependent on age, family, and presenting concerns.

3. **Participation also includes routine out-of-session activities.** Out-of-session practice is essential to reinforcing and generalizing lessons taught in session. Call external work something other than "homework." Draw parallels to other examples from the youth's life. For example, how do they learn math, clarinet, or softball? They may receive instruction in school from a teacher, instructor, or coach, but there is only so far one can get if they do not practice on their own time.

Self-Monitoring

Anxiety and depression often seem unmanageable because they feel diffuse and all-encompassing. Various tracking exercises (e.g., thought tracking, functional assessment, parent–child interaction trackers) help the youth become more aware of their own experiences and begin to connect their thoughts, feelings, and actions. Self-monitoring exercises and home practice also help youth become more specific about their experiences, the events that trigger them, and the consequences that follow. Knowing the youth's cognitive–emotional–behavioral patterns helps the youth and therapist better tailor CBT interventions to the youth's personal needs.

Affective Education

Affective education generally includes four key components: (1) normalizing anxious and sad feelings; (2) learning how to identify, distinguish, and label feelings; (3) distinguishing a range of intensity in emotion; and (4) connecting emotions to internal and external behavioral reactions.

The first task for a therapist is to *normalize the experience* of anxious and sad feelings. Anxious and depressed children often worry that the intensity of their emotions means that something is seriously wrong with them. It helps them learn to see emotions as natural experiences that serve important functions. For example, we often feel anxiety (e.g., increased heart rate, rapid breathing) when there is real risk (e.g., crossing a busy street) or an upcoming challenge (e.g., an important test). Anxiety helps us prepare for the big test or become more alert when potential danger exists. Sadness comes in response to realistic disappointment (e.g., getting cut from the team) or loss (e.g., a friend moving away, a death in the family). Sadness indicates that it is time to mourn or to reflect on how you would like the situation to change. These are natural processes that we do not want to eliminate. It is when emotional intensity begins to interfere with the youth's functioning that we want to regulate moods.

Building the youth's *emotional vocabulary and understanding* is the next task. The therapist helps the youth brainstorm a list of feelings, working to generate increasingly refined labels for feelings. For example, an initial brainstorm of feelings may include "happy," "sad," or "angry." The therapist helps the youth elaborate to include emotions like "loved," "embarrassed," "disappointed," "jealous," "discouraged," and so on. The therapist can do this by providing examples of situations that would evoke such feelings and having the client guess which feelings match. The therapist might say, "What might you feel if you were trying out for the school musical and didn't get the part?" (disappointed, sad, etc.). This exchange lets the youth understand that events can have a recognizable impact on feelings. At the same time, when children feel multiple emotions simultaneously, it can be confusing for them. "How would you feel if you did not get the part in the play, but your best friend did?" ("Disappointed for me, but happy for my friend"). These activities help the youth learn to identify, distinguish, and label feelings so that they can express themself more effectively.

The third step of affective education is understanding that emotions extend across a wide range of *intensity*. The therapist helps the youth learn that feelings do not come as "all or none" or "on or off." Instead, the therapist helps the youth build a rating scale (e.g., 0–10, 0–100) that communicates the dimensionality of intensity. Youth can be oriented to the use of rating scales with general fun-filled and interest-specific examples, for example, "On a scale from 0 to 10, how much do you like ice cream?" "On a scale from 0 to 10, how funny do you think this picture is [insert an amusing dog meme]?" "On a scale from 0 to 10, how excited are you to watch the Women's World Cup?" Then we find it helps to have the youth anchor problem-specific real-life events to each rating. For instance, building a "sadness" rating scale with a youth using scores from 0 to 10, the therapist and youth start by labeling each score with a descriptor (e.g., "Zero equals no sadness; feeling comfortable"; "Five equals feeling down and discouraged"; "Ten equals crushing depression"). Next the therapist helps the youth recall different events where they have felt different intensities of sadness (e.g., "I was at 0 last summer when we went to the shore"; "Was a 5 when I heard about not getting the part in the play"; "I've never felt this bad, or been a 10, but I can imagine this will happen when my parents get divorced, something that's coming up"). Figure 2.3 (a blank version is available as Worksheet 4 in Appendix A) gives an example of a completed feelings rating scale, called a "feelings thermometer," for younger clients. During this step in affective education, the therapist can gather data and provide feedback on how youth report the intensity of their emotions (e.g., everything is a 10).

Fourth, clients often benefit from exercises designed to help connect emotions to internal and external behavioral reactions. External expressions of emotions can be illustrated by reviewing magazines, movie clips, memes, gifs, or YouTube videos (with the volume turned down)—especially if these are tied to the youth's areas of interest. The youth can try to identify what the person in the image is feeling based on posture, facial expression, and actions. For younger clients, games like *Feelings Charades* or building a *Feelings Dictionary* (e.g., Kendall & Kedtke, 2006) can make the same point. To connect clients to internal expressions of feelings, the therapist helps the youth identify how different body parts react to different situations. For example, a youth might experience a racing heart, shortness of breath, a stomachache, dizziness, or sweating in response to feeling anxious before going to an unfamiliar social event. Another youth might feel a weight on their shoulders, a pit in their stomach, and a headache when feeling depressed after a fight with a friend.

Gaining fuller awareness of one's own physical and behavioral reactions to emotions leads naturally to retraining breathing and teaching progressive relaxation. (See the "Physical Interventions" section later in this chapter.)

WORKSHEET 4. Feelings Thermometer

Pick a feeling to describe (e.g., sadness, nervousness, anger). Then try to think about that feeling on a 0–10 scale. What words would you use to describe each rating? Can you remember a time when you've felt that way?

What feeling you are rating:

Mood rating	How intense is it? (0 "Not at all" to 10 "the worst")	Describe the feeling (in your own words) for each level.	Describe past times you've felt this way.
100	10	Total pain	Don't think I've been there.
	9	Lost, totally hopeless	I've felt this way, but don't remember when.
80	8	Alone and empty	When I was bullied in the hallway and no one stuck up for me
	7	So sad and crying	When my dad forgot my birthday
60	6	Isolated	When my friend told me I was being stupid for feeling sad
	5	Hating myself	When I got a bad grade and couldn't study.
40	4	Tired	Most afternoons
	3	Blah. Why bother?	Most mornings
20	2	Bored	Doing homework
	1	Slightly tired	Typical day
0	0	OK—not good, not bad	

FIGURE 2.3. Completed Feelings Thermometer with personalized anchors.

COGNITIVE INTERVENTIONS

Self-Talk and Cognitive Restructuring

Cognitive restructuring is a flexible set of techniques that has been found useful across a wide range of youth problems (Peris et al., 2015; Shirk, Crisostomo, Jungluth, & Gudmundsen, 2013). It is designed to help the youth become more aware of the impact that unrealistically negative thoughts have on emotions and to learn that they themself have the power to challenge and change their thought patterns. Cognitive restructuring can be broken down into several core skills, including thought tracking, connecting thoughts to emotions, identifying thinking traps (cognitive distortions), challenging unrealistic assumptions and expectations, and generating more realistic, encouraging coping thoughts. Behavioral experiments can then be used to challenge unrealistic assumptions, and home practice can be assigned to reinforce and generalize lessons.

Step 1: Track Events, Thoughts, and Mood

First, the therapist helps the youth notice the connection between their thoughts, mood, and the events that precede them. For younger children, these internal thoughts can be explained as "things you say to yourself in your thought bubbles, as in comic books." For adolescents, the thought process can be described as an inner dialogue or private thoughts that may be just below the surface of awareness. The teen might be attending to these "automatic thoughts" like background music or background chatter at a party—barely audible but subtly influencing one's mood or attention. Indeed, the content of our thoughts can also have a powerful impact on our subsequent mood. Negative thinking tends to precede sad feelings, threat-based thoughts precede anxious feelings, optimistic thoughts precede hopeful feelings. Thus, the first major skill in cognitive restructuring is to teach the youth how to identify the thoughts that surface in different situations and the impact those thoughts have on mood. The completed Thinking Traps Tracker in Figure 2.4 (a blank version is available as Worksheet 5 in Appendix A) can be used to help the youth monitor triggers (events, interpersonal interactions, internal memories), the thought that surfaces in response to the trigger, and the mood (and intensity) that follows. In the office or over telehealth, the therapist can teach and practice this skill with a game like *Catch the Thought*, where the therapist prints or draws a thought bubble outline for the client and themself and each takes a turn imagining different scenarios, with the other raising the thought bubble over their head and both having to name the thought they were thinking. Each chapter provides examples of problem-specific automatic thoughts.

Step 2: Identify Unrealistic Assumptions and Label Thinking Traps

The thinking patterns of anxious and depressed youth are characterized by a high degree of self-criticism and other criticism, negative outlook, and helplessness in the face of threat. These thoughts rarely reflect the objective evidence in the youth's immediate experience; rather, they reflect distortions of the external world, false conclusions based on partial information, and premature assumptions about future events. After tracking automatic thought patterns, the therapist leads the youth in a series of questions to examine if their conclusions and expectations realistically reflect the evidence. For example, a youth who discloses that a friend does not want to attend their party after the friend fails to text beforehand may be jumping to unfounded conclusions. The

WORKSHEET 5. Thinking Traps Tracker

What thinking traps do you fall into when feeling sad, anxious, or distressed? For each situation, describe and rate how you feel. Describe your automatic thought (the first thought that comes into your head). What thinking trap might you be falling into? How does that make you feel (the result)?

Trigger	Feeling (Rate 0–10: "not at all" to "excruciating")	Thought	Thinking Trap	Result?
I hear the alarm go off on the day of a big test.	Fear, panic (7)	"I'm not ready for the test!" "This will kill my grade!"	Fortune-telling, catastrophizing	Felt worse (9)
Missed a pass during practice. Other team stole it for a point.	Frustrated (8) Embarrassed (6)	"I suck at this." "I've lost my touch."	Catastrophizing	Frustrated (9) Angry at myself (8)
Couldn't sleep because of spelling test	Tense, nervous (8)	"I won't remember all of the spellings." "What if I'm awake all night?" "I won't be able to concentrate for the test and will fail."	What if/tell me, catastrophizing	Got out of bed 3 times, went looking for mom, she got mad at me

FIGURE 2.4. Completed Thinking Traps Tracker worksheet.

34

therapist asks open-ended questions to help the youth self-evaluate the veracity of their assumption. For example, "Did your friend tell you they didn't want to come to your party?" If the youth can provide evidence to support their conclusion (e.g., the two friends recently had a fight, and the friend told the youth they did not want to come to the party), then cognitive restructuring may not be warranted. Other options like assertiveness, conflict resolution, or acceptance skills may apply. If the youth cannot provide evidence for their conclusion, then they are likely jumping to conclusions and "filling in the blanks" from partial information. In these cases, the youth is likely falling into one of several thinking traps.

Some of the most common cognitive distortions (unrealistic assumptions) are summarized in Table 2.2 (a reproducible version is available as Handout 2 in Appendix A). After identifying automatic thought patterns, the therapist helps the youth recognize if each reflects a common "thinking trap." Such traps serve to keep the youth stuck in feelings of sadness or anxiety when alternative interpretations exist. The teen in the party example above may be falling prey to the thinking trap of "mind reading" unless they had invited their friend and were told directly that the friend did not want to attend their party. A teen who is overly self-critical after a poor sports outing one day may be "disqualifying the positives" by ignoring their typical performance or the fact that they had made the varsity team as a sophomore. It is not clear why some youth fall into these thinking traps more than others; with practice, clients can become skilled at identifying their own thinking traps, which can then help them distinguish realistic from unrealistic evaluations of situations.

Step 3: Generate More Positive, Realistic Coping Thoughts

The therapist next helps the youth develop more realistic and adaptive coping thoughts. Ideal coping thoughts directly address the specific thinking trap the youth is stuck in. In the above party example, a helpful response to the mind reading trap might be to adopt this coping statement: "I can't assume I know what my friend thinks until I ask." In the sports disqualifying the positives example, a useful coping response might be "One bad day a soccer career does not make," "Even the pros have bad days," or "It wasn't even the whole match, I played decent defense the second half."

Coping thoughts should also not be *unrealistically positive*. Novice CBT therapists often misunderstand the goal of cognitive restructuring and encourage unvarnished "positive thinking" or dismissive responses like "Don't worry about it," or "It will be fine." However, adopting the coping thought "Why am I worried? Everyone at the school gets along and wants to come to my party" is as equally unrealistic as the initial negative thought and may set up the youth for disappointment. Furthermore, it is not very believable. Pushing this kind of Pollyannaish agenda can quickly damage the therapist's credibility and the value of the strategy. Instead, the goal is to encourage the teen to adopt a more balanced, flexible point of view that enables them to push forward without ruminating on false negativities. Adopting a coping thought like "All I can do is plan a great party and hope people want to come" may not protect the youth from all possible negative outcomes, but it keeps them from dwelling on negativities that have not yet happened.

Mindfulness Training

A complementary intervention to cognitive restructuring is mindfulness training. Cognitive restructuring focuses on identifying and challenging troublesome thought patterns by generating

TABLE 2.2. Common Thinking Traps That Get Us Stuck

1. **Mind reading (Mind Reader):** You assume you know what other people think without sufficient evidence of their thoughts. "He thinks I'm a loser." "Everyone can see what cheap clothes I'm wearing."

2. **Fortune-telling (Fortune Teller):** You're positive you know what will happen in the future, but you don't have enough evidence! "I won't know anyone at the party." "I have no chance making the basketball team."

3. **Catastrophizing (Doomsday Predictor):** All you see are the worst-case outcomes! "Now I'm going to fail this class because I got this 'B' on my test." "Everyone will know what a loser I am after I got rejected for the prom."

4. **Jumping to conclusions (The Assumer):** You assume you know something, but you only have a little amount of information. "No one's going to show for my party" (after receiving one or two declines). "My boyfriend is going to break up with me" (after not return a phone call).

5. **What if's (Tell Me, Tell Me):** You keep asking question after question because nothing seems to answer the question. "What if they give a pop quiz tomorrow?" "What if they test us on new material?" "What if a substitute doesn't know how the teacher does things?" No answers seem to reassure you, no matter how many times you ask.

6. **Discounting the positives (Nothing Special):** You minimize the positives of a situation or minimize your contributions. You claim the positive actions you take are trivial (e.g., "Anyone could have helped my friend study"). You disregard positive events that may have occurred (e.g., "They invite everyone who's in the honor society to that dinner").

7. **Looking for the negatives (Walking with Blinders On):** All you can see are the negative things happening around you. You can't see the positives. "I couldn't even find anything fun to do while my friend was here." "School is nothing but fake people."

8. **Overgeneralizing (The Big Snowball):** One bad thing happens, and everything will turn out the same. "See? Other kids don't give you a chance to be yourself." "I'm not very good at school—I don't think I have much to look forward to."

9. **All-or-nothing thinking (Black-and-White):** Everything's either all good or all bad. All perfect or all a failure. "If I don't get an 'A,' I'm a failure." "If you miss one party, people will forget about you."

10. **Should statements (Must/Has-to-Be):** You see events in terms of how things should be, rather than simply focusing on how they are. "I should ace all my exams." "I need to be available to my friends all the time." "My parents don't care about me if they make me go to school [my parents ought to let me stay home]."

11. **Taking things too personally (The Self-Critic):** If something goes wrong, it must be your fault. "We lost the game because of me." "I'll never get better." If someone says anything a little bit negative, it feels like the world is crashing.

12. **Blaming (Hot Potato):** You focus on the other person as the source of your negative feelings, because it is too difficult to take responsibility. "Why won't you let me stay home from school?" "Why is everyone against me?"

more realistic and adaptive coping thoughts. Mindfulness, on the other hand, helps the individual identify troublesome thought patterns and learn how to gain *distance* from them without necessarily altering the content of their thoughts. Extensive research has shown that anxious and depressed youth often experience intrusive thoughts, characterized by significant worry and rumination. Evidence suggests that when youth attempt to suppress or distract themselves from intrusive thoughts, this can decrease their distress in the short term but often leads to increased return of the distressing thoughts over time (Pettit et al., 2009). These thoughts occupy increasing cognitive attention and contribute to increased impairment (e.g., elevated somatic complaints, internalizing symptoms, externalizing behavioral problems) (Greco, Baer, & Smith, 2011).

Mindfulness exercises help interrupt ruminative cycles by providing an alternative to thought suppression, distraction, or cognitive restructuring (Greco, Blackledge, Coyne, & Ehrenreich, 2005; Kallapiran, Koo, Kirubakaran, & Hancock, 2015). They start with *noticing* the thought. One mindfulness exercise is to envision placing each intrusive thought on a leaf floating in a stream, and then to let it flow gradually down a stream away from yourself. Another is to envision your thoughts being placed on pieces of luggage as they circle around a conveyor belt at the airport. (See Figure 2.5 for an exercise script; a reproducible version is available as Handout 3 in Appendix A.) You can also have a youth imagine the thought as a cloud drifting by. The goal of mindfulness exercises is to accept that a whole range of thoughts (negative and positive in valence) enter our minds continuously throughout the day. Overattending to any one thought gives that thought too much "power" over one's mood, choices, and beliefs. Mindfulness helps clients treat their thoughts as not literal—as thoughts, no more, no less. It is as if you could place your thoughts on a cloud that is tethered to one's hip; allow the thoughts to rest there without giving into urges to pull the cloud closer or push it further away. In this way, you acknowledge that thoughts will always be there, but they do not necessarily compel us to act.

BEHAVIORAL INTERVENTIONS

Problem Solving

Teaching effective problem-solving techniques is an integral part of evidence-based treatments for anxious and depressed youth. The goal is to help youth gain control over the situations for which they have control and become more flexible in how they approach problems. We teach problem solving (see Chapter 6 for a case example) using the STEPS approach (Chorpita & Weisz, 2009; Weisz, Thurber, Sweeney, Proffitt, & LeGagnoux, 1997):

S: Say what the problem is.
T: Think of solutions.
E: Examine each solution. (List pros and cons for each solution.)
P: Pick one solution and try it.
S: See if it worked. (If "yes," great! If "no," try another solution!)

S: Say What the Problem Is

In the first step, the therapist asks the youth to concretely describe the problem they are facing. Clients often give overgeneralized descriptions, (e.g., "anxious feelings," "fighting with my mom")

This script is to be used by the therapist to help practice mindfulness with their teen client.

For the next several minutes, we're going to be trying something. It may seem a little different, or even unnatural, but I want you to give it a try. Sometimes, our thoughts get the better of us, and today, we're going to try and just let go of them a little bit.

For this exercise, I'm going to ask you to simply notice your thoughts as they naturally come. The aim will be to watch any thoughts—whatever they may be—come into our mind, notice that they're there, but then allow them to pass through you without a fight. We will try to "accept" your thoughts for what they are, just thoughts. Sometimes, the more we fight our thoughts, the stronger they become.

So, for the next several minutes, I'd like you to imagine a conveyor belt in front of you; just like one you'd see at an airport. Think about how a conveyor belt works—luggage comes down from the chute, lays down on the conveyor belt, and then circles around and around. Each piece of luggage gently slides down the chute and then begins its trip around the belt. If you just watched from afar, you'd see that if nobody came to pick up the luggage, the luggage would just go around in circles . . . coming around the front end, circling around, and disappearing around the back end. As you wait, you see the same luggage going around the front end and then back around the back end, slowly but surely circling around.

Well now, as you think of the luggage on this belt, I'd like you to start putting each thought that comes into your head onto a piece of luggage. Just like a label that gets stuck on the luggage. Each thought: gently stick it on the luggage and watch as the thought just stays on the belt, circling around and around. You may feel the urge to do something with the luggage or the thought. You may want to pick it up, put it down on the ground, stop it from circling around and around. You may feel the urge to turn away or distract yourself, to get bored by the circling luggage. When you notice this happening, just turn your attention back to the thought and just appreciate that it is circling gently on the belt in front of you. Sometimes, thoughts will suddenly disappear from the belt. When this happens, simply let them go. No reason to keep a thought on a belt when it doesn't want to be there.

You can either then observe silence as the client practices this, or you can facilitate by asking the client to describe their thought and helping them envision placing it on the luggage and circling around.

Now keep going. I will let you know when to stop. It may seem like a long time, but just allow your thoughts to come as they do.

FIGURE 2.5. "Luggage on a Conveyor Belt" mindfulness script.

that need to be specified further. The youth might feel "anxious all the time," but to solve this problem, it is necessary to identify a specific *context* (e.g., "nights before tests") and *outcomes* that they want to see happen (e.g., "to be able to get to sleep"). Thus, a solvable version of "anxious feelings" might be "I can't fall asleep on nights before a test." Another version might be "Feeling tense and on edge all throughout the day." This version may not offer a specific context, but it localizes a specific *target* (muscle tension) the youth wants to solve. While these translations do not promise to solve everything associated with feeling anxious all the time, they provide a specific target over which the youth can gain some control and that will move toward the ultimate goal: feeling less anxious throughout the day.

T: Think of Solutions

In the second step, the youth learns to brainstorm as many solutions as possible to solve the problem without prejudging any. Once idea generation starts, the therapist must prevent the youth from interrupting the brainstorming process with evaluative criticisms of solutions. This list is just a preliminary list of possible solutions. Anxious and depressed youth often interrupt the process by listing why a particular solution will not work or because they are anxious about choosing the "right" solution. It is the therapist's job to refocus the youth on freely brainstorming without evaluation. The brainstormed solutions do not need to be logical. For example, if a child or adolescent experiences the problem of "not being able to find their homework," problem-solving solutions could be to "ask my parents if they have seen the homework," "post flyers around my neighborhood asking people to send information about the missing homework," or "search the Internet for leads about the missing homework." The goal is to help the child learn they have the ability to be creative about their problems and are not limited to the typical, logical, or socially acceptable options. Youth should be encouraged to continue to identify multiple alternatives as they may stop after naming 2 or 3. One of us has a rule that brainstorming can only stop when 10 to 12 ideas have been generated, at first collaboratively, and then independently by the youth. This *process* as well as the content of this skill may need to be shaped. For some clients at first, this "brainstorming rule" seems daunting, but over time with practice and as they become familiar with the expectation, their hesitancy or tendency to stop after a few options diminishes and they develop the capacity to name successively more potential solutions.

E: Examine Each Solution

After exhaustively generating ideas, the therapist and youth evaluate the pros and cons of each potential solution. Therapists should be careful not to push their agenda toward a favored solution at this point. This can damage the credibility of the strategy. Instead, the therapist's job is to objectively help the youth think through the realistic consequences (both good and bad) for every given solution. If one of the solutions to getting to sleep at night is to "play video games all night until I feel sleepy," the therapist simply helps the youth identify all possible outcomes of that choice. Pros might include wearing the teen out, distracting the teen from their upcoming test, increasing confidence in one area of life. Cons might include limiting the amount of sleep the teen gets, increasing tension and anxiety because games can be activating, and preventing any review of test material. If the therapist and teen execute this process faithfully, the preferred solutions tend to reflect the ones that promote the youth's well-being.

P: Pick One Solution and Try It

Once the pros and cons of each solution are identified, the youth is ready to select one to try first. Again, the therapist adopts a neutral posture, allowing the youth to weigh the pros and cons of generated solutions. The therapist encourages the youth to select their first choice to try, emphasizing a trial-and-error approach. Prepare the youth that the first solution may not work. (We can't expect to solve difficult problems on our first shot!)

S: See If It Worked

The youth attempts the selected solution and evaluates its outcomes. The therapist and teen evaluate the success of the solution (including partial successes) and how and why it could have worked better. The therapist and youth evaluate whether it makes sense to refine the solution and try again, or to move on to another solution from the original brainstormed list.

Activity Monitoring and Behavioral Activation

Activity monitoring and behavioral activation are two core behavioral interventions that have received significant support for improving mood symptoms in youth with depression and broad applicability to youth with anxiety and other disorders (Chu et al., 2016; Cuijpers, Van Straten, & Warmerdam, 2007; Hopko, Robertson, & Lejuez, 2006). Activity monitoring consists of tracking the youth's events and activities over the course of a day or week and their corresponding mood. Behavioral activation is a group of strategies that aim to increase the youth's physical activity and emotional engagement. The two work hand in hand in an assessment–intervention feedback loop.

Activity monitoring is designed to increase awareness of the natural fluctuations of mood across the day and week, and it helps identify the events that trigger changes in a youth's mood (from positive to negative). By keeping track of the people and scenarios that naturally reinforce or discourage, youths can consciously incorporate more enriching elements in their lives and help themselves prepare for challenges. This can be especially important for youth who report flat mood or experience low self-efficacy in bringing about positive experiences. Activity monitoring helps them to see that mood fluctuates more than they may realize and to notice patterns, and provides target goals for the youth to work toward (i.e., increase valuable experiences). Figure 6.5 (a blank version is available as Worksheet 12 in Appendix A) provides an example of a completed activity–mood worksheet, on which the teen was asked to rate mood on a scale from 0, "The worst mood I ever felt," to 10, "The best mood I've ever felt." Activity trackers are generally assigned for home practice so that the youth can monitor events and mood in real time or at the end of each day.

When reviewing activity–mood trackers, the therapist highlights several themes, looking for trends both within and across days:

1. Increase awareness of automatic behaviors: Are there certain habits that contribute to negative moods that escape the youth's awareness (e.g., sleeping all weekend; watching TV all night long; scanning social media for hours; skipping lunch)?
2. Connect mood with events, activities, and people: Do certain settings, people, or interactions reliably lead to negative feelings? Do others consistently promote positive feelings?

3. Identify fluctuations of mood and what events trigger mood changes: What events, activities, and people have the power to change a negative mood to positive, or even to "less bad"? How about the opposite? Triggers that can change mood are some of the most powerful antecedents we can attend to.

Behavioral activation directs the youth to increase contact with meaningful experiences, including pleasant and mastery experiences. It can also be used to decrease a youth's avoidant responses to distress and anhedonia-related withdrawal from previously enjoyed activities, and to increase goal-oriented approach behavior in valued life domains. The therapist and young client use the activity–mood trackers to identify activities and people that reliably improve the youth's mood. These may be factors that increase physical activation (e.g., exercise, sports, recreation, walks), activities that are enjoyable or comforting (e.g., hobbies, social interactions, listening to music or reading), or those that build a youth's sense of mastery (e.g., skills-based activities). The therapist can assign the youth to increase the frequency of pleasant and mastery activities over the course of a week and also help the youth practice utilizing activation as a coping strategy (seeking out pleasant activities when the youth is feeling sad or down).

Behavioral activation can also be used to decrease the frequency of avoidant responses the youth resorts to in the face of stressors. Research has identified behavioral avoidance as a common behavioral mechanism that maintains anxiety and depression in youth. When activated by a stressful trigger, anxious and depressed youth are prone to avoid or withdraw from a situation as a way to eliminate their negative feelings, even at the expense of long-term consequences. For example, when a youth has an argument with a friend, they might think it is easier to avoid the friend than to confront them and reconcile the disagreement. The avoidance might limit distress in the short term since it removes the teen from the immediate conflict. However, failing to approach their friend allows bad feelings to linger and fester, lowering the chances for ultimate reconciliation. We summarize this avoidance cycle using the acronym TRAP (T: Trigger, R: Emotional Response, AP: Avoidance Pattern; Jacobson et al., 2001) to highlight how avoidance can perpetuate distress and impairment in the long run. We then use functional assessment worksheets to help the teen track their own avoidant responses to triggers and its subsequent short- and long-term consequences (see Figure 1.4). Once avoidant and withdrawal patterns are clear, problem solving can be used to direct the youth toward goal-oriented solutions that counter avoidance.

Challenge Hierarchies, Exposures, and Behavioral Experiments

Exposure exercises are behavioral experiments or practice sessions designed to help youth approach a situation that is difficult so that they can learn to (1) manage the distress they feel when they're in that situation, (2) practice skills that will help navigate that situation, and (3) challenge unrealistic assumptions they typically experience in the situation. Exposures can be conducted as imaginal exposures (using imagery and recall to envision oneself in the challenging situation) or *in vivo*, which means "in life." *In vivo* exposures aim to re-create the real-life scenario as closely as possible to give the client a chance to challenge themself in difficult situations with the support of an encouraging coach. For example, a socially anxious youth may avoid giving class presentations for fear of stuttering and being unprepared. One example of an imaginal exposure would be to have the youth envision themself giving their next required presentation, focusing on all of the details (who, what, where) of the situation that usually activate the youth. For an *in vivo* exposure, a therapist might arrange a group of confederates to serve as a real-life audience to observe the presentation and ask questions. Throughout the therapist coaches the youth to use their coping skills to manage distress and become more confident and competent in the situation. The therapist can also encourage the youth to imagine themself stuttering in the middle of the presentation, slowing down, and coaching themself to keep going.

Building a Fear or Challenge Hierarchy

Designing exposures starts with an examination of the youth's (and parent's) treatment goals and brainstorming relevant challenges that would activate fear or distress for the child. The therapist and youth rate the difficulty or distress experienced in each scenario and rank-order them in a challenge hierarchy (for younger children, a challenge or fear ladder analogy may help). In the above social anxiety example, one appropriate challenge hierarchy might look like the following:

Challenge Hierarchy A: Oral Presentation

1. Read a scripted short passage to the therapist.
2. Read a longer scripted presentation to the therapist.
3. Read a scripted passage while stuttering on purpose.
4. Present a semi-scripted presentation and allow the therapist to ask questions.
5. Present an impromptu presentation on a topic of the therapist's choosing.
6. Repeat a scripted short presentation with a small audience of family members.
7. Read a scripted short presentation with a small audience while stuttering at least two times.
8. Repeat a scripted short presentation with a small audience of same-aged peers.
9. Present a scripted long presentation to peers and allow questions.

Notice that each exposure on the challenge hierarchy represents a step of increasing difficulty. This is reflected in the length of the presentation, how much structure is allowed (scripted vs. impromptu), and how many challenges are included (familiar vs. unfamiliar audience; allowing questions; including one of the youth's main feared outcomes, stuttering). This variation allows the youth to gain confidence and competence across a diversity of contexts and challenges and to face varying levels of distress. Traditionally, exposure exercises were pursued in a hierarchical fashion; exposures would proceed in order of difficulty from easier to harder. Recent evidence suggests that it may be beneficial to alternate between easier and more difficult tasks (Craske et al., 2008) to optimize emotional activation during exposures and enhance retention of learning. Nonetheless, it is helpful to lay out the spectrum of youth challenges to provide an organized approach to exposures.

For depressed youth, the types of scenarios that are most distressing do not necessarily revolve around fearful encounters. Frequently these youth feel stuck because the experience of pushing through a challenge feels like too much effort or they expect the outcomes to be punishing. As an example, a depressed youth might have difficulty reaching out to friends for support when their parents are fighting. To help gain confidence in these situations, a therapist could build a challenge hierarchy that helps the youth practice accessing social support in increasingly vulnerable situations.

Challenge Hierarchy B: Accessing Social Support

1. Text a close friend to just say, "Hi."
2. Text a close friend to talk about a favorite topic (e.g., YouTube channel, class, celebrity).
3. Message an acquaintance and ask for information about a class assignment.
4. Call a close friend and engage in small talk (review the day at school).
5. Message an acquaintance from a school club and arrange to go together to the next meeting.
6. Call a close friend and tell them about a difficult experience you had that day.

Any of these situations may provoke a mix of anxiety and sadness (described as skepticism). The goal for each is to provide the youth with an opportunity to overcome these fears and to note the positive outcomes that result from challenging oneself. Importantly, we encourage therapists to stay flexible in planning and executing exposures. Each exercise should be seen as a *collaborative experiment*. There are always ways to design exposures to be easier or more challenging. If one is minimally activating, the therapist and client can brainstorm ways to make it more challenging. If the youth cannot complete a task because they freeze or refuse to initiate it, future exposures and experiments can be broken down into smaller increments to reach the goal of optimizing the challenge but ensuring a sense of success for the client.

How Do Exposures Work? What Am I Targeting?

Some scholars make distinctions between *in vivo* exposures and behavioral experiments. Traditionally, exposures are referenced when the target emotion is fear or anxiety, and habituation is the desired outcome. Behavioral experiments tend to refer to opportunities where the client is practicing instrumental skills or challenging unrealistic expectations and assumptions. In behavioral experiments, challenges are seen as ways to identify and change cognitive distortions and thinking traps. Given the recent deemphasis on habituation as a key mechanism of change in exposures (Craske et al., 2008; Craske, Treanor, Conway, Zbozinek, & Vervliet, 2014), the difference between these two therapeutic interventions is fading. As discussed here, there are a number of goals and targets that exposures and behavioral experiments should have:

1. **Building distress tolerance.** Youth learn to tolerate the distress they feel when they are in a challenging situation. Unpleasant feelings are the primary reason people avoid difficult situations. If they get to practice "sticking with it" in a supportive, safe environment, they will begin to learn that they can push through the distress, and will subsequently find it easier to handle the distress when they are in such a real-life situation. A therapist can communicate this concept to a client with phrases like "handling, managing, tolerating, or accepting distress," "riding the waves," "letting things roll off your back," and "building a tolerance muscle."

2. **Habituation.** In addition to tolerating distress, youth may notice that distress actually decreases over time with practice. After engaging in *in vivo* exposures and learning that they are able to cope with triggering situations, their sadness, anxiety, and anger may start to gradually decrease over time.

3. **Challenging thinking traps and assumptions.** Talking in a room or via telehealth with a therapist can help a client begin to detect where their thinking traps lead to assuming the worst

in neutral situations. When cognitive restructuring is a goal of exposures, a therapist will help the youth lay out their thinking traps, generate more realistic coping thoughts, and practice challenging negative assumptions. Engaging clients in real-life scenarios provides direct evidence that their worst fears are unlikely to come true. This can result from noticing that the child's performance is better than expected. It can also come from getting positive or constructive feedback from confederates. Objective feedback can increase the child's sense of self-efficacy and provide strong evidence to counter typical thinking traps.

4. **Violating expected outcomes.** Research suggests that the more one's expectations are violated, the more that learning is enhanced (i.e., expectancy violation; Craske et al., 2008). Expectations can be verbally mediated, but they do not have to be expressed in negative thought content via thinking traps or cognitive distortions. Beyond anxious and negative thoughts, youth can have expectancies about how they will react, how they will feel, how others will respond, or assumptions about outcomes. To violate expectancies, the therapist helps the youth identify key outcomes they expect ahead of time and then reviews which of those outcomes occurs during and after the experiment.

5. **Practicing skills.** One reason people avoid difficult situations is because they do not know what to do under such circumstances (e.g., they don't know how to start a conversation at a party). Practicing these situations will give them a chance to "try out" different skills (e.g., different ways to start and maintain a conversation) and figure out which strategies work best for them. Sometimes people do not even realize that certain worries can be successfully addressed by "practice-able" skills.

6. **"The pleasant surprise."** Sometimes the most rewarding outcomes are those that we are not expecting. Youth go into feared situations expecting so many catastrophic outcomes that they can't imagine anything going right. They avoid a situation because the potential "reward" does not seem to match the risk. However, it is impossible for any of us, particularly youth who are prone to anxiety or depressed mood, to anticipate all the possible neutral or positive outcomes that await us in any given situation. The truth is, none of us knows exactly what will happen in a specific situation. You could go to a party expecting to not know anyone and to be left in a corner all by yourself staring at your smartphone. What you could not know is that other partygoers would be playing your favorite game and asking you for help. Or, maybe another guest is new to town and you spend the whole time talking to this teen and realize you have so much in common with them. None of these pleasant surprises would have happened if you had decided to stay home. A famous sportscaster always says, "That's why they play the game—it's the only way to find out what happens!" Peter Lewinsohn (Lewinsohn & Libet, 1972; Lewinsohn & Graf, 1973) referred to this as taking advantage of "opportunities for reinforcement found in natural environments." However you convey this concept, the idea is the same: half the contest is simply putting yourself in the game.

Planning and Executing an Exposure Exercise

Once a challenge hierarchy is created, the therapist and youth are ready to try one out. As much as possible, we encourage conducting experiments live in session in addition to assigning follow-up exercises at home for practice. To help set up a live exposure in session, we use the *In vivo* Exposure/Behavioral Experiment worksheet (see Figure 2.6; a blank version is available as Worksheet

WORKSHEET 6. *In Vivo* Exposure/Behavioral Experiment

> Complete this worksheet with the youth as you are preparing for a behavioral experiment.

1. Situation (What's the situation?):

Impromptu speech of therapist's choosing.

2. Feelings: **Distress Rating:** __85__

Anxious, sweaty palms, butterflies in stomach.

3. Anxious/Negative Thoughts:

Anxious/Negative Thoughts:	**Thinking Traps (See list below.)**
a. "I won't know what to say."	a. Fortune-telling
b. "You're going to think I'm stupid."	b. Mind reading
c. "Everyone can do this and I can't."	c. Overgeneralizing; all-or-nothing
d. "I'm going to stutter and mumble."	d. Fortune-telling, looking for the negatives

Thinking Traps: mind reading, fortune-telling, catastrophizing, jumping to conclusions, what if's, discounting the positives, looking for the negatives, overgeneralizing, all-or-nothing thinking, should statements, taking things too personally, blaming.

4. Coping Thoughts (How do you respond to your anxious thoughts?):

"If my mind goes blank, I can just pause and take a deep breath."
"You've been supportive so far. You're not here to judge me."
"Most people get anxious during speeches."
"If I stutter or mumble, just keep going."

Challenge Questions: Do I know for certain that _____? Am I 100% sure that _____? What evidence do I have that _____? What is the worst that could happen? How bad is that? Do I have a crystal ball?

5. Achievable Behavioral Goals (What do you want to accomplish?):

Goal	Accomplished?
a. Just keep going if I get stuck—avoid 10 sec pauses.	
b. Last 5 minutes.	
c. Make eye contact at least 10 times.	

6. Rewards:

Reward	Earned?
a. Earn open talk time at the end of session.	
b. Get a new bitmoji app for phone.	
c.	

FIGURE 2.6. Completed Behavioral/Exposure Experiment worksheet using a social anxiety example.

6 in Appendix A). This worksheet can help the therapist and client prepare the technical aspects of the experiment as well as rehearse coping skills the youth will use.

1. **Describe the situation.** The therapist and youth collaboratively select a situation from the challenge hierarchy. The goal is to select a scenario that will be sufficiently activating for the youth (e.g., youth rates their distress as a 7 on a 10-point scale), but that is manageable enough that the youth will be willing to engage in the challenge. This is not to say that any youth will be excited to enter a feared situation, but they must be willing to participate. Still, we never *make* youth participate in exposures—we plan, encourage, identify skills, and reinforce. Sometimes a youth will offer a statement like "My therapist made me give a speech," or say something to this effect, and we suggest correcting this each time: "We planned for it and I coached and supported you, but you decided to try it!" It may help for the therapist to offer two or three scenarios from which to choose, and role-plays can be used to warm up the youth. Furthermore, they can gain a sense of control by contributing to the planning—identifying the specific setting, the structure, the initial supports. In the current example, the therapist and youth have progressed midway through their oral presentation hierarchy and so choose an impromptu speech for the youth to practice with the therapist. To make the situation as real as possible, you want to get as many details about how this scene (trigger, situation) would play out. This helps plan out the most realistic exposure possible. In this case, the youth's history class requires students to give a "current events" presentation when the teacher calls on them. The timing is unpredictable, so the therapist and youth agree to practice being "caught off guard" and to conduct an impromptu speech on a topic the therapist chooses.

2. **Arrive at a feelings and distress rating.** Solicit from the child what kind of emotional responses and physical symptoms they might expect. This may signal what kind of breathing or relaxation strategies could help. In this example, mindfulness techniques to stay grounded, and focused relaxation of the youth's stomach muscles, may help them. The distress rating of 85 indicates that the experiment is sufficiently activating to the youth but still do-able.

3. **Identify anxious/negative thoughts.** Have the youth describe the anxious and negative thoughts associated with their distressing feelings. Have them try to be as specific as possible, using "I" statements. Then help them identify any potential thinking traps. Have them notice the connection between their thoughts and feelings, and watch for urges to avoid.

4. **Generate coping thoughts.** Help the youth brainstorm coping thoughts that can respond to the anxious and negative thoughts and counter thinking traps.

5. **Outline achievable behavioral goals.** In an experiment like this, it's always helpful to identify concrete goals that the child is aiming to accomplish. It can be particularly helpful if these goals are observable so that the therapist (or any confederates) might provide objective feedback afterward. In this example, the youth fears they will have interminable pauses of 10 seconds or more. Note this as a goal and then provide feedback later on. It is unlikely that the youth will have many pauses lasting that length of time. Try to avoid picking goals that require long, involved steps that will overwhelm the youth. Also avoid unrealistically ideal goals that the youth is unlikely to accomplish (e.g., "I won't make any mistakes or say anything wrong"); rather, it may help to have a goal related to a feared outcome (e.g., "If I make a mistake or stutter, I will take a deep breath and keep going"). We want to emphasize outcomes that result from the youth's attempts to cope.

6. **Establish rewards.** It is important that the youth become accustomed to evaluating themself positively for attempting challenges and trying to cope. Any efforts at approach can be reinforced, and therapists can encourage desired behavior with positive, specific labeled praise (e.g., "I'm so proud of you for being willing to practice this even though you are feeling nervous"). The therapist can also help the youth select rewards that can be obtained immediately or shortly after successful exposures.

7. **Now, do the exposure!** Once planning has been completed, the therapist can then lead the youth through the exposure. In this case, the therapist would set up a mock classroom setting and give the youth a topic to present extemporaneously (e.g., "For the next 5 minutes, describe what you would do if you won the lottery!"). As the youth enacts the exposure, the therapist can monitor distress ratings, asking for a rating every minute or so. This will help to determine if any habituation occurs or if the youth is able to persevere through distress. The therapist can also prompt the youth to report their anxious and coping thoughts periodically through the exposure. This can help remind the youth to use coping thoughts throughout. All the while, the therapist acts as a supportive coach, encouraging the youth to push through the experiment while using the most useful coping strategies.

Exposures can be quick (3–4 minutes) or last the entire session, depending on the goals and task. Quick exposures can be repeated several times in order to have the child get initial feedback, try it again, get additional feedback, and try it again. It's not uncommon to repeat the same exposure 3–4 times or more before moving on to the next exposure. If a youth rolls their eyes at completing the exposure again out of boredom, this is a good sign and can be reflected back to them as data ("I notice this has become really easy for you now, but the first time, it took a lot of convincing to get you to even begin").

8. **Review the results (How did it go?).** The therapist solicits general comments from the child: How did the exposure work? Was it like they expected? Easier than they thought, harder than they thought, or about the same? How would they do it differently? If there were some easy-to-modify technical issues that interfered with the exposure, feel free to redo the exposure. Otherwise, review the completed exposure worksheet (see Figure 2.6) and evaluate the success of the youth's coping skills, highlighting expectancies that were violated, pleasant surprises, and take-home messages that challenge unrealistic assumptions.

9. **Determine distress ratings.** The therapist can graph distress ratings obtained during the exposure to determine if habituation occurred or if the youth persisted through distress.

10. **Generate feedback.** Constructive and supportive feedback is provided regarding the specific goals defined at the beginning. Did the child achieve their behavioral goals? Did they fall into any thinking traps or avoidance patterns? Did they notice urges to avoid or escape but kept going? Did they use coping thoughts or relaxation? Were there pleasant surprises? The youth and therapist should explore what made accomplishing certain goals difficult. The therapist also provides feedback about the youth's evaluation of their own performance. Is the client being overly harsh? Troubleshoot alternate ways to meet the youth's goals next time. Remember to focus on providing specific labeled praise for the youth's efforts and willingness to approach challenges rather than achieving specific outcomes.

11. **Formulate a take-home message.** At the end of the exposure, it can be helpful to generate a so-called take-home message. This helps consolidate the experience so the child can draw

on the experience in the future. So, for example, if the child realized via the exposure that "Other people don't expect you to say something genius, you just have to say one or two interesting things," then the take-home message might be "Just be yourself—the rest will work itself out" or "Being a perfectionist only holds me back." It doesn't matter really what the message is as long as it helps the youth remember that engagement is better than avoidance and that coping skills can help manage distressing emotions (even if these strategies do not produce perfect results every time!).

12. **Assign home practice and plan for future exposures.** After completing the in-session exposure, it is important to create a home assignment that matches the theme. Outside practice is critical for continued comfort with coping skills and for greater generalization to diverse scenarios. At the same time, the therapist and youth can plan for future in-session exposures, arranging to bring in props or make other preparations as necessary.

Home Practice

Practice outside of session is essential for improving coping skills and helping to generalize them to diverse settings. Practicing skills solely in session limits the chances that lessons will transfer in personalized and novel situations the youth faces. Some tips on assigning home practice:

- *Home practice should relate to lessons learned in the current session.* Assignments can be active experiments (e.g., "Test out your new coping thoughts by approaching three people this week and starting a conversation"); self-monitoring (e.g., "Fill out this activity–mood tracker"); or any other task that provides a real-life demonstration of the current skills.

- *Do not overload!* It is better to assign a couple of thoughtful home assignments that the youth is likely to complete than to overwhelm them.

- *Keep it simple and clear.* Assignments should be simple enough that the youth could recall them by memory rather than relying on extensive to-do lists. While writing down the home practice assignments helps, they should not be so complicated that the youth require detailed analysis to recall and execute them. Also make sure youth understand what is expected of them before they leave session. For younger children, it may be necessary to coordinate with their parents.

- *Check completion of home practice at the beginning of the next session.* It is critical to reinforce the importance of home practice by addressing it at the beginning of each session and by providing a reward and praise when the youth completes it (even if they only partially complete it). Tracking home practice completion in a chart can help monitor progress and plan for concrete rewards. (See Chapters 6, 8, and 11 for examples of reward charts.)

Reward Charts and Self-Rewards

When working with the individual youth, the CBT therapist tries to incorporate positive reinforcement principles wherever possible. Anxious and depressed youth tend to be overly critical of their performances, minimize successes, and set perfectionistic standards for self-reward. One of the goals of CBT is to reset expectations such that youth place an emphasis on effort and less on the outcomes achieved. As an example, the CBT therapist cares less about whether a teen gets a hit, walks, or strikes out in a baseball game. The therapist communicates to the teen that their willingness to get up to bat, utilize coping skills, and attempt the at-bat is deserving of credit. The teen is not always open to this concept as their own perfectionism refuses to settle for good effort. To counter such a response, the therapist can communicate that a person will never succeed if they do not put themself in the position to succeed. In the words of the great Wayne Gretzky, "You miss 100% of the shots you don't take." And succeeding often includes learning to embrace mistakes and failing,

Reward charts emphasize orienting goals around efforts to cope and reinforcing "success" with rewards the youth finds meaningful or satisfying. Chapters 6 and 11 (Figures 6.6 and 11.12) provide examples of basic reward charts that identify behaviors or goals the youth is trying to achieve and the rewards they are promised. Importantly, rewards can be self-rewards or those arranged by parents. Remember that rewards do not always have to possess monetary value. Allowing oneself privileges or treats can often be as rewarding as obtaining consumable products. For example, giving oneself a break to call friends after attempting a difficult math homework. Or similarly, allowing oneself to spend an hour on YouTube after pushing oneself to text friends whom one has been avoiding. Some youth may need instruction in self-praise and "patting themselves on the back" for their efforts. For many teens self-reward is possible, but it can be helpful to involve parents when the most reinforcing rewards will be privileges that are controlled by the parents (e.g., driving the teen to the mall to meet friends, giving the teen the right to choose a family activity). Parents can also be helpful when the youth is reluctant to self-reward. This will often require providing the same education about effort and outcome given to the youth.

PHYSICAL INTERVENTIONS

Progressive Relaxation

Progressive relaxation is a technique used to loosen muscle tension, a common symptom of anxiety and depression. To emphasize the impact that muscle tension can have on our emotional state, the therapist can have the youth make a fist for several seconds, taking note of the generated tension, and then release the fist and notice how much more relaxed and comfortable the hand feels. The therapist may direct the youth to repeat this action several times to show how the fist becomes increasingly relaxed with repeated contractions and relaxations. The therapist can then lead the child through an extended script that progressively relaxes all core muscle groups (see Figure 2.7 for a sample relaxation script). To illustrate this concept with younger children, have the child switch between acting like a rigid robot and a loose ragdoll or jellyfish.

Breathing Retraining

Breathing retraining can aid progressive relaxation as breathing often becomes shallow and rapid when one is anxious. Breathing retraining helps the youth focus on breathing from the diaphragm in slow measured breaths. To practice this, the therapist can have the client lie on the floor, identify their diaphragm just below the base of their rib cage, and practice breathing by imagining a string pulling their diaphragm up with each breath and releasing with each exhalation. For extra practice, the youth can place a light book at the base of the rib cage and lift the book evenly with each breath. Diaphragmatic breathing helps use full lung capacity in measured rhythms to limit

PROGRESSIVE RELAXATION

Go ahead and settle in so you feel comfortable. Let all your muscles go loose and heavy. Close your eyes and take three deep, slow breaths. As you breathe in, breathe in through your nose, noticing how the cool air passes through your nostrils. As you breathe out, breathe out slowly through your mouth, letting the warmed air pass gently over your lips. With each breath, take a brief pause at the top of the breath. In through the nose, pause, and out through the mouth.

Now, I want you to clench your right fist as tight as you can, and hold it while I count down from three . . . pay attention to the tight feeling in your fist as I begin to count . . . 3 . . . 2 . . . 1 . . . relax your fist and notice the feelings of warmth and relaxation that flow through your fingers into your arm. . . . Let's do it one more time. Right fist . . . 3 . . . 2 . . . 1. Now, clench your left hand into a fist and hold it while I count down from three . . . pay attention to the tight feeling in your fist . . . 3 . . . 2 . . . 1. . . . Release your fist and notice how the tight feeling leaves your fingers, hand, and arm. Notice how it is replaced by the warm heavy feeling of relaxation. Let's repeat it again . . . 3 . . . 2 . . . 1. . . .

OK, let's move to your shoulders. Take both of your shoulders and PULL them up to your ears—like you're trying to touch your ears with your shoulders. Let's hold for a count of three . . . 3 . . . 2 . . . 1. . . . Now, let them drop. Notice the feeling of tension drop out. Let's do it again. Hunch your shoulders up to your ears. What do you notice? Feel that tension and stiffness. 3 . . . 2 . . . 1. . . . Relax your shoulders. Pay attention to the warm soothing feelings of relaxation that run down your head, neck, and shoulders.

How do we relax our stomach? Imagine you want to squeeze your belly so that your belly button touches your spine. Can you try that. Squeeze in—don't hold your breath—and just try to touch your spine with your belly button. Hold it, 3 . . . 2 . . . 1. . . . And release. Feel that tension in your stomach, back, and sides release. Let's do it again, hold, 3 . . . 2 . . . 1. . . . Release. Feel the tension release as you let go.

Let's try your legs and feet. Imagine you have your feet at the banks of a muddy brook. Push your legs out as if you're trying to push the mud as far away as you can. Hold, 3 . . . 2 . . . 1. . . . And relax. Letting your legs come back to you. Let's do it again. This time really try to imagine pushing your legs out as far as you can—even extending your toes out as far as possible, pushing the mud through your toes. Ready, push! 3 . . . 2 . . . 1. . . . And release. Letting your legs relax and feeling free.

When you're ready, we're going to slowly return to the room. All the while focusing on your breath as you sit relaxed. With each breath, slowly open your eyes. 5 . . . breath in through your nose. 4 . . . out through your mouth. 3 . . . open your eyes a little bit more. 2 . . . in through your nose. 1 . . . out through your mouth. And welcome back.

FIGURE 2.7. Sample relaxation script.

hyperventilation and shallow breathing. Younger kids can be taught this as belly breathing; they can pretend they are trying to fill a balloon in their bellies by inhaling through their noses. Then they exhale through their mouths to let the air out of the balloon.

Sleep Hygiene

Sleep disruptions are a frequent and significant symptom in many anxious and depressed youth (Brand, Hatzinger, Beck, & Holsboer-Trachsler, 2009; Rao, Hammen, & Poland, 2009). Anxious youth may become preoccupied with the past day's events or worried about the upcoming day's events and have trouble initiating and remaining asleep. Depressed youth often end up shifting their sleep cycle such that they end up going to sleep later, experience disrupted and restless sleep, and have difficulty rising and feeling unrested. Sleep hygiene includes doing an assessment of the youth's sleep routine, providing education about good sleep hygiene, and incorporating a plan to improve sleep habits. The therapist can use the Facts about Sleep Hygiene handout (Handout 4 in Appendix A) to educate youth and parents. The therapist helps the youth establish a regular sleep routine by picking a standard bedtime, with the youth agreeing to avoid caffeine, computer screens, homework, and other stressful tasks prior to bedtime, and to make the sleeping environment as pleasant as possible. If the youth wakes in the middle of the night, they will rise from bed and not lie awake for more than 15–20 minutes. The teen chooses a light activity to relax (e.g., listening to music; light reading, just not onscreen; journaling) until drowsy enough to return to bed. The teen must establish a regular wake time and adhere to it. If they routinely adhere to a standard wake time, their body will begin to regulate.

SUMMARY AND KEY POINTS

CBT therapists can avail themselves of many interventions and strategies that adhere to the central model while tailoring them to the individual youth's needs, interests, and abilities. It is not expected that a therapist will use each strategy for each case; a therapist uses case conceptualization to identify the key maintaining factors and youth processes that need addressing. The therapist then selects interventions that target key maintaining factors to achieve youth and parent goals. In treatment planning, the therapist also maps out the expected time course. Each phase of therapy may consist of separate but related goals that require unique or overlapping interventions. Treatment starts with building a strong working alliance and psychoeducation. The key categories of intervention then match the three sections of the CBT model:

- Cognitive interventions
- Behavioral interventions
- Physical interventions

CHAPTER 3

Later Treatment Phase and Termination

The later phase of treatment typically is a continuation of interventions carrying over from the middle phase of treatment, including exposures, activity scheduling, skill rehearsal, and generalization of skills across multiple identified situations (see Chapter 2). Later-phase sessions include reminders of earlier psychoeducation regarding the CBT model and course of treatment, such that it is goal- and assessment-driven and is intended to be time-limited.

Early in treatment, the therapist will have assessed caregiver and youth expectations regarding course, duration, and potential effects of treatment. This is important for later-phase work, especially since caregiver expectations regarding their child's therapy may affect outcomes (Nock & Kazdin, 2001). A preparatory question that therapists can discuss early in treatment to prime later collaborative decisions regarding terminating treatment is: How will we know when we are ready to end treatment?

KNOWING WHEN TO END TREATMENT

Rapport building shifts to rapport growing and rapport maintaining, with the therapist continuing to coach, cheerlead, and positively reinforce youth and families. A foundational aim is to help caregivers step into these roles more effectively and to help youth become their own therapists and self-coaches. Therapy can begin to transition when there is evidence of transfer of these skills in homework, exposures, activity scheduling, and functional improvements (e.g., attending school, joining activities, making friends, etc.).

The assessment–treatment dialectic (Weisz et al., 2011) calls for the continual modification of treatment planning and also informs termination planning. Deciding *when* to terminate treatment is intended to be a collaborative process, and when working with youth, there are more participants in this process. Termination includes multiple considerations regarding timing; progress and outcomes; therapeutic alliance between the therapist, youth, and family; and relapse prevention (Vidair, Feyijinmi, & Feindler, 2016). Progress monitoring and ascertaining input from multiple reporters across domains will inform such decision making. Such monitoring may have its own intervention effects (Bickman, 2008; Lambert, Harmon, Slade, Whipple, & Hawkins, 2005). By merely observing and tracking something systematically, we may change our understanding of and reaction to that something. Youth and families frequently note this observational effect.

In then answering the question of how we will know when it is time to end treatment, the therapist can thus consider the following interrelated, sometimes overlapping indicators:

1. **Symptom change on assessment forms across multiple reporters and domains.** As noted, we encourage routine administration of clinical symptom measures for youth and caregivers (e.g., Revised Children's Anxiety and Depression Scale or RCADS). Self-reported and caregiver-reported changes and reductions can be noted to inform progress in symptom presence, intensity, and/or frequency. Teacher report forms may also provide this information for clinical decision making. Notably, beyond numerical review of these forms, graphic representation may also aid the therapist in optimizing treatment response (Nadeem, Capella, Holland, Coccaro, & Crisonino, 2016). Absence of change or discordant reporting of change among reporters, of course, also informs treatment and termination planning. In-session observations of a youth's mental status are data upon which clinicians determine progress over the course of treatment (e.g., improved eye contact, engagement, more consistent brightening of affect, reductions in reported self-harm urges and behaviors).

2. **Goal achievement based on the target problem lists.** CBT case conceptualization drives development of target problem lists that for youth likely include caregiver and youth goals. Reliance on these target lists to drive treatment requires that these goals be collaboratively operationalized and converted to language that makes them specific, observable, and measurable for progress monitoring. As discussed, since youth rarely self-refer for treatment, it may be necessary to address discordant goals between a youth and caregiver and reconcile these as the youth progresses through treatment. This does not mean that goals need to be fused or a goal from one reporter is necessarily better; rather, it requires keeping the multiple perspectives in mind.

3. **Skill building.** Early- and middle-phase treatment includes teaching the youth a variety of skills that seek to aid in symptom reduction, functional improvements, and goal attainment. Therefore, the therapist can note the youth's acknowledgment of skills taught (and hopefully learned) via in-session and at-home practice of these skills. For example, is the youth practicing mindfulness-based skills, relaxation, deep breathing, distress tolerance, and/or problem solving? Are there associated reductions in nonsuicidal self-injury (NSSI) behaviors? Is the youth demonstrating skill use (e.g., "In school today, I took three deep breaths before my test")? Are caregivers demonstrating increased use of specific labeled praise? Are caregivers using empathize and encourage statements?

4. **Behavior change.** Are there increases in youth and caregiver adaptive behaviors and decreases in maladaptive behaviors? Essential behavioral interventions include behavioral activation guided by activity monitoring, exposures guided by fear or challenge hierarchies, behavioral experiments, and behavior reward charts. Is the youth approaching and not avoiding formerly avoided anxiety-provoking situations? Are they engaging in developmentally appropriate and prosocial activities? Given the primacy of the school domain for youth in particular, the therapist can also gauge treatment progress via the youth's in-school functional targets, such as attending school consistently, staying in school, reduced visits to the school nurse, academic participation, extracurricular participation, seeking help from available school-based supports, and the like. Again, the therapist will want to gather collateral information from key school personnel. Other sources of collateral information also can signal treatment progress. For example, one of us received a writ-

ten letter (yes, a letter sent with a stamp!) from the aunt of a patient who wished to express her gratitude for "having my niece back." Family members reporting observable behavioral changes in a youth is good data.

5. **Changes in self-talk.** Cognitive changes may seem difficult to track given their very nature. However, as the therapist and youth work on developing cognitive skills, for example, identifying negative self-talk and associated anxiety or depression, demonstrating comprehension of the link among thoughts, feelings, and behaviors via home practice and in-session discussions, labeling thinking traps) therapists can work with youth to notice improvements and salient changes in such skills. The therapist can note if a youth is expressing more coping-focused self-talk, acknowledging processes of change including habituation (e.g., "I was really nervous when I started giving my presentation but felt a lot less nervous by the end"); expectancy violation (e.g., "I thought I would totally freak out during the presentation, but I didn't and was able to finish it," or "I freaked out a little bit but I got the job done"); and behavioral activation (e.g., "I was so tired and didn't want to go to the park, but then I told myself I had to go and, while I was there, noticed I felt better. I was proud that I went"). This last example exemplifies another potential progress marker for which therapists may want to listen—a youth's ability to express self-praise and reward. Early in treatment, youth with anxiety and depression may evidence cognitive distortions that hinder their ability to acknowledge incremental progress. For example, the youth will show all-or-none or perfectionistic thinking; they may overemphasize outcome over effort and may need to be taught and reinforced to note incremental improvements rather than dichotomous good-or-bad evaluations of performance.

6. **Changes in targeted parent/caregiver behaviors.** Functional assessment will reveal caregiver and system variables that may be reinforcing maladaptive youth behaviors. Optimizing youth CBT will require targeting these caregiver-level behaviors and teaching caregivers new or expanded skills. The extent to which caregivers are involved will depend on several variables, such as the youth's age (see Chapter 5). As therapy progresses, the therapist can note increases in parental use of skills, for example, the use of empathizing and encouraging talk as self-reported by caregivers and possibly noted by the youth; consistency in implementation of behavior charts that provide the youth with reinforcement; active follow-through on the execution of out-of-office exposures especially for younger children; reductions in accommodating behaviors that negatively reinforce the youth (e.g., allowing them to avoid or escape anxiety-provoking situations, parents rescuing the youth from bad situations).

In the context of goal-based therapy, the therapist, youth, caregivers, and other providers as appropriate (see Chapter 5) can measure progress across many contexts and indicators. Ideally, termination can be decided naturally, collaboratively, and in advance. Progress itself organically may dictate the final phase of treatment. For example, not infrequently, formerly withdrawn youth begin to reengage extracurricular after-school activities; this demonstration of therapy progress may begin to present scheduling conflicts with session appointment times—what a terrific problem to have!

As youth and families continue to demonstrate improvements across varied indicators, the therapist and families can assess the pros and cons of the current treatment frequency. The decision can then be made to begin to end treatment.

TERMINATION AND RELAPSE PREVENTION

Optimally, the therapist prepares the youth and family for the discontinuation of therapy in the context of behavior change that has generalized. Consideration may require discussion with referring providers (e.g., pediatricians) and other treating providers (e.g., child psychiatrists). The conclusion of acute treatment can be conceptualized as termination, graduation, or a therapy break, depending on the particular needs of youth and families. In the final therapy sessions, which may be tapered as appropriate to ascertain maintenance (e.g., moving from weekly to biweekly, and then perhaps monthly), the therapist can work with the youth and family to do the following:

1. **Review the indicators of progress.** What has changed over the course of the early and middle phases of treatment? Such a review can include explicit comparison of each of the indicators noted above. Depending on the duration of treatment, youth and caregivers may not remember earlier levels of distress or dysfunction.

2. **Consolidate treatment skills, strengths, and gains.** Over the course of treatment, youth and caregivers have been introduced to and worked on a multitude of skills, often via trial and error. The later phase of treatment allows for the accumulation of these skills. Specifically, the therapist works with a youth to identify their most effective skills, strategies, coping self-talk, and meaningful take-home messages. Similarly, the therapist works with caregivers to identify their most effective skills, strategies, coping self-talk, coaching self-talk, and meaningful take-home messages.

3. **Reflect on the difficulties encountered in treatment.** What were some of the biggest challenges faced over the course of treatment? How did they turn out? How did the outcomes compare to what was anticipated? Were there any exposure "disasters"? Were they really "disasters"? What were the pleasant surprises? Were there instances in which the youth surprised caregivers?

4. **Reflect on rapport and the therapeutic alliance.** Therapists serve many roles over the course of treatment (e.g., expert, provider of unconditional positive regard, coach, listener, cheerleader, mentor, hope-instiller). Therapists, youth, and families have likely spent consistent time together and built a meaningful relationship over time. The end of treatment offers an opportunity to look back on this relationship as a model for the positives associated with seeking help.

5. **Normalize the likelihood of future triggers.** In addition to reflecting on the course of therapy, the final phase of treatment allows the therapist to look ahead with the youth and their family for opportunities to continue to maintain and generalize treatment gains. During this phase, furthermore, therapists can provide psychoeducation on the distinctions among a lapse, relapse, and collapse. Whereas a single slip to former behavior represents a *lapse* (e.g., missing one day of school because of anxiety), several lapses can turn into a *relapse* to the previous state of functioning (e.g., refusing to go back to school for several days). A relapse can then turn into a *collapse* with consequences that are significantly more difficult to address (e.g., missing a full year of school). Therapists can utilize a relapse prevention model that prepares families for situations that may prove challenging. As such, therapist and families can work on predicting and planning for potential future triggers of anxious or depressive responses (e.g., transition to middle school, a prom, *quinceañera*, school field trips, college entrance exams or applications, a parent's work travel, holidays, summer camp). For some youth and families, it may be helpful to utilize a

calendar to look ahead and start considering themes (e.g., social issues or separation), time of year (e.g., summer, specific holidays or dates), or events (e.g., bar mitzvahs, graduations, school dances). Therapists will also want to consider planning for meaningful anniversaries that may be especially difficult and a trigger for difficult emotions (e.g., anniversary of a loved one's death or suicide attempt, the last time a patient engaged in NSSI) as well as potentially celebratory events.

6. **Prepare caregivers for extinction bursts and setbacks.** Relatedly, the therapist will want to prepare caregivers for the likelihood that a youth may demonstrate a former problematic behavior that they believed had been successfully extinguished (e.g., behavioral outburst at a separation) and prime them for potential despair if this occurs. In priming caregivers for such a possibility in advance, they can then hopefully access more positive thoughts in the moment (e.g., "OK, we talked about how this might happen") rather than a more negative or catastrophic response (e.g., "Ugh, here we go again. I can't believe this is happening again!). While validating a caregiver's possible future frustration, therapist and caregiver can work to review the appropriate empathize and encourage responses, coaching, and behavioral limit-setting approaches that have been effective in the past and can be applied again.

7. **Collaborate with other providers as appropriate.** Termination of the CBT portion of treatment also includes consideration of collateral sources and other providers. For example, if school personnel had been engaged in treatment, therapists may want to work with the youth and their caregivers to identify an in-school counselor who can be identified in relapse prevention planning as a support. Referring and other treating providers also should be included in end-of-treatment planning to coordinate care. For example, if a youth experienced medical correlates (e.g., headaches, GI distress) for which they were referred to behavioral health services, these same providers can be enlisted to monitor posttreatment symptoms and assess response maintenance at their appointments. Care coordination is especially key if youth are continuing with psychotropic medication; the therapist and prescribing psychiatrist or psychopharmacologist can establish a plan for later phase and post-psychotherapy monitoring (see Chapter 4).

While the word "termination" is commonly applied to the conclusion of therapies, therapists can work with families to conceptualize an acute phase of the initial treatment with booster or follow-up sessions as either prescheduled or as needed. A helpful analogy can be dental health models: youth likely are accustomed to having regularly scheduled dental health check-ups, with additional appointments for acute needs (e.g., fillings, orthodontics). Mental health can be framed this way, too: regular check-ups with additional sessions as needed or to prepare for particular challenges (e.g., pandemic-related life disruptions, high school transition, stress from a caregiver's job loss, summer camp) or acute issues that emerge (e.g., an episode of NSSI). Adding booster sessions to CBT for youth with anxiety and mood disorders has been shown to be effective for improving treatment effectiveness (Gearing, Schwalbe, Lee, & Hoagwood, 2013). Longer-term follow-up of youth who received CBT for anxiety disorders in one randomized controlled research trial indicated that some youth could likely benefit from ongoing booster sessions (see Ginsburg et al., 2018). Scheduling longer-term follow-ups with youth and families may aid in maintaining the behavioral changes made over the course of therapy (see Foxx, 2013).

To better consolidate treatment gains and skills in the final phase of treatment, the therapist and youth can convert the take-home messages to an *actual* take-home product that summarizes the most effective skills and components of the treatment and captures elements of the relapse prevention strategies identified. Having a tangible take-home product may be especially helpful for younger patients. This is likely an accumulation and consolidation of previous skills and can be packaged in various ways, such as a "commercial" at the end of treatment where a youth can creatively present their learned skills (e.g., Kendall & Hedtke, 2006). Another option is a take-home coping toolkit that can be gathered in a box and decorated; it includes coping self-statements, somatic management tools, and skill reminders. Caregivers can also create a toolkit. The therapist, youth, and their family can find various way to summarize this information (see Figure 3.1; a blank version is available as Worksheet 7 in Appendix A).

Given the ubiquity of smartphones, the therapist and youth can create a "Notes" section on their phones or tablets dedicated to coping Support that is creatively named, with a list of coping strategies and identified sources of social support. For a youth with previous safety concerns, this section can include a safety plan with contact information for the National Suicide Hotline (988) and text line (text the word "CONNECT" to 741741).

A reminder to therapists: What *we* therapists suspect may be the most memorable take-home message for a child or caregiver may not match *their* perceptions of treatment. For example, a young boy and his two parents traveled weekly from the suburbs to an urban area for CBT for his previously impairing social and separation anxiety. This family had wonderfully set up a multitude of exposures over the past several weeks and seen benefit in the boy's mood, engagement with peers and activities, and overall functioning. The boy himself reported how proud he was for "being brave" and "killing the butterflies" in his stomach. During one final session, when asked to summarize their take-home message, both parents spoke of their ability to coach their son through their anxiety and encourage and reinforce his new behaviors. They spoke of their own improved abilities to cognitively coach themselves when they noticed their anxieties increasing in anxiety-provoking situations for their son. Excellent! When the attention shifted to the youth for his take-home message, he stated confidently: "It was fun to come here AND I got to pick which restaurant we ate at after we left here." While we are confident this youth learned a host of skills and clearly demonstrated improvements during exposures (in which he did not always appear to be having fun), *his* take-home message in that moment was connected with fun and the likely positive reinforcers of picking a restaurant and experiencing special time with his parents. Therefore, a meaningful aspect of relapse prevention was to target how the family could maintain a version of this practice. Including maintenance tips for both a youth and their parents in a take-home toolkit can help.

THE "FINAL" SESSION

However the timeline has been determined, there can be an agreed-upon end date for the acute phase of treatment. In the context of all the therapeutic work, progress, and improvements in functioning, the final session can be a celebration of the effort and time invested. Therapists can also model how to say goodbye. They can acknowledge and validate a range of sometimes mixed emotions, as therapy can be a formative interpersonal experience (Vidair et al., 2016). The therapist can further reinforce and praise the work and progress of the youth and family with pride and happiness, while also appropriately expressing sadness in not meeting regularly. For some youth for whom check-ins and boosters may be prescribed, the goodbye may be a "see you later" and "keep me posted" exchange and encompass discussions regarding how to maintain contact.

WORKSHEET 7. Coping Reminders Success Summary

> You have learned a lot of great skills during our work together. Take a moment to think through the strategies that work best for you.

Key Negative Thoughts to Watch For:

1. *"I'm weird, awkward, or an idiot."*

2. *"I can't bear it; I need to get out of here."*

3. _____

My Thinking Traps:

1. *Mind reading*

2. *Looking for escape hatch*

3. _____

My Key Coping Thoughts:

1. *"I don't know what they're thinking."*

2. *"I'll feel better if I at least try. I feel like I want to escape and I can handle sticking it out."*

3. *"I can choose not to use the escape hatch. I don't want to miss out on dance anymore."*

People Who Can Help Me:

1. *Mom, Dad*

2. *My aunt*

3. *My ELA teacher, my dance instructor*

Actions and Behaviors that Help Me:

1. *Remind myself of my values and goals for making friends and doing dance.*

2. *Set goals about showing up and talking to new people.*

3.

I Remember When I Struggled with <u>*all the negative worries*</u>   .

What Helped Me Most was: *Giving myself a break and hanging in there.*

What I Need to Keep Practicing: *Talking to people; showing up at dance class; sending the first text; catching the self-judging thoughts; using nicer language about myself when I try stuff.*

My Therapy Take-Home Message: *It's usually not as bad as my anxiety tells me it will be.*

What Is a Sign That I May Want to Check In: *If I give in to the urges to use the escape hatch and am avoiding things.*

FIGURE 3.1. Coping Reminders Success Summary with the Shelby example discussed in Chapter 9.

SUMMARY AND KEY POINTS

The later phase of CBT includes all of the elements of earlier phases and proceeds from ongoing assessment, progress monitoring, and collaborative planning with youth and families. The therapist tracks various indicators of functioning across domains, reporters, methods, and settings to determine transition from middle- to later-phase treatment. The later phase includes ongoing skill practice and transitions to consolidation and review of skills; furthermore, it includes collaborative relapse prevention planning. When able to collaboratively reduce and end treatment, the therapist and families can discuss different models that may include planning for booster sessions for longer-term maintenance of behavioral responses to therapy. Preparation for termination includes:

- Review of the indicators of progress
- Consolidation of treatment skills, strengths, and gains
- Reflection on any difficulties in treatment
- Reflection on rapport and the therapeutic alliance
- Normalizing the likelihood of future triggers and preparing ahead of time for them
- Parent preparation for extinction bursts and setbacks
- Collaboration with other providers as appropriate

CHAPTER 4

Psychiatric Referral and Collaboration

Pragmatic Recommendations

with Uri Meller

This chapter will review pharmacotherapy efficacy in treating children and adolescents with anxiety and mood disorders. It then will focus on pragmatic recommendations for collaborating with psychiatrists and psychopharmacologists to ensure the best possible health outcomes for youth and their families.

What are some signs and symptoms that would indicate a psychiatric evaluation? When do vital points to communicate with the prescribing physician occur? What are the essentials to communicate to the youth and family? In this book, we will also focus on how to formulate effective treatment plans that incorporate psychotherapists and prescribing providers, account for changes in treatment, monitor progress, and weigh the risks and benefits of treatments. For a more comprehensive overview, see Birmaher, Brent, and AACAP Work Group on Quality Issues (2007) and Connolly and Bernstein (2007), both published by the American Academy of Child and Adolescent Psychiatry.

EVIDENCE FOR PHARMACOTHERAPY

Research consistently demonstrates that for many youth, combined psychotherapy and psychopharmacological treatment are superior to CBT alone or medication management alone in the treatment of mood and anxiety disorders (March et al., 2004; Walkup et al., 2008). The two psychopharmacological and psychotherapeutic interventions can synergize to advance treatment. For example, Walkup and colleagues (2008) found an 80% response rate in combined treatment compared to a 55–60% response rate in medication or CBT alone in 7- to 17-year-olds. Similarly, Piacentini et al. (2014) determined in the Child/Adolescent Anxiety Multimodal Study (CAMS) that combined CBT psychotherapy and medication were superior in the treatment of anxiety

Uri Meller, MD, is a board-certified adult psychiatrist and child and adolescent psychiatrist and Assistant Professor at Albert Einstein College of Medicine. He is also Medical Director of the Child and Adolescent Training Clinic at Montefiore Hospital, Albert Einstein College of Medicine. Dr. Meller has been developing curricula for training mental health professionals, with a focus on intersectionality, global psychiatry, and the cultural components of mental health. He has presented workshops and posters at multiple national conferences.

compared to both monotherapies alone. Likewise, the Treatment for Adolescents with Depression Study (TADS) Team (2009) found comparable rates of response for adolescent depression across combined (82%), fluoxetine (75%), and CBT (70%) interventions in 12-month naturalistic follow-up after acute intervention. The above evidence supports the combining of psychotherapy and psychopharmacology to aid in symptom reduction and disorder remission in the treatment of youth anxiety and depressive disorders.

REFERRING A PATIENT FOR A PSYCHIATRIC CONSULT

Case Vignette: Jesse

Jesse is an 11-year-old Caucasian cisgender girl currently in the fifth grade who lives with her two mothers and older brother. She has always been a diligent and attentive student who receives high marks and is highly regarded by her teachers and peers as intelligent, caring, and hard-working. Jesse has two close friends with whom she interacts in and outside of school, and she restricts her social interaction to these two friends. For the past year, Jesse has been complaining of stomachaches most mornings and refuses to go to school. Getting her to school is especially a challenge on Mondays and after longer school holidays. She reports that her distress and associated behaviors became exacerbated after one of her classmates did not invite Jesse to their party, an event attended by many of her peers—something she learned about on social media. Jesse describes her fear of being ridiculed and often does not speak in class or engage with her fellow students.

At the recommendation of the school guidance counselor and teacher, Jesse's mothers brought her to a psychologist who completed a comprehensive intake evaluation that included semi-structured interviews with Jesse and her mothers as well as child and caregiver report forms. Jesse was diagnosed with social anxiety disorder, which had become increasingly severe given her worsening somatic distress and school avoidance. Jesse began CBT targeting the school avoidance secondary to her social anxiety. Her therapist collaborated with her caregivers and the school guidance counselor. Although Jesse was initially guarded and had difficulty engaging with her therapist, the two were able to form a rapport and worked slowly on the first phase of skill building and exposure planning. After several weeks, however, there was limited progress on her functional social and academic impairments and daily symptoms of anxiety. Furthermore, Jesse's reported level of anxiety and somatic complaints remained very high, and her willingness to engage in therapeutic exposure activity was minimal. Her parents were very supportive and collaborative, and worked to implement a behavioral plan, but they expressed concern about Jesse's tardiness and missed school days and the prospect of her repeating the academic year.

What Signs and Symptoms Indicate Psychiatric Referral?

As a therapist conducts the initial assessment with a new client, several factors indicate whether pharmacotherapy would be potentially useful. These might include chronicity and severity of the concern. The therapist would also want to assess past treatment history to determine if prior behavioral treatments failed to achieve sufficient outcomes. Knowing that a youth is experiencing moderate to severe impairment across multiple domains, which has been present for an extended period, should signal to the therapist that a new client might benefit from a psychiatric consultation early in therapy.

However, the need for a psychiatric consult may not become apparent until later in therapy. Evidence suggests that clients who experience the greatest improvement via CBT will show signs of response early in therapy (Renaud et al., 1998; Tang & DeRubeis, 1999). This is not always the case and depends on when key interventions (e.g., exposures) are introduced. Nonetheless, if the youth is slow to respond to behavioral intervention, even after exposures and behavioral challenges have been introduced, pharmacotherapy may be considered. Deteriorating conditions and emergence of new risk behaviors (e.g., suicidal ideation, severe absenteeism from school) are also indicators that a medication consult might be beneficial.

Talking with Families about the Psychiatric Referral

Given Jesse's limited progress, her therapist suggested that the family consider taking Jesse to a psychiatrist for an evaluation and other treatment considerations, including a medication intervention. Although Jesse's parents confirmed that she had already been seen by her pediatrician regarding her gastrointestinal upsets, the therapist wanted to also consider and rule out any medical conditions that might be affecting her symptoms.

Like many parents, Jesse's mothers had multiple concerns about this proposition and initially did not favor medication as a treatment option. Echoing the concerns of many, they raised the following issues:

1. They inquired about the available evidence on medication treating this condition in children.
2. They expressed concern about the potential short- and long-term side effects.
3. They were health conscious and wanted to avoid exposing their child to any toxins.
4. While they recognized the impairments associated with Jesse's significant anxiety and wanted what was best for her treatment, they did not wish to change who she is and worried about altering her personality.
5. They voiced concerns that Jesse would become addicted to any prescribed medication and would not be able to function without it.

Raising the issue of medication tends to be overwhelming for a youth's family members. They may have a strong emotional response to and reasonable reservations about such an approach. Adding medication management to the youth treatment plan can be a charged topic. At the start of any discussion, explore the thoughts, emotions, and narratives families may have about psychiatric medications. Despite progress in the de-stigmatization of mental illness, some families and clients may experience underlying feelings of shame and guilt. Figure 4.1 illustrates common concerns and lists the steps a therapist can take to introduce the possibility of medication treatment. Therapists can provide psychoeducation about the efficacy of combination treatments while creating a nonjudgmental space to discuss youth and caregiver concerns and beliefs about medication interventions. Such discussions can impact the chances of the youth following up with a prescribing physician or adherence to a recommended course of treatment. Using metaphors and cognitive restructuring techniques can help families engage in hearing about the risks and benefits of medications. It can also foster discussions regarding the potential harm and risk of not utilizing medication when needed. For example, we often use the metaphor of corrective glasses to explain how psychotherapy and medications can be useful. When individuals with impaired vision wear prescription glasses, they see their surroundings differently and that, in turn, allows them to

---

- Provide evidence-based information on monotherapy and combined treatment and discussed practice guidelines.
- Elicit questions, concerns, and positively and negatively valenced beliefs about medications. Discuss history and experiences with any psychotropic medications contributing to these.
- Validate concerns and provide corrective information as needed within the scope of expertise.
- Discuss the rationale for considering medication as well as potential consequences of not utilizing medication.
- Discuss psychiatric referral as information gathering and option building.
- In case of ambivalence, create a framework and milestones when family will accept a psychiatric referral.

FIGURE 4.1. Introducing and discussing medication referral with a patient and their family.

be more engaged in those surroundings. The glasses do not see *for* the person; they are tools that promote improved vision and the possibility of greater engagement. Engagement can then lead to developing skills and knowledge that are independent of the glasses.

To use another metaphor, the presenting symptoms a youth experiences can feel like a very loud song stuck streaming through one's headphones; medication may help to turn down the volume. A reduction in symptoms can allow the youth to engage in treatment-related activities and targets that include self-monitoring, mindfulness, cognitive restructuring, behavioral activation, and exposures. Once learned, these skills can become independent of the medication and psychotherapy. Empirical data have found lower symptoms' relapse secondary to medication and psychotherapeutic intervention and the synergistic effects of medication and psychotherapy to treat mood and anxiety disorder resulting in better outcomes 24 and 36 weeks post treatment (Piacentini et al., 2014).

A prescribing physician may also screen the client for medical conditions that cause or exacerbate mental health symptoms. Some medical issues that can induce mood and anxiety symptoms include: endocrine imbalance (e.g., thyroid dysregulation), infectious disease (e.g., Lyme disease, mononucleosis), neoplasm and other forms of cancer, as well as sleep disorders, to name just a few. Involving a medical provider offers benefits in this regard. Such medical conditions can have various forms of treatment that ultimately will improve one's mental health outcome directly or indirectly. Lastly, it is important to consider the cultural identity or identities of the youth and family. Often learning about their culture and the narratives about mental health and medication management is very useful in providing compassionate and competent care.

Exploring Caregivers' Knowledge of and Beliefs about Medication

The therapist can open the discussion with caregivers about the possibility of seeking a psychiatric consultation with the intention of gathering information from them.

Jesse's therapist scheduled a parent-only session with Jesse's mothers and elicited some of their concerns and beliefs about psychiatric medications. For example, one of Jesse's mothers described that their mother had been given psychiatric medication at the end of her life, which caused many side effects including sedation and blunting of her usual lively personality. As such, they worried that the medication had changed their mother and the same thing might happen to Jesse. Her mother also expressed worry that Jesse would have to be on medications for "the rest of her life."

Figure 4.2 provides a summary of common concerns and beliefs related to medication treatment that a referring therapist should keep in mind (a reproducible summary for laypeople is available as Handout 5 in Appendix A).

Validating Concerns and Providing Corrective Information as Needed

The therapist can validate how some medication may indeed have negative side effects and that such decisions may be anxiety-provoking. The therapist's goals are to work with the family to consider all possible evidence-based therapeutic options for easing Jesse's worsening anxiety and ongoing functional impairment, particularly school avoidance. The anxiety was significantly impairing Jesse's social and academic developmental trajectory. While medications can have side effects, not taking medication can also have negative consequences by allowing serious disorders to go

Broad concern and example cognitions	Discussion points that may be helpful
Addictive "My child will never be able to stop taking them." "They will become addicted."	Most children and adults taking psychiatric medications for mood and anxiety symptoms eventually stop taking the medications and do so successfully. In fact, a discussion about stopping the meds should take place before any meds are prescribed. Most approved pediatric medication do not cause tolerance, which is the hallmark of an addictive substance (needing more of a substance to experience the same effect).
Long-term consequences "Taking drugs will affect their growth or development."	Side effect profiles vary between different medications and will be considered on a case-by-case basis.
Side effects "What if I gain a lot of weight?" "I heard that these drugs make kids think about suicide."	As noted, side effects may occur and are a reason to change course of treatment if they are not tolerated. Offer data about a black box warning with respect to antidepressant use in children.
Afraid it will change their child's personality "What is the drugs make them a different person?" "Will it change who they are?"	Psychiatric medications should make someone feel more like themselves, not less so. A medication that changes a child's personality is a reason for a prescribing physician to stop the medication.
Shame/judgment "It kind feels like I'm a bad parent and I did not do something right if my kid needs meds like this."	Give support, reserve judgment, and offer positive cognitions for the family.
Medication "meaning" "I don't want my child to think she's disabled." "Normal people don't take psych drugs."	A medication won't usually make a child feel disabled. Experiencing loss in function (which is the reason for prescribing meds) will.
Not organic	Some organic substances may be highly addictive and toxic to our body, and some nonorganic substances may be life-saving. Each situation should be considered case by case, weighing the risks and benefits.

FIGURE 4.2. Common concerns and beliefs about medication interventions.

untreated. Furthermore, it is critical to communicate that the choice always remains in the family's hands: even if the prescribing psychiatrist recommends medication, the family may decide to either hold off or not heed the recommendation.

Discussing the Rationale for Medication

Explain why you believe the youth might benefit from medication. The level of symptom severity and the youth's—and family's—functional impairment are considerations for making a psychiatric referral. A related consideration in Jesse's case is the initial response to the behavioral intervention, which was limited. The therapist can describe the research evidence as well as practice guidelines for treating youth with anxiety and mood disorders. Additionally, examination by a medical provider may be indicated to be sure that medical conditions are not being overlooked. These may be exacerbating the youth's symptoms, or even be the primary cause of the presenting symptoms. The referral may be framed as having another set of clinical eyes to assure nothing is missing from the clinical picture.

The therapist can provide the rationale and frame the medication referral as option building and being a good medical consumer. Together with the parents, gather information, determine options, and conduct risk–benefit analysis to weigh the pros and cons of various alternatives.

Jesse's therapist worked with her parents to acknowledge that listening to available options did not necessarily mean they needed to accept a specific intervention. Also, agreeing to an intervention did not necessarily mean long-term commitment to that intervention. Every treatment (medication or otherwise) has potential side effects and benefits; we always want to make sure that the benefits outweigh any adverse effects. The therapist assured the family she would process these options and weigh the risks and benefits of other treatment options with them to assure that treatment was individualized for Jesse and the family's goals.

REFERRAL CONSIDERATIONS: WHOM TO SELECT? HOW TO REFER?

Although some communities and families have ample child and adolescent psychiatrists trained as medical doctors, this is not always the case. Some psychiatrists are doctors of osteopathic medicine (DOs), while other prescribing physicians are neurologists, pediatricians, and primary care providers, as well as psychiatric nurse practitioners or physician associates. The degree of training and experience with mental health issues should be considered case by case, as well as community and family resources. Another consideration is whether or not the provider has training and expertise in working with youth. When collaborating with providers, be sure to assess resources, insurance coverage, geographic location, and availability prior to giving a referral. Providing a referral to a provider with no availability, or whom the family cannot afford on an ongoing basis, will likely lead to frustration, lack of compliance, and disrupted care. Working consistently with the same prescriber offers continuity of care and a more systematic and methodological approach. It also makes for more time-efficient collaboration. Therefore, hours spent finding the right prescribing physician up-front may save time and improve outcomes in the long term. Various resources to obtain psychopharmacology referrals exist (e.g., the American Academy of Child and Adolescent Psychiatry, local academic centers, National Alliance on Mental Illness [NAMI]) or can be found via additional organizations listed as resources in Appendix B. Table 4.1 enumerates the pros and cons of using various sources to identify a consulting physician. As illustrated, frequently the

TABLE 4.1. How to Identify a Prescribing Physician: Pros and Cons of Common Referral Sources

Source	Pros	Cons
Direct referrals form colleagues	Has firsthand experience working with them.	May be full or have a long waitlist for new patients.
Primary care physicians and other subspecialties	Is readily available resource; may assist with in-network referrals.	May not have as much experience with collaboration as occurs between a therapist and prescribing physician.
Patient or family insurance panel	In-network; cost-effective.	Insurance will generate a long list of providers that may not be in-network or may not accept new patients.
Reputable academic and other mental health centers	Has a good reputation; may accept a variety of insurances.	May vary between clinicians and may not have firsthand accounts of specific providers.
Commercial or not for profit listservs for prescribing physicians (AACAP, APA, Psychology Today)	Lists many providers who can be searched based on specifics (gender, insurance, location, rate, etc.).	May be challenging to verify firsthand accounts of provider.

therapist and family will have to balance a number of factors, including accessibility, cost, experience, and expertise.

Knowing the prescribing provider allows therapists to assess if they would be a good fit with the family and client. CBT clinicians will likely begin to assemble a list of trusted local colleagues with whom they can collaborate effectively within the cognitive-behavioral frame. Speaking to the prescribing provider after the initial assessment, and reviewing the diagnosis, formulation, and possible modification of the treatment plan, will assure a solid collaborative framework. It is vital to make sure that both providers take ownership of the treatment plan and that neither is working against the other. Of course, different providers may have varying ideas about the formulation of case and treatment strategies; this can promote a more inclusive and holistic approach and enrich the treatment plan. Again, the goal is to create a framework of communication between providers, family, and youth in order to improve care and outcomes.

Initial Communication with the Prescribing Provider

Jesse's therapist contacted a child and adolescent psychiatrist with whom she had previously collaborated. The therapist believed she would be a good fit because this psychiatrist has expertise with youth, Jesse's particular psychopathology, and the expressed family concerns. The psychiatrist was known to be collaborative and communicated well with therapists and families alike. Her availability worked with the family's schedule. Although it was determined that the psychiatrist was an out-of-network provider, the family's health plan would reimburse them with half the expenses for this service and Jesse's mother agreed to make an appointment with her.

The Most Important Information to Provide When Referring

After obtaining the parents' written and oral consent to speak with the psychiatrist, Jesse's therapist discussed the case with her, providing the following:

- Chief complaint
- History of presenting disorder
- Course and progression of symptoms
- Pertinent past history; developmental, family, and social history; notable medical history
- Assessment: highlights and diagnosis, main areas of impairment
- Cognitive-behavioral case formulation
- Course of current psychotherapeutic treatment
- Reason for psychopharmacological consultation at this time
- Expectation from the consultation
- Notable patient and family concerns communicated to therapist

Figure 4.3 (a reproducible version is available as Worksheet 8 in Appendix A) provides a checklist of questions to ask a potential consulting physician and a list of topics to discuss during and after any psychiatric evaluation. Therapist and psychiatrist should agree that there is a good fit in order to move forward. After the psychiatrist's initial consultation with Jesse and her family, and upon family consent, the doctor scheduled a phone call with the therapist to obtain further collateral information and assist in developing a collaborative treatment plan.

Discussing the Case Formulation and Treatment Plan

An advantage in collaborating with another provider is that it introduces another expert from another system with whom one can partner in case formulation and treatment planning. For the CBT clinician, finding prescribing providers with whom they may discuss systematic and functional assessment, development and family factors, and CB case formulation is optimal.

When Jesse's therapist and psychiatrist spoke, they discussed how the family and Jesse have been responding to the therapeutic intervention provided to date and the possibly expanded CB case formulation. They agreed on the primacy of the social anxiety disorder, but were also considering a diagnosis of attention-deficit/hyperactivity disorder (ADHD), inattentive type, given a developmental history of inattention and difficulty organizing tasks. While Jesse excels in school, she needs to be reminded multiple times to complete tasks and often procrastinates with assignments until the last minute. According to her parents and teacher, she often fails to pay attention to small details, forgets about books and other assignments at home, and has lost various items, such as her phone and keys. In fact, a high level of anxiety seems to help her complete some tasks and keep up with her academic work. As reflected in the psychiatrist's assessment and review of systems, she noted no major red flags indicating the need for further medical workup. With the parents' consent, the psychiatrist had also communicated with Jesse's pediatrician, and based on recent labwork and a physical exam, they had ruled out major medical illnesses.

Jesse's therapist and psychiatrist discussed a clarified functional assessment of the interaction between Jesse's anxiety and attentional difficulties. As such, they expanded the case conceptualization and modified the current treatment plan. To do so, both professionals highlighted key

WORKSHEET 8. Coordination Checklist: Consulting with a Prescribing Physician

Pre-referral
About Physician
Full name (and how the providers would like to be addressed)
Years of practice (with kids)?
Subspecialty in psychiatry or otherwise (addiction, forensics, etc.)?
Is referral for psychopharmacology alone or in conjunction with psychotherapy? You want to be clear that the referral is for psychopharmacological evaluation
Office location
Time/day availability
Pricing for intake and follow up sessions.
Any commercial or other health insurance that is accepted
Types of cases with whom they will not work (eating disorder, suicidal, self harm, etc.)
Preferred method of communication
Offer to present the patient (briefly) and see if the provider thinks they may be a good fit.
Be prepared to answer any of the above questions about yourself.
About Patient
Consent/release of information signed by caregiver?
General patient information and family demographics
Chief complaint
History of presenting disorder
Course/progression of symptoms
Pertinent past history; developmental, family, and social history; notable medical history
Assessment: highlights and diagnosis, main areas of impairment
Cognitive-behavioral case formulation
Course of current psychotherapeutic treatment
Reason for psychopharmacological consultation at this time
Expectation from the consultation
Notable patient and family concerns communicated to therapist

(continued)

FIGURE 4.3. Collaboration Checklist: Preparing for consultation with a physician.

WORKSHEET 8. Coordination Checklist: Consulting with a Prescribing Physician (p. 2 of 2)

	Post-referral
	Ask for provider's formulation.
	Obtain specific recommendations.
	Understand potential side effects and benefits of offered treatment (or lack of).
	Further medical work up recommended?
	Other diagnostic consideration that may require additional evaluations.
	In case of medication recommendation, ask for titration schedule and end goals.
	Collaboration schedule: When would the therapist like to be contacted (increased risk, change in medications, etc.)?
	When would the prescribing psychiatrist like to be contacted?

FIGURE 4.3. *(continued)*

impairments and identified triggers and maintaining functions. In the case of social anxiety, Jesse's isolation was maintained by the negatively reinforcing reduction of distress by avoiding social gatherings. Jesse's ADHD could be viewed through a similar lens, in that she would avoid any task that required too much effort. Initiating and persevering through difficult homework created too much tension for Jesse to bear, leading to "quitting" behavior. Using this conceptualization, and consistent with earlier psychoeducation, the psychiatrist recommended fluoxetine (Prozac) or sertraline (Zoloft) to address the anxiety and ADHD symptoms. The rationale offered to the parents was consistent with our eyeglass metaphor: the medication was intended to support Jesse's natural abilities to learn and to socialize by helping to focus her efforts. Her tension was making it difficult for her to reach her goals. In this way, the medication would support the CBT conceptualization by helping Jesse withstand the tension that comes with difficult tasks. As Jesse approaches new challenges, her ability to complete each one with increased confidence (e.g., telephoning or texting new classmates, getting through math homework) will provide the positive feedback she needs to gain renewed confidence and mastery. A time frame was discussed to set appropriate expectations, and follow-up measurements were introduced to monitor how the interventions are working. Additional screeners and symptom assessments were suggested to capture Jesse's current symptoms as well as the effectiveness of the medication intervention.

What Therapists Should Know about the Prescribed Medication

Jesse's psychiatrist discussed with the therapist the medication options they would be recommending to the family. They would explain the rationale for these medications (in this case, Zoloft and Prozac), including their potential benefits and some of their potential side effects. They would specifically describe the anticipated timeline within which the medications should have an effect, as well as how they should be administered. In advance of their dialogue with the family, the therapist asked the psychiatrist (1) to inform them of any changes they should expect to notice as a result of the medication, what side effects they should also look out for, and (2) to clarify if the medications could potentially get in the way of the CBT plan.

Therapist as a Source of Feedback

Jesse's therapist and psychiatrist agreed to communicate more regularly in the immediate short term. In particular, the therapist would communicate to the psychiatrist any observed or reported significant changes, both positive and negative. The therapist would also communicate any concern that she or the family might have, given their regular meetings, her observations, and her close rapport with the patient and family.

PSYCHOPHARMACOLOGICAL INTERVENTIONS

This section offers a brief review of some of the most commonly prescribed medications for child and adolescent mental health concerns, along with their drug class, typical dosage, and FDA-approved and off-label use. It is in no way a comprehensive resource on psychopharmacological intervention for youth anxiety and depression. Table 4.2 provides a summary of the medications discussed below.

In this chapter, we highlight two major classes commonly considered for youth with depression and anxiety: selective serotonin reuptake inhibitors (SSRIs) and benzodiazepines. We will review how these agents work, the risks and benefits of these interventions, as well as evidence supporting their use or nonuse in the pediatric population. Remember that any intervention has risks and benefits, but not using an intervention has risks and benefits, too. Table 4.2 summarizes the key side effects of the main classes of drugs. Therapists will want to discuss these with families as they consider a medication. Such side effects are notable because they raise concern, but that does not mean they are necessarily common in youth who take these medications.

Common questions, discussed further below, include:

- What factors are considered when selecting a particular medication?
- Why would a provider pick a medication that is not an FDA-approved agent?
- For how long should a patient be on medication?
- When should a dose be increased? What is a "therapeutic dose"?
- How long does it take for a medication to have a therapeutic effect?
- How should the medication be stopped if desired by the patient and or their family?
- What other options exist?

Our nervous system utilizes various chemicals to communicate and generate neuronal activity. These molecules are called neurotransmitters. Some of the neurotransmitters include dopamine, serotonin, GABA, glutamate, norepinephrine, among others. Our peripheral senses transmit information to our brain by chemical and electric impulses guided by the molecules listed above. When someone suffers from severe depression and anxiety impairing their functioning and emotional well-being, modulating neurotransmitters through cognitive-behavioral psychotherapy and/or medications can improve daily life and emotional experiences. As a long-term goal, all interventions should allow recipients to feel more like themselves; medications are not intended to alter someone's core personality.

Selective Serotonin Reuptake Inhibitors

Most medications used to treat the pediatric population for depressive and anxiety symptoms are SSRIs. These medications include agents such as fluoxetine (Prozac), sertraline (Zoloft), and escitalopram (Lexapro), to name a few. The SSRI medications affect the presynaptic pump, which removes the neurotransmitter serotonin from the synaptic cleft back to the presynaptic neuron. In other words, an active pump decreases serotonin's activity by decreasing its stimulation of the postsynaptic pump. By inhibiting the pump, the medication generates more serotonin activity in the synapse and increases postsynaptic activity. The therapeutic effects of SSRIs, however, are more complex than simply increasing central nervous system (CNS) serotonin activity; otherwise, the effect of the medication would be immediate and not take days to weeks to occur, as discussed by Stahl (1998). It is believed that the initial increase in serotonin generates neuronal receptor modulation and affects neuronal communication. This process takes longer and is thought to be responsible for the therapeutic effect. While the exact mechanisms of action causing therapeutic benefits are unclear, there are data linking low serotonergic activity to depressive and anxiety symptoms, as well as suicide (Pandey, 1997; Underwood et al., 2018).

Studies offer ample evidence of the safety and effectiveness of these agents in both anxiety and depression diagnoses in the pediatric population. For example, in a comprehensive meta-analysis of 27 studies, Bridge and colleagues (2007) demonstrated that over 60% of youth responded to the first SSRI trial compared to 50% of the placebo. In another comprehensive study, the Treatment of Adolescent Depression Study (TADS; March et al., 2004), the response rate increased to 70% when combined with CBT. This rate was the highest among the three study arms of placebo, CBT alone, and SSRI alone after 12 weeks. The response rate increased to 86% after 36 weeks in the combined CBT + SSRI arm. Similarly, Walkup and colleagues (2008) have shown that combined CBT and SSRI treatment in children has an 80% acute response rate compared to 55–60% treatment with either medication or psychotherapy alone. Furthermore, there appears to be a correlation between initial response and overall effectiveness of treatment (Walkup et al., 2008). This suggests that early effective treatment can yield a better response.

Although the U.S. Food and Drug Administration (FDA) has only approved fluoxetine (8–17 years) and escitalopram (12–17 years) as treatment for major depressive disorder in youth, there is ample evidence that other SSRIs are effective and may be used to treat anxiety disorders with an excellent response. Some of the considerations taken into account when selecting an SSRI have to do with the medication's properties and the potential side effects of each agent. For instance, some of the SSRIs such as fluoxetine are more activating compared with others (i.e., sertraline). Each medication has a particular half-life, which signifies the length of time it takes our body to eliminate the medication. Other factors that come into play may have to do with family experiences, including a family history of positive response to a specific SSRI with limited side effects or a family member's particularly favorable attitude toward a medication. Medications may also interact with one another, and it is therefore important to assure that no negative interaction is anticipated. While some patients respond to an SSRI within a few days, a 2- to 6-week time period is expected for a full response. If a medication is not having the desired antidepressant or anxiolytic effect, the first step would be to increase the dose. If there are intolerable side effects that do not remit with time, or no therapeutic benefits are observed, another SSRI should be tried.

Some of the common side effects of SSRIs include gastrointestinal symptoms such as nausea, headache, insomnia and other sleep disturbances, drowsiness, and agitation, to list but a few.

TABLE 4.2. FDA–Approved and Common Psychotropic Medications for Pediatric Populations

Medication	Brand	Class	Dose	Pediatric FDA indication	Off-label use	Key side effects
Alprazolam	Xanax	Benzodiazepine	Safety not established	Adult anxiety disorders	Pediatric anxiety symptoms	Sedation, paradoxical disinhibition, cognitive impairment, tolerance
Lorazepam	Ativan	Benzodiazepine	Safety not established	Adult anxiety disorders	Pediatric anxiety symptoms	Sedation, paradoxical disinhibition, cognitive impairment, tolerance
Clonazepam	Klonopin	Benzodiazepine	Safety not established	Adult anxiety disorders	Pediatric anxiety symptoms	Sedation, paradoxical disinhibition, cognitive impairment, tolerance
Sertraline	Zoloft	SSRI	25–200 mg	OCD	MDD, anxiety disorders	Increased suicidal ideation
Fluoxetine	Prozac	SSRI	10–80 mg	OCD, MDD	Anxiety disorders	Increased suicidal ideation
Escitalopram	Lexapro	SSRI	5–20 mg	MDD	Anxiety disorders	Increased suicidal ideation
Duloxetine	Cymbalta	SNRI	40–120 mg	GAD	MDD; neuropathic pain; urinary incontinence	GI symptoms, increased suicidal ideation
Clomipramine	Anafranil	TCA	25–200 mg	OCD	Enuresis, ADHD	Arrhythmia
Bupropion	Wellbutrin	Atypical anti-depressant/NEDRI	150–450 mg	MDD, SAD, nicotine addiction	ADHD	Seizures
Olanzapine	Seroquel	Antipsychotic	25–800 mg	Psychosis	Mood symptoms	Metabolic (weight gain, hypercholesterolemia)
Aripiprazole	Abilify	Antipsychotic	2–30 mg	Schizophrenia	Aggression	Metabolic effects, akathisia.

Lithium	Lithium	Mood stabilizer	Based on blood level	Bipolar	MDD	Ataxia, tremor, renal impairment, thyroid dysfunction, seizures
Valproic acid	Depakote	Mood stabilizer	Based on blood level	Seizure/bipolar	N/A	Teratogen, sedation, liver toxicity, weight gain
Lamotrigine	Lamictal	Mood stabilizer	100–200 mg	Epilepsy	Bipolar	Steven Johnson syndrome, allergic skin reaction, vision changes.
Methylphenidate ER	Concerta	Stimulant	18–54 mg	ADHD	N/A	Cardiac
Methylphenidate IR	Ritalin	Stimulant	10–60 mg	ADHD	N/A	Cardiac
Dexmethylphenidate hydrochloride	Focalin	Stimulant	2.5–20 mg	ADHD	N/A	Cardiac
Dextroamphetamine mixed salt	Adderall	Stimulant	5–40 mg	ADHD	N/A	Cardiac
ALisdexamfetamine	Vyvanse	Stimulant	20–70 mg	ADHD	N/A	Cardiac
Guanfacine	Intuniv	Alpha agonist	1–2 mg	ADHD/HTN Tic D/O	N/A	Change in blood pressure
Atomoxetine	Strattera	SNRI	40–100 mg	ADHD	Treatment-resistant depression	Fatigue, cardiac, potential increase in suicidal ideation
Clonidine	Catapres	Alpha agonist	-0.1–0.6 mg	HTN	ADHD, Tourette's syndrome	Dry mouth, fatigue, hypotension

Note. SNRI = selective norepinephrine reuptake inhibitor; NEDRI = norepinephrine dopamine reuptake inhibitor; SSRI = selective serotonin reuptake inhibitor; TCA = tricyclic antidepressant; ADHD = attention-deficit/hyperactivity disorder; HTN = hypertension; OCD = obsessive compulsive disorder; MDD = major depression disorder; SAD = seasonal affective disorder; GAD = generalized anxiety disorder.

Recently, especially when utilizing polypharmacy (multiple medications), metabolic effects have been noted, which might include weight gain, increased cholesterol, as well as other related side effects. Some of these side effects may stop after a short time, while others may persist. It is thus important to discuss such side effects with the prescribing physician. A "black box" warning was issued in 2004 regarding increased suicidal ideation associated with SSRI use in the pediatric population. This has been a major concern among providers, clients, and families. It is crucial that we as mental health providers understand the complex data responsible for the issuing of the black box warning in order to support our clients and their families in understanding the risks and benefits of SSRI interventions.

SSRIs and the Black Box Warning

Data looking at SSRI prescriptions in early 2000 showed a correlation between increased suicidal thoughts and behaviors, but not suicide attempts or completed suicide, and the use of SSRI medications. Specifically, there was a 4% incidence of suicidal ideation and associated behaviors in comparison to 2% in the placebo (no SSRI) group (Friedman, 2014). However, there have not been sound studies supporting the relationship between suicide attempts or completed suicides and SSRI use (Cuffe, 2007). National Institute of Mental Health (NIMH)-funded trials of SSRI use in the pediatric population suffering from internalizing conditions, such as depression and anxiety, indicate the potential significance of their therapeutic benefit (Walkup et al., 2017). For example, the Treatment of Adolescent Suicide Attempters (TASA) Study that explored treatment of severely depressed adolescents with psychotherapy and antidepressant medication demonstrated lower suicide rates compared to the community at large (Brent et al., 2009). In sum, while requiring consistent assessment and monitoring, utilizing SSRIs may provide major benefits that mitigate the risks.

Researchers continue to try to find evidence to account for a small but significant increase of reported suicidal ideation with SSRI use in the pediatric population. There are some prevailing theories, one of which suggests that the various symptoms of major depressive disorder (MDD) include both physiological experiences (lack of energy, fatigue, cognitive impairment, etc.) and other symptoms that more closely relate to mood and emotional experiences (sadness, irritability, etc.). It is believed the SSRI medications affect physiological experience first and only later assist in improving mood. In other words, an adolescent who is suffering from MDD and treated by SSRIs has improved energy and cognitive functions but continues to experience mood symptoms, so they may be more likely to vocalize these emotions, resulting in increased expression of suicidal ideation (Nischal, Tripathi, Nischal, & Trivedi, 2012). Either way, data do not support a causal link between suicide and SSRI use (Simon, Savarino, Operskalski, & Wang, 2006), though a positive correlation between decreased SSRI use and increased completed suicide and attempted suicide has been established (Hamilton et al., 2007; Cuffe, 2007). The most important take-home message of the black box warning is that any youth who is being prescribed an SSRI needs to be followed appropriately by trained professionals to monitor any potential side effects, knowing that the large majority of SSRI interventions can be safely applied in pediatric populations.

The most frequent SSRI side effects in adults that are responsible for discontinuation of medication treatment are the sexual ones. These may include a delay in sexual climax and decreased libido. Clinicians, caregivers, and patients (especially adolescents) may avoid speaking directly about sex. Providers need to explore these issues as they might contribute to noncompliance or worse—the adolescent may blame something else for the sexual side effects. While there are few data exploring sexual side effects in adolescents, it is a good idea to speak with them about sex in general and how it relates to their functioning and experience of self, as well as the potential side effects of medications.

Making a Collaborative Decision

After conferring with the therapist and psychiatrist, Jesse and her mothers decided to proceed with combined psychotherapeutic CBT and medication management. The psychiatrist suggested starting with a low dose of sertraline (Zoloft) in the hope of decreasing her anxiety symptoms and thus producing greater engagement with exposure work in therapy. The range of therapeutic dose was discussed in depth; however, it was made clear that the interventions were going to be driven by Jesse's response, rather than statistics. Furthermore, the psychiatrist fully addressed the potential side effects, including the black box warning on SSRI use in the pediatric population, with her and her family. A timeline of expected outcomes was highlighted for Jesse, her mothers, and her therapist, in addition to creating a roadmap of what to do if she experienced a lack of response or intolerable side effects. All parties involved in Jesse's care agreed to the proposed plan. Some of the therapist's screening tools were utilized to assess Jesse's progress and response to treatment in concordance with her regular visits with the prescribing physician. The psychiatrist instructed the mothers on how to administer sertraline and, to ensure safety, they were asked to restrict access to the medication as younger children might come into the home.

In the first few days of taking sertraline, Jesse reported symptoms of nausea throughout the day. She consulted with her psychiatrist, who recommended taking the medication with food and a wait-and-see attitude. Administering the medication at mealtime alleviated some of the symptoms, and within a week the nausea had completely disappeared. During the next scheduled meeting with her psychiatrist, 2 weeks later, both Jesse and her parents were excited to report a reduction of symptoms. Jesse noted: "The heaviness in my chest is not as bad when I wake up in the morning, sometimes it takes a few hours for me to even think about my anxiety. Before it was nonstop." After a few more weeks and appropriate titration, further symptom improvements were confirmed by her parents: "Jesse has been showing more emotions and been more engaged." Some anxiety symptoms persisted, as did the associated behavioral avoidance, but overall the intensity and functional impairment of symptoms had greatly remitted. At the next meetings, Jesse, her caregivers, the prescribing psychiatrist and therapist decided that the current dose struck a good balance between symptom reduction, and limited side effects and engagement in therapy. A continued follow-up plan was established by the family, therapist, and psychiatrist. The therapist also noted that Jesse's exposure exercises had been more productive, yielding great clinical and subjective progress. Regular sessions, CBT, and home practice resulted in greater progress toward achieving the treatment plan.

Jesse had benefited from her first SSRI trial with a good response and limited side effects, a result similar to that of approximately 60% of pediatric patients treated with an SSRI for anxiety symptoms. However, some pediatric patients don't respond adequately, show only a partial response, or have intolerable side effects when treated with SSRIs for depressive or anxiety symptoms. The standard of care is to first titrate the medication dose to the maximum indicated for a minimum of 8 weeks followed by a trial of a different SSRI.

Augmenting Agents and Other Antidepressants

If there is a partial response, the prescribing physician can consider augmenting agents such as lithium (a mood-stabilizing agent), bupropion (Wellbutrin, an atypical antidepressant), or aripiprazole (Abilify, an antipsychotic with strong serotonin action). Different classes of antidepressants, such as tricyclic antidepressants (TCAs), monoamine oxidase inhibitors (MAOIs), selective norepinephrine and serotonin reuptake inhibitors (SNRIs), may also be considered for partial responders or those who do not respond at all (Connolly & Bernstein, 2007). Please see Table 4.2 for more information.

Benzodiazepines

Many adults utilize benzodiazepines for treating anxiety. Benzodiazepines are a class of medications that potentiate the neurotransmitter receptor Gamma-aminobutyric acid (or for short, GABA), which is the major inhibitory neurotransmitter. GABA causes a sense of relaxation sedation and at times disinhibition, similar to the initial intoxicating effects of alcohol. Examples of some medications in this class include alprazolam (Xanax), lorazepam (Ativan), and clonazepam (Klonopin). While benzodiazepines have an immediate anxiolytic effect, people may develop tolerance, which is the phenomenon of needing a higher dose of a medication to achieve the same therapeutic effect. In other words, benzodiazepines could result in an addiction. The data do not support long-term and daily use of benzodiazepines for the treatment of anxiety disorders. If and when benzodiazepine agents are used in the pediatric population, it should be only for the short term, as when the primary anxiolytic agent, such as an SSRI, is taking effect. Benzodiazepines may also be used short term to allow initial engagement in psychotherapeutic work, such as exposure (Connolly & Bernstein, 2007). When utilizing benzodiazepines, close monitoring by the caregiver and prescribing physician should always be a priority. Benzodiazepines are off-label use for anxiety symptoms in the pediatric population and may have some side effects, including sedation, paradoxical disinhibition, and cognitive impairment. Long-term use may result in addiction and significant withdrawal symptoms when the medication is suddenly stopped. Furthermore, they are contraindicated in adolescents with a history of addiction.

Other Options for Treating Resistant Depression

There are other options for treatment-resistant depression, but these only should be considered as a later resort after appropriate and specialized consultation. Transcranial magnetic stimulation (TMS) has been studied predominantly in adults and has demonstrated significant improvements compared to controls. The treatment consists of applying varying intensities of magnetic fields to various CNS regions. Multiple sessions are required, and this treatment can be quite costly if not covered by insurance. It also carries the risk of significant side effects including seizures (Allen, Kluger, & Buard, 2017).

Another treatment is a ketamine IV infusion. Ketamine is a medication used frequently during anesthesia. Evidence has shown that ketamine infusion in adult population suffering from treatment-resistant depression (TRD) results in a reduction of depressive symptoms (Wan et al., 2014). Protocols vary from a single infusion to multiple infusion frequencies. Data for utilizing ketamine infusion for TRD in the pediatric population are limited. Some studies have shown that while a complete response is associated with treatment in a small group of patients, overall response rates may be lower compared to the adult population (Cullen et al., 2018). Again, ketamine infusion for TRD should be cautiously considered as a later option and after consultation with a specialist. These treatment options are relatively new with limited data supporting their use in the pediatric population; therefore, their longer-term risks have not yet been established (Cullen et al., 2018).

Various supplements have been advertised for the treatment of anxiety and depression in the pediatric population and new products are advertised regularly. There is some good research to demonstrate the efficacy of agents such as omega-3 fatty acids and other supplements (Osher & Belmaker, 2009). These substances are not governed by the same standards as medication imposed by the FDA; it is thus challenging to determine their psychoactive ingredients. Note that an agent's efficacy means that it has a better response compared to a placebo and not compared to other medical options. The research supporting some of these products lacks scientific rigor and conclusions are questionable. Another consideration is that some of the supplements may interact with other medications, and they might have significant side effects. While supplements are marketed as natural products, some are processed like pharmacological agents. Providers and families should be cautious. Providers should review the evidence for utilizing or avoiding supplements to treat anxiety and depression; families should also do so in consultation with a mental health professional.

For the next few months, Jesse continued to work with her therapist on building therapeutic skills to cope with her symptoms of anxiety, which were creating morbidity and dysfunction. Jesse made great progress and during the last several weeks had not missed any school days. She reported consistently having only minor and tolerable symptoms of anxiety. Although the anxiety symptoms greatly improved, some of the attention deficits and executive function issues became more visible in her everyday life. At this stage, her family declined a medication intervention to assist with the ADHD symptoms as psychotherapy had resulted in a positive response. The family asked when it would be appropriate for Jesse to stop taking medication for her anxiety. But they also expressed concern about the reemergence of her previous behaviors and symptoms if she stopped taking her medication and they wanted to minimize any emotional and functional hardships. The mothers wanted to know the risks associated with stopping the medication and what they should expect.

Many families have concerns with a child utilizing medication to treat mental health problems and worry that once a medication has been started, they will always need it or "be addicted to it." Once a patient responds positively to a medication and psychotherapy interventions, as providers, we hope they learn skills that may be used in the future, even in the absence of direct interventions. We may think of these interventions as a bicycle's training wheels that will provide supports and teach children how to do without them. Therefore, after a positive response to a medication, it is reasonable to see how a patient responds to its removal under psychiatric supervision. The relapse rate is 30–40% (Donovan, Glue, Kolluri, & Emir, 2010), but this depends on the initial severity of symptoms, level of response to intervention, comorbidity, and other factors as well. The standard of care is to consider titrating off a medication 9–12 months after a full response (Walkup et al., 2008). When titrating off medication, it is important to do so slowly in order to minimize the symptoms of discontinuation syndrome and symptom relapse. Discontinuation syndrome involves emotional and physiological symptoms that occur when stopping SSRIs abruptly or too fast. It may include GI symptoms, headaches, and a temporary increase in anxiety and irritability. These usually do not last longer than 2 weeks. It is therefore important to continue follow-up with the prescribing psychiatrist 6–12 weeks after the medication has been discontinued. Some providers prefer to discontinue a medication during the spring to not disrupt the beginning of an academic school year. This also allows observation before any sleep-away summer programs.

Titration of medication should be done via close communication between providers. This will allow all parties to know of progress and to react quickly if any changes in emotional well-being and behaviors occur Even after the medications have been stopped, it may be advisable to continue communicating with the prescribing physician and provide updates. Similarly, if major events take place that may trigger anxiety, these could be considered with the prescribing physician.

SUMMARY AND KEY POINTS

Psychopharmacological intervention is another avenue for achieving treatment goals and there is ample evidence of its effectiveness and safety. Collaboration between the primary therapist and prescribing physician can empower both CBT and psychopharmacological intervention and allow the family and youth to feel supported. Different families have different beliefs about medications, and this will be vital to consider as part of the conceptualization and during treatment. If a family refuses to go for a psychiatric consultation, the therapist can set goals and benchmark dates with the youth and family and propose that if these goals are not met by a certain date, they will reconsider the psychiatric evaluation. Progress monitoring aids in this decision making. Sharing the care of a challenging patient can also broaden the scope of the treatment plan and offer additional support not only to the family, but also to the therapist. Research shows that combined psychotherapy and psychopharmacological interventions work synergistically to advance treatment plans and achieve treatment goals in children and adolescent patients with diagnoses of anxiety and depression. In summary:

• Evidence-based treatment for moderate to severe depression and anxiety in children and adolescents supports considering selective serotonin reuptake inhibitors (SSRI) such as sertraline (Zoloft), fluoxetine (Prozac), and escitalopram (Lexapro).

• Psychopharmacological interventions may have significant side effects. The incidence of these are low, and usually the benefits outweigh the risks. Pediatric patients receiving psychopharmacological intervention should always be appropriately followed by a prescribing provider.

• Creating a nonjudgmental and empathic therapeutic space, while utilizing cognitive reframing, may be the best way to allow families and patients to explore risks and benefits of including or excluding psychopharmacological interventions.

• Creating a collaborative interdisciplinary team allows providers to enrich the treatment plan, support families and patients, and improve outcomes of care.

CHAPTER 5

Working with Caregivers and Families

How can therapists best partner with caregivers to enhance the treatment of a child or teen? As youths' families and caregivers often form their most immediate environment, CBT therapists will want to use their own observational and conceptualization skills to identify consistent family interactions that impact the youth. The therapist will then want to make caregivers partners or direct targets of treatment, depending on the case. How does one do this while keeping the primary focus on the teen? This chapter answers this question.

THE CAREGIVER'S ROLE IN YOUTH ANXIETY AND DEPRESSION

Parent and caregiver behaviors have been associated with the development and maintenance of youth anxiety and depression (McLeod, Weisz, & Wood, 2007; McLeod, Wood, & Weisz, 2007; Sander & McCarty, 2005; Wood, McLeod, Sigman, Hwang, & Chu, 2003; Yap, Pilkington, Ryan, & Jorm, 2014). Substantial research has identified the common family and parenting factors that influence the maintenance of anxiety and depression in youth. Such research has focused on family environment, general parenting (caregiver) styles, and specific parenting practices (DiBartolo & Helt, 2007; Sander & McCarty, 2005; Wood et al., 2003). "Family environment" refers to the quality of the overall family context (e.g., cohesion, conflict, independence, organization, control, achievement orientation, focus on recreation). "Caregiver style" refers to a global set of parental attitudes, goals, and patterns of parenting practices, and it contributes to the emotional climate of the caregiver–youth relationship. Examples include the extent to which the youth perceive caregiver warmth, autonomy granting, or criticism. "Caregiver practices" refer to specific kinds of caregiver–youth interactions in certain situations. For example, we might want to observe how a caregiver encourages autonomy ("I believe you have the right judgment to make these decisions") in a specific situation (e.g., the youth making a difficult choice). Therapists often focus most of their attention on the level of caregiver practices, because they are the most concrete processes to observe and they offer the most direct ways to intervene.

The most consistent parenting factors to be linked to youth anxiety and depression include parental control and rejection (McLeod, Weisz, et al., 2007; McLeod, Wood, et al., 2007; Yap et al., 2014). "Parental control" is broadly defined as excessive regulating of their child's activities, instructing a child or teen on their cognitions or affect, which can result in the hindering of their child's growing independence. In contrast, efforts to grant autonomy and teach independence help youth become emotional copers. One highly cited dimension of parental overcontrol is "parental intrusiveness," which refers to caregivers who will perform tasks for their children, even if their child can do it independently, leading to impairment in the youth's self-efficacy. Such caregivers are not likely to acknowledge or foster their child's autonomy. As a result, children with anxiety disorders may not believe in their ability to effectively manage a novel situation without parental assistance (Wood et al., 2003). In contrast, the more parents encourage the youth's opinions and choices—even if they result in mistakes and failures—and solicit their teen's input into decisions, the less risk we see for later distress. One reason offered to explain high degrees of control is the parent's own distress intolerance at witnessing their children struggle in a distress-provoking situation (Tiwari et al., 2008). Caregivers also step in to help or rescue children prematurely, partially because of doubt in their child's ability to perform. In depression, caregivers may exert control by using coercive, hostile parenting techniques to intrude on the teen's experience or choices.

Parental "rejection" is often described as a caregiver's coldness, disapproval, and unresponsiveness toward their child (McLeod, Wood, et al., 2007; Yap et al., 2014). It can include parental hostility, like criticism, punishment, and conflict, that communicates a lack of parental acceptance. Rejection can also include a lack of pleasant interactions, lack of interest and involvement in the youth's activities, low emotional support, and even withdrawal. Maternal depression, low maternal emotional availability, and high parental control are consistently predictive of depression in teens and teens with low self-esteem (Sander & McCarty, 2005). Maladaptive cognitive styles in the caregiver can also influence a youth's negative views of the self, world, and future. In contrast, parents who exude warmth, interest, and investment help youth develop confidence in managing the challenges surrounding them.

Additional parenting factors that have strong associations with youth anxiety and depression include interparental conflict, low monitoring, and erratic discipline (Yap et al., 2014). The frequency of parental conflict, marital dissatisfaction, and expressed hostility between caregivers has been associated with greater anxiety and depression in longitudinal studies. An authoritarian parenting style, paired with minimal monitoring and inconsistent discipline, has also been uniquely associated with depression. Similarly, lower levels of anxiety have been linked to parental encouragement of sociability through modeling and verbal encouragement. Together, the strongest evidence in the development and maintenance of internalized distress in youth suggests a central positive role for warmth (positive regard, involvement) and negative roles for aversiveness (parental hostility, criticism, punishment, conflict), interparental conflict (marital dissatisfaction, expressed hostility), and overinvolvement (interference with autonomy, psychological control). Caregivers should be encouraged to keep conflict to private quarters and model problem-solving and effective conflict-resolution skills in front of their children.

Because caregivers play important roles in helping their children manage anxiety and distress, therapists should include caregivers in the assessment process. Therapists gather information about the caregivers' own distress and obtain multiple perspectives of family functioning. Valuable information can be gathered about the family's emotional atmosphere, general parenting styles and attitudes, and specific practices. We then encourage clinicians to work directly with parents in order to reduce parental rejection and overcontrol, and promote warmth and autonomy granting. Additionally, caregiver involvement can be leveraged to promote skill generalization and reinforce approach behaviors. To make the most of caregiver participation in the therapeutic process, we focus on several concrete skills that can supplement the youth's work:

1. Include caregivers as partners or agents of change.
2. Provide psychoeducation and normalize emotions.
3. Identify problematic patterns using functional assessment.
4. Practice communication skills that foster active family problem solving.
5. Develop reward-focused contingency management (CM) systems.

Caregivers as Partners or Agents of Change

The first decision a CBT therapist will need to make is how much to involve the caregivers as *partners* or as *agents of change* (Sander & McCarty, 2005). Caregivers can be engaged as partners in the therapy process by educating them about relevant disorders and providing them with summaries of youth skills (e.g., problem solving, cognitive restructuring). The frequency of meetings could range from one session, to monthly, to as needed, as well as attending portions of some sessions with the teen. The goal is to partner with the caregivers so they reinforce therapy lessons at home with the youth and to help generalize skills by arranging the youth's practice outside of session. This way, caregivers can also enhance their coaching skills.

Alternatively, caregivers can be included as co-clients or agents of change, learning the same lessons the therapist teaches the youth. In this approach, therapists include caregivers more explicitly in therapy. Meeting frequency can range from every session to less frequently, sometimes separately from, or conjointly with, the teen. The goal of this approach is to teach caregivers the same anxiety management and positive coping skills that the youth learns. This can help the caregiver apply strategies to their own distress and the youth practice skills at home. This approach may prove very beneficial given that caregivers often find it difficult to manage their own distress during challenging moments with their youth (Sander & McCarty, 2005; Tiwari et al., 2008). Parents might also need assistance with management training skills to implement consistent behavior plans, which include instruction on how to identify behavioral patterns, to use clear communication strategies, and to implement structured CM programs.

When working with caregivers, the CBT therapist directs attention to youth/family interactions that are contributing to youth symptoms and functioning (Barmish & Kendall, 2005). Some patterns to watch for include caregiver responses that may *inadvertently reinforce* anxious or depressive behaviors in the youth (avoidance, withdrawal, shutting down, negativity). You can also teach caregivers how to *model appropriate coping behaviors,* such as active problem solving, demonstrating realistic coping thoughts, and approaching problems with minimal avoidance. You may additionally identify *family conflict* as a problem and work directly with affected family members to enhance communication and practice family problem solving. Identifying and addressing these systems-level family interaction patterns can help reinforce anxiety and depression-specific coping skills.

PSYCHOEDUCATION FOR CAREGIVERS: NORMALIZING EMOTIONS

The first goal in helping anxious and depressed youth is establishing a supportive environment where intense emotions are normalized and where anxiety and sadness are seen as natural responses to scary situations and disappointments. When providing education to caregivers, therapists focus on sending messages that normalize intense emotions and concentrate on issues of avoidance. Therapists also work to minimize the blame and guilt parents may feel for contributing to their youth's distress and provide a pathway to help them out. To do this, therapists can meet with the parent at or near the beginning of treatment to provide psychoeducation around these issues and then confer periodically to reinforce such messages. In Chapters 6 through 11, we provide psychoeducation therapists can give to their clients and families for specific disorders and problems.

In general, we teach that emotions, sometimes even intense feelings, are natural and often serve useful functions. Emotions can be distressing, but they are not dangerous. Youth can use the coping skills they learn in therapy when their emotions feel overwhelming and know they can keep moving forward even in the face of distress and challenge. Caregivers can learn this, too. They can help their teen by reinforcing this message through the words they speak and the actions they model. Below we summarize the key points therapists can emphasize for caregivers and highlight the central messages (see Handouts 6 and 7 available in Appendix A).

Key Points about Anxiety

1. **Normalize anxiety.** Anxiety is a natural emotion that all people feel when they confront something scary, threatening, or challenging. Sometimes anxiety can be helpful, such as when a teen needs motivation to study for a test. However, anxiety can get a youth in trouble when it becomes so intense that it interferes with their typical ability to handle a situation (e.g., anxiety makes them so distracted that they do poorly on a test).

2. **Avoidance hurts more than it helps.** Behavioral avoidance, such as procrastination, withdrawal, and escape, can seem like a natural response in the face of new unpredictable challenges. Avoidance might be appropriate when there is a real threat (e.g., avoiding a dark alley late at night). But avoidance can be a problem when youth turn down opportunities because they misinterpret or exaggerate threat cues (e.g., turning down an invitation to a party because most of the attendees will be strangers). Consistently taking the *safe* option means losing opportunities to learn, grow, and make the most of pleasant activities.

3. **Learning coping skills helps.** While intense feelings are natural, a youth can learn how to manage their anxiety or sad feelings. To do this, you will help the youth identify the triggers (e.g., situations, people, thoughts) that prompt anxiety and teach them how to recognize when the anxiety reaches interfering levels. Second, a youth can learn coping skills (active problem solving, brave approach behaviors, activity scheduling, and coping thoughts; see Chapter 2) that will help them push through their distressing feelings and pursue desired goals. When a teen is standing at the foul line trying to make the game-winning shot, it is natural to feel anxious. Thinking that one has to be free of anxiety before taking such a shot would cause just about any person to freeze. You can reference the experiences of professional athletes who frequently describe how to use anxiety to enhance performance. One principle to communicate is that anxiety is not life-threatening in, and of, itself. The more a youth can learn to tolerate and live with their anxiety, the more they can keep doing the things they enjoy (playing basketball) even while feeling emotional ups and downs.

4. **Parents can help.** A number of caregivers come to therapy worried and expressing guilt that their own anxiety has contributed to their youth's anxiety. There's good research to suggest that young children have their own anxiety. In one line of work (Whaley, Pinto, & Sigman, 1999;

Moore, Whaley, & Sigman, 2004), observations of mother–child dyads showed that key parenting styles (warmth, catastrophizing) were linked to child anxiety more than maternal anxiety status. Whether a mother was diagnosed with an anxiety disorder or not, playing with an anxious youth evoked a tendency to be overprotective. Thus, anxious youth carry their own anxiety, eliciting responses from their environments, and many parents are just trying to be responsive to their youth's needs. Caregivers are not necessarily causing anxiety in their children. At the same time, there are stances and behaviors that caregivers can adopt that will help ease their child's anxiety. As reviewed earlier, parental warmth, granting of autonomy, and minimal criticism can minimize a child's anxious reactions. The strategies you will be teaching the parent can help the family stay on the right path.

Key Points about Depression

1. **Distinguish sadness from depression.** Sadness is a natural feeling that all of us experience when difficult things happen (e.g., a friend moves away, the loss of a loved one, arguments with friends) or when situations do not go our way (e.g., receiving a poor grade on a test, not getting selected for the school play or team, having a privilege restricted). Sadness should draw adult attention when a youth's behavior begins to interfere with their typical functioning (sleeping, eating, socializing) or stops them from pursuing goals and activities they care about because of isolation, withdrawal, and inactivity.

2. **Avoidance hurts more than it helps.** As with anxiety, behavioral avoidance can seem like a natural response to sad feelings. When a teen is feeling sad or lethargic, it might seem natural for them to withdraw to their room, ignore texts or calls from friends, and not go to school or participate in activities. It may seem like the only way for them to deal with their feelings is to let the day pass and *reset* the next day. Giving into this temptation to shut down relieves distress in the short term, but repeated avoidance can become a hard habit to break. Avoidance deprives the teen of opportunities (every missed soccer practice puts the child further behind). They also miss chances to cope and see if they can handle the challenge when confronted by it. Avoidance is different from self-care or nurturance (e.g., being realistic about demands, evaluating oneself fairly, taking planful breaks with fulfilling activities) that is restorative and promotes continued action. Therapy will help a youth distinguish between avoidance and self-care.

3. **Coping skills can help.** Depression can feel intense (painful sadness, irritable anger) or deflating (low energy, weight on shoulders). Therapy will help the youth learn skills to manage intense pain with emotion regulation skills and evaluation of negative self-critical thoughts. Deflated avolition is countered with the scheduling of pleasant activities, active problem solving, and approach behaviors. With caregiver assistance, the youth will be taught to push through the sadness that defines depression.

4. **Parents can help.** Caregivers come to therapy often frustrated or scared because of their child's inactivity. They don't know how to help, motivate, or encourage their child. Parents might find themselves swinging between overaccommodating the child's negative moods or being harshly critical when they see their child depressed. It may be difficult to distinguish depression from developmentally appropriate "teen moodiness" or a preference to seek increased privacy. Therapy helps caregivers to make this distinction, to understand that the youth's depression is not necessarily a reflection of the child's innate personality or of the family. With this perspective, you

help caregivers practice active listening and encourage active approach behaviors when responding to their child.

IDENTIFYING PARENT–CHILD INTERACTION PATTERNS

The first step in managing challenging youth behavior is to identify the behavioral patterns and unique roles of caregivers and youth. Early in therapy, it is helpful to inform parents of the vital role they play in modeling and sending the right messages to their teen or child. Conducting functional assessment does not only help the individual youth who is trying to understand and change their own behavior. It can also be used to understand how, as a system, different members of the family influence each other. As stated above, a number of caregiver styles and practices have been found to be associated with increased anxiety and depression. Below we list several of these patterns and describe them in language that highlights the interactive and reciprocal nature of family interactions.

The Accommodation Spiral

The Accommodation Spiral describes a pattern in which caregivers respond to a child's distress by accommodating, encouraging, or facilitating avoidance. A teen's refusal to go to school in the morning provides an example of this (see Figure 5.1; a reproducible version is available as Handout 8 in Appendix A). The alarm goes off in the morning; the youth says he feels sick, and the mother asks if he is well enough to attend classes. The teen protests, and his mother suggests that he go to school after lunch. The teen returns to bed and sleeps through the morning. Caregivers can slip into this spiral because they experience their own distress at witnessing their child confronting an anxiety-provoking challenge (Tiwari et al., 2008). Rescuing the child or solving their problems is the quickest way to resolve the child's distress (the problem is solved for the time being), but it limits the youth's chance to practice their own coping skills and learning to ride out discomfort. In the long run, the youth's anxiety persists and reliance on the caregiver intensifies. Your goals are to help increase the caregiver's awareness of this pattern of interaction, validate the discomfort parents may be feeling, and devise an alternative approach-oriented solution.

The Passivity–Discouragement Spiral

The Passivity–Discouragement Spiral describes a pattern in which caregivers respond to youth fatigue, lack of motivation or interest, and hopelessness with passivity and accommodation that reinforces the youth's lack of efficacy. Figure 5.2 (a reproducible version is available as Handout 9 in Appendix A) shows how a caregiver could concede to a teen who is struggling to follow through with social plans. The teen's depression raises the threshold for activation, and it is often easier for them to stay home and exert less effort. The parent's passivity in this case reinforces the youth's belief system that staying home is the best way to manage fatigue. Caregivers can resort to this kind of pattern due to some of the same negative reinforcement cycles that perpetuate the Accommodation Cycle. Allowing the teen to escape the social obligation takes the caregiver off the hook from pushing the youth to make the effort. Given the familial links to depression across generations, depressed teens may have caregivers who have limited pro-approach coping skills of their own.

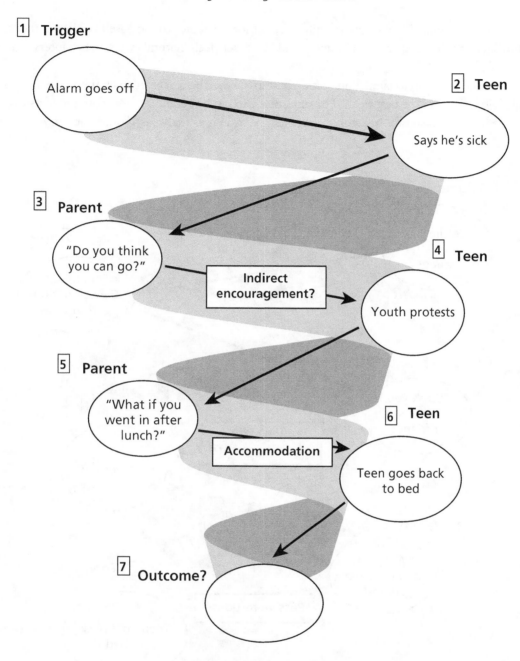

FIGURE 5.1. Parent–child interaction pattern: The accommodation spiral.

The Aggressive–Coercive Spiral

The Aggressive–Coercive Spiral describes a pattern in which caregivers respond to oppositional behavior with anger and criticism, which leads to escalated aggression. In one school refusal example, the caregivers attempt to compel the youth to go to school with threats and criticism (see Figure 5.3; a reproducible version is available as Handout 10 in Appendix A). This approach is ineffective because shame and criticism only discourage the teen further, making it less likely for them to comply or initiate active problem solving. Punishment, or the threat of punishment, can sometimes compel immediate compliance, but it contributes to increased family conflict and diminished future compliance. However, this approach feels natural when other interventions have failed.

To draw attention to family interaction patterns, have the caregiver track their own and their teen's behaviors over the past week. The objective is to identify common hot spots and to assess for possible interaction spirals. In Figure 5.4 (a blank version is available as Worksheet 9 in Appendix

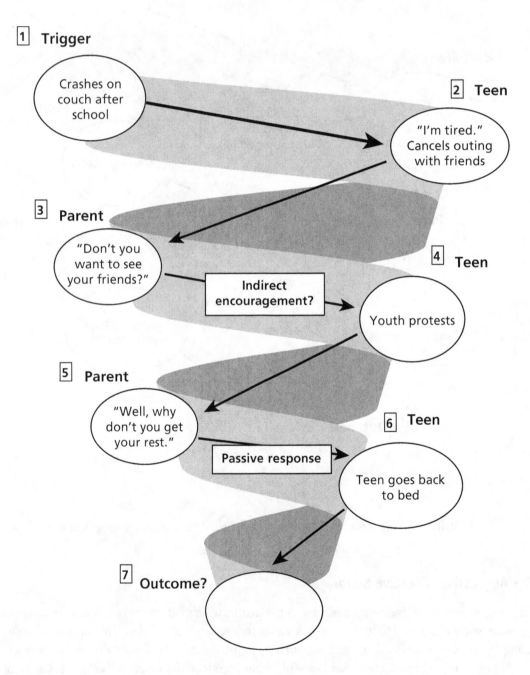

FIGURE 5.2. Parent–child interaction pattern: The passivity–discouragement spiral.

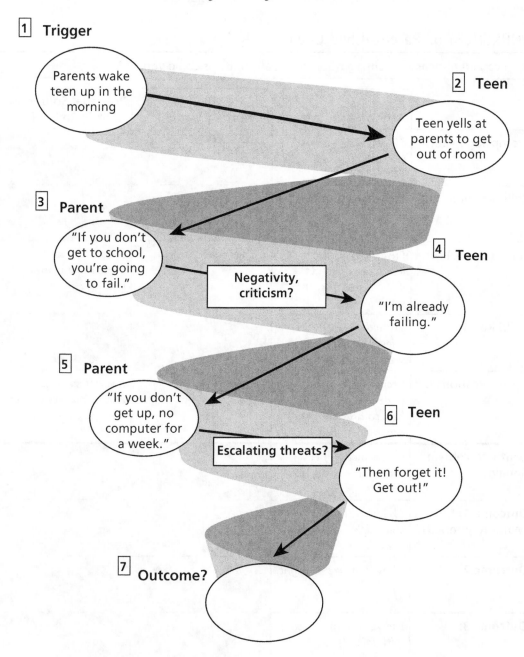

FIGURE 5.3. Parent–child interaction pattern: The aggressive–coercive spiral.

A), the caregiver resorts to aggressive–coercive reactions to motivate the youth initially. When that does not work, the caregiver concedes and falls into the passivity–discouragement cycle. Alternative solutions could have included approach-oriented interventions, such as empathize and encourage (see next page) and reinforcing any reward plans that have been designed to encourage new behaviors. We describe these interventions below in more detail. Handout 11 in Appendix A describes common parenting traps and alternative approaches that can help.

WORKSHEET 9. Parent–Child Chain Analysis

Can you identify any parenting traps? What alternatives could you try?			
	Action/Response	**Parenting Trap**	**Potential Solution or Skills to Use?**
Prompting Event:	Ch was invited to a party by friends.		
Child Action:	Ch was acting mopey and didn't want to go.		
Parent Response:	I (mom) told her she'll lose all her friends if she doesn't accept some invites.	Aggressive–coercive	Empathize and encourage; planned ignoring
Child Reaction:	Ch said she feels like a loser when she goes; she cries at night.		
Parent Response:	I told her I understood—maybe best to find another group of friends.	Passivity–discouragement	Empathize and encourage; remind of reward plan
Conflict/Problem Behavior:	Ch crashed in her room; didn't call/text anyone.		
Outcome 1 (What happened)?	Ch looked miserable that night; down on herself.		
Outcome 2:	Ch was awake all night.		
Outcome 3:	Didn't end up meeting with friends.		

FIGURE 5.4. Parent–child chain analysis completed by parent.

COACH AND APPROACH: LABELED PRAISE, ACTIVE LISTENING, AND ENCOURAGING APPROACH BEHAVIORS

The second critical component of parent management is to teach caregivers how to use clear communication strategies that incorporate active listening, reinforcing desired behaviors, and setting a tone of encouragement. Before a youth will listen to direct instructions from a caregiver, a positive parent–youth relationship is required. Such thinking is supported in research on parent management techniques with defiant behaviors. For example, in clinical research on parenting skills for managing defiant behaviors (e.g., the "incredible years," parent–child interaction therapy), the initial phase of treatment focuses on establishing positive relations with children before any directive instruction (limit setting, CM) is introduced. Positive relationships are fostered via active listening, joint attention on the child's interests, labeled praise, and labeled feelings. These strategies help to demonstrate both a parent's regard and positive attention.

Within the context of a positive parent–child relationship, directive strategies like limit setting and CM can take place. For example, a common strategy to reduce aggressive tantrums in the household is to establish a reward plan that spells out concrete rewards (e.g., points) for specific goals (e.g., completing a task demand, such as doing homework). However, reward plans often fail if the right groundwork has not been first established; the parent needs to be able to identify when the child is behaving favorably and can let the child know when they approve—hence, a reward is earned.

Working with anxious and depressed youth may not require the full-scale parent management interventions reflected in the work with oppositional children, such as creating detailed token economies or using bug-in-the-ear coaching (real-time coaching through wireless earbuds) for parent-directed commands. However, CM will be important when creating reward schedules to encourage active approach behaviors. Ignoring may be helpful for removing attention from "whiny" communication. Limit setting may be useful when dealing with the irritability of depression or defiance associated with school refusal. To set the foundation for this, we teach the skills of labeled praise, active listening, and directive parenting to educate parents in creating a positive baseline for parents and youth.

Labeled Praise: Catch Them Being Good

One key skill we teach parents is to become trained spotters of their child's good behavior. It becomes an active mission for parents. Consider this situation: a typically rambunctious child is playing quietly in the den by himself. What do you do? Go over and let the child know how pleased you are with his play, or leave the child to play on his own? (e.g., "Ah ha! I caught you being good!") Conventional wisdom commonly convinces parents to "let sleeping dogs lie" and leave the child alone as long as they are playing quietly. This advice leads one to believe that paying any attention to the child would disrupt a desirable pattern and trigger the feared attention seeking and demands. So, you leave the child to play alone until the child starts to play rough, throws toys, and demands new activities. You quickly respond and lecture the child for playing aggressively and making demands. What is learned?

Research shows that children are keenly sensitive to a parent's signals, and social attention is one of the strongest reinforcers to motivate behaviors (Brinkmeyer & Eyberg, 2003; Rapee, 1997).

Unfortunately, negative attention (yelling, overly structured directions, complaints) is still attention, even if it's less positive than praise. In the above scenario, the parent makes the common mistake of ignoring the desirable behavior (playing quietly) while providing (negative) attention when the child acts out. Unfortunately, this only perpetuates the undesirable sequence whereby the child only gets social reinforcement (the most powerful kind) when they act aggressively. The same cycle can be seen in anxious and depressed teens. When a worried teen is doing their homework quietly, we leave them alone. When they repeatedly ask for reassurance wondering if they can complete the assignment on time, we might get annoyed and criticize the repeated questions. Why not reinforce the youth's independent work ("You're working so hard on that homework")?

For depressed teens, it is key for parents to reinforce any attempt the teen makes to get going or to persevere. The prospect of failure or rejection is too intense to confront, so the teen withdraws. Likewise, motivation may be hard to muster. When a challenge presents itself, the amount of effort it would take to overcome that challenge seems overwhelming. The teen shuts down instead. The challenge could be a long homework assignment or confronting a friend with whom they just argued. To move the teen forward, a parent may need to provide an initial "push" to get their child started ("I know this is difficult, and I know you can push past the first question"). Once started, we advise the parent to reinforce any efforts the youth makes to approach the problem ("I like how you pushed past the initial hump").

It is essential to remind parents to limit inadvertent criticism whenever possible. When a teen is procrastinating or withdrawing, it can be easy to fall into the trap of trying to motivate through criticism or shame: "If you don't get going on that homework, you'll never catch up!" "If you stay in that bedroom all day, your friends will forget about you!" Remind parents that criticism and shame rarely motivate and often instill greater hopelessness. At other times, criticism can inadvertently provide the social reinforcement that the child needs but for the wrong behavior. When advising parents, we follow the Hippocratic Oath: "First, do no harm." If parents can avoid harmful, demotivating statements, they can make progress toward shaping more desired behaviors. At times, we assign parents the home practice of catching their own urges to make such statements; even disrupting the automatic cycle that parents and children fall into is a start! The strategy is for caregivers to ignore the youth's reassurance seeking and isolation, and instead use approach-oriented behaviors. When an isolating teen finally leaves their room, parents should provide reinforcing attention ("Hey, come over here and take a look at this. . . ."). When the youth finally attempts a challenge they have been avoiding, a parent might make a validating and reinforcing comment (so-called labeled praise) such as "That must've been hard to call up your friend." Specific labeled praise is more impactful than general praise (e.g., "good job"). *Catching the positive* has to become a part of the family culture; thus, caregivers are asked to practice this skill early and often.

Active Listening and Positive Encouragement: Empathize and Encourage

Labeled praise helps parents observe their children's behaviors and notice how they are acting and feeling. That skill forms the basis for a second intervention parents can use to promote forward behavior, called *empathize and encourage*. Empathize and encourage combines attentive observation of the youth's emotional state (e.g., "I can see this is really hard for you") with reinforcement of approach-oriented efforts to cope (e.g., "I know you can stick through this. Why don't we try using a coping thought?"). We recommend using a statement with both validation and change elements, because even well-meaning parents can unintentionally lean too heavily on validation or commands to cope.

The steps of empathize and encourage are as follows:

1. **Empathize.** Actively listen to the youth's expressed emotions. Parents provide a labeling statement showing the youth they have heard their distress. For example, "I know getting to school in the morning is really difficult for you." "I see how much pain you are feeling right now." Parents may jump to problem solving or encouraging too soon, so validating what the teen is feeling is a good starting point. Parents can aim to validate the feeling even if they do not understand or agree with it.

2. **Encourage.** Provide calm encouragement to move forward, emphasizing the youth's ability to cope with the situation. For example, "I know you can push yourself over this hump." "And I wonder if any coping skills you're learning can help in this moment." Parents can reference previous examples of coping: "The last time you experienced this, I remember you said that mindfulness exercise really helped you."

3. **And Then . . . Stop!** After repeating empathizing and encouraging statements three times, the parent must stop and walk away. The statement can be repeated verbatim or can be changed to reflect the natural progression of the conversation, as long as the statement does not move prematurely to problem solving or questioning. The aim is to simply show that you are listening. The purpose of stopping after three iterations is to disrupt the typical escalation of a conflict that results from repeated negotiations.

Active listening must precede active encouragement, and both precede planned ignoring. Therapists can work with parents to catch their urges to respond, to slow down and more carefully consider specifically what they will say. Then they should practice this type of responding with more intention. The goal is not to simply neglect or ignore a child's distress. Rather, we encourage parents to listen actively to their child's emotional state and practice actively communicating their understanding in empathetic statements. It is critical that these empathic statements are genuine and accurate. This intervention can become robotic if parents rely on generic "listening" statements (e.g., "I'm sure this is hard" "You must be anxious"). The statement should be as specific as possible ("I know you struggle with math homework" "It's confusing when your friend doesn't respond") to communicate that the parent actually *gets it*.

Caregivers who tend to be rejecting (e.g., exhibiting low warmth) or critical will need extra practice at providing descriptive, empathic statements. They may require actual scripted statements to consider and practice. After a series of complaints or acts of defiance, it is not unexpected for a parent to respond to a youth's negativity (e.g., "Why do you make such a big deal over this?") with an accommodation that rescues the teen (e.g., solving the homework problem for the youth). Instead, we ensure that parents repeatedly practice actively listening and reflecting their youth's distress before practicing approach statements. Likewise, approach statements can focus on encouraging the youth's own attempts to cope: "I know you can take this one step at a time." We also carefully make use of "and" statements rather than "but" statements (e.g., "It's hurtful that your friend hasn't texted you back . . . and I imagine that reaching out to them will help"). The temptation is to insert a "but" in the middle of the statement ("It's hurtful, but you can do this"). Using "and" statements reorients solutions from an "either-or" perspective to a "both-and" (one can be distressed and still do it) perspective. This helps reinforce validation and approach over time.

The instruction to stop intervening after three attempts falls under the Hippocratic Oath described earlier. The three steps provide a balanced approach that encourages the youth to move forward while avoiding the negative consequences of escalating conflict that often occurs with anxious and depressed teens. Consider this example of escalating conflict as a mother tries to encourage their teen to make plans with friends:

> MOTHER: You've been spending a lot of time at home. Why don't you go meet up with some friends?
>
> ABBY-LYNN: Nah, no one's around. Besides I'm beat.
>
> MOTHER: I'm sure someone's around. What about the girls from the team? Why don't you call one of them up?
>
> ABBY-LYNN: And do what?
>
> MOTHER: I don't know, practice some shots?
>
> ABBY-LYNN: Practice some shots? What am I, in 3rd grade? That's what practice is for. I'm not calling people to "practice shots."
>
> [*This type of exchange continues for minutes, until frustration grows. . . .*]
>
> MOTHER: Look, Abby-Lynn, this is what always happens. If you don't do anything, you'll just end up sitting home and doing nothing.
>
> ABBY-LYNN: So what?
>
> MOTHER: If you don't see your friends, they'll go on and do things without you. You won't have anyone to call.
>
> ABBY-LYNN: Who cares—just leave me alone. Why do you care so much?!
>
> MOTHER: Fine! But if you keep this up, you really won't have any friends!

This exchange is sadly a common scenario for many families. Caregivers start off with the right intentions ("Why don't you meet up with friends?") and even reflect some recommended encouraging statements ("I'm sure someone is around"). The mother even identifies a problem the teen might relate to ("You've been spending a lot of time home"), even if she is not technically empathizing with Abby-Lynn's apathy. Unfortunately (and as one would expect), the mother demonstrates little empathy, and the interaction does not stop there. Abby-Lynn protests, and instead of simply reinforcing the recommended "empathize and encourage" message, the mother escalates her attempts to convince Abby-Lynn to act. As a result, conflict increases and the mother resorts to shaming and critical statements to push Abby-Lynn, but the teen moves no closer to calling her friends, and the last thing she hears is her mother claiming she will no longer have any friends before long.

Consider this alternative scenario where the mother adheres to the three-statement limit:

> MOTHER: You've been spending a lot of time at home [empathize]. Why don't you go meet up with some friends [encourage]?
>
> ABBY-LYNN: Nah, no one's around. Besides I'm beat.

MOTHER: It's tough getting out when you're tired [empathize]; and I think spending time with friends can bring some energy [encourage].

ABBY-LYNN: You've got to be kidding.

MOTHER: It's always hard calling up a friend when you're tired [empathize], and I think you can push yourself over that hump [encourage].

ABBY-LYNN: Mom! You're not listening!

(Mom gets up from the bedside and walks out of the room.)

In this exchange, it appears that Abby-Lynn may *still* not call any friends, but at least this approach avoids an escalating conflict and its associated power struggles that entrench both parties. Furthermore, the last thing that Abby-Lynn hears (in fact, the only thing) is "I understand, and I still think you can call some friends." This approach may not produce immediate results in terms of proactive socialization. However, if delivered consistently, it begins to communicate a changing mentality in the family that the parents can honor the youth's pain and distress (empathizing) while also encouraging the youth to push through painful challenges. As parents increasingly limit their responses to empathize and encourage statements, there is less room for problematic parent–youth spirals. Walking away after delivering statements three times is essential even though it is one of the most challenging skills a parent can master.

CONTINGENCY MANAGEMENT

Reward Plans and Goal-Oriented Behaviors

Anxious youth often need external rewards to get them to move forward and commit to doing something difficult. Depressed youth typically need something concrete to give them a reason to change. A meaningful reward chart (contingency management or CM strategy) incentivizes specific behaviors and goals achieved by the youth. While one might think it would be ideal for these youth to be intrinsically motivated to work toward goals, anxiety and depression interfere with their natural goal orientation. It can be difficult for these youth to see that achieving the goal will be worth the required effort or the fear they have to endure up front. To help motivate change, individualized reward programs are necessary. Likewise, CM programs can help extinguish disruptive behaviors (such as defiance and aggression) that can interfere with successful anxiety and depression treatment.

When initiating a reward program, we draw analogies to other areas of life where the youth and caregivers set goals for themselves. We ask both to recall times when they learned a new skill or made a New Year's resolution. "When you promised yourself you would go to the gym three days a week, how did you get yourself to go?" For the most part, individuals need some incentives to sustain effort to overcome challenges. If achieving goals were easy, people would not need to wait for New Year's Day to make resolutions! Pushing oneself to overcome anxiety or depression requires the same kind of reward structure. Some activities come easier for some people than others. For an anxious child, going to social activities, separating from a caregiver, or feeling confident about decisions is difficult. For a depressed youth, following up on commitments and being positive are challenging. In these cases, it is essential to reinforce any effort to change with meaningful, personalized rewards until pro-active behaviors become more natural.

At that point, the extrinsic rewards can be phased out. A reward plan can be built following four critical steps.

Step 1: Define Goals

The first step to building a reward plan is to identify a concrete, achievable goal that is a specific target for the youth and parent. In other words, what behavior do each want to encourage or extinguish? Tips for establishing effective goals include:

Brainstorm widely at first, but then narrow down the goals to focus on. Working on goals is challenging enough; start by focusing on a limited number of them so the family can track success and modify the system before adding more goals.

Keep the goals behavioral (observable). It always helps to start with behaviors that parents can observe the youth doing. This will make it easier to for them know when to reward their child, and it will also be easier to identify when the behavior has changed (success!). For example, "Getting out of bed by 6:30 A.M." is a more observable behavior than "Feeling motivated to go to school each morning." "Calling up one friend a week" is more observable than "Trying harder to reach out to friends." Focus on what can be observed.

Keep the goals concrete and specific. Relatedly, focus on goals that are clear to both caregiver and youth. "Finishing your math homework within 30 minutes" is more specific than "Doing your homework more consistently." "Using three coping statements before you ask Mom for reassurance" is more specific than "Trying to cope yourself before asking Mom." "Staying in the classroom through period 1 each day" is more concrete than "Getting to your morning classes each day," just as "Getting on the bus" is simpler and more specific than "Getting on the bus, feeling OK, and talking to three friends." Focus on one thing at a time and build success. Parents and youth can learn to ask themselves, "Am I able to observe and measure this goal, and if not, how do I make it so?"

Focus on behaviors you want to encourage, not the behaviors you want to extinguish. It is often the case that parents will take a reward plan as an opportunity to identify all of the behaviors they want to extinguish (and by translation, "punish"). Remind them that this is an opportunity to shape and reward good behaviors. Although punishment can lead to a decrease in negative behavior, that behavior often returns, and the punishment frequently inflicts damage on the caregiver–youth relationship. Parents should focus on the goals they want to encourage (e.g., "Text a friend each day") rather than the goals they want to discourage (e.g., "Stop hanging out in your room all day by yourself"). Focusing on undesired behavior inadvertently results in more attention to it than the desired behavior, which can lead to coercive cycles between parent and youth.

Step 2: Establish a Reward: A Daily Renewable Reward

To motivate challenging behaviors, a reward must be *meaningful* and *rewarding*, above all else! Brainstorm with the youth to arrive at rewards that can be incentivizing and realistic. Ideally, these rewards are easily available and nonmonetary, and can be delivered in increments. Tips for identifying effective rewards include:

Ensure the reward is meaningful to the youth. Do collaborative brainstorming with teens to make sure that the rewards you select are meaningful to them. Identifying a specific and personally meaningful reward is more important than suggesting rewards that the teen already has access to or ones that other teens might like. Once several potential rewards are identified, it is helpful to involve caregivers to garner buy-in and ensure feasibility.

Be creative when devising rewards. A reward can be any item or privilege the youth is willing to change behavior for. However, *a reward does not have to consist of monetary incentives or purchased goods!* Parents often worry that reward programs will end up costing them money, but typically family privileges make better rewards. Offering the ability to choose what the family eats for dinner, what they watch on the family TV that night, what movie the family goes to see on the weekend, staying up an extra hour on weekends, inviting friends to come over or sleep over, going to a special place with friends—all can be better options than simply giving the youth cash or purchasing the latest favor. Remind caregivers that social attention can be among the strongest reinforcers, so the best rewards often take a little extra time, effort, and creativity on the family's part, but the investment is well worth it. Teens may be more willing to work (by way of behavioral changes) for money than younger children, as their independence becomes increasingly important and money can represent independent decision making. If money is considered as a reward and the family can afford it, try to set up an incremental savings account for a specific prize that has special meaning. With each client, think creatively about rewards.

It's not bribery when you develop a plan. Parents sometimes resent having to *pay* for the youth to do something they *should* be doing. This is another reason why money is not always the most effective reward. In these cases, you may want to return to psychoeducation if the parent voices concern and reiterate how some tasks or challenges are easier for youth than others, and how incentives help everyone start something new or difficult. You can also tell the parents that the plan will be to fade out the incentives as the youth becomes better at meeting challenges. As they become more accomplished, the requirements for attaining certain rewards are increased and eventually the rewards are phased out.

Do not make one reward contingent on accomplishing a different goal. It is best if a reward is not something that you and the family are targeting as another goal. For example, if we have set increased socialization as a goal for a socially anxious teen, we should not make social activities a reward for accomplishing a different goal. The parent of that same teen might suggest a goal and reward such as this: "If you ask the teacher for help in class, then I will take you and your friends to a movie." Even if the teen finds going to a movie rewarding, we would want their attendance with friends to be its own goal that receives a different reward. If we made seeing friends contingent on achieving some other social goal, we might be depriving the youth of necessary opportunities to find reinforcement in social situations.

Create a reward schedule that works. The reward schedule can include the delivery of a concrete reward or privilege immediately after achieving a goal, or the youth can earn points that accumulate to a larger reward. Use the schedule that works for the particular goal and reward, but do remember that more immediate reinforcement tends to be stronger than rewards delivered further into the future. These decisions can be made based on the age and developmental and cognitive level of the child as well as the pragmatics surrounding a family's schedule (e.g., certain rewards may be more realistically given on the weekend).

Daily renewable rewards: Encouraging daily behavior change. When the goal is to encourage changes to daily routines and behaviors, like school attendance, we have found it useful to incorporate *daily, renewable privileges* that are meaningful to the youth (see Figure 5.5; a blank version is available as Worksheet 10 in Appendix A). Access to mobile phones is a perfect example. No teen needs a cell phone, but most will work very hard to ensure continued access to their phone. Consider making phone usage contingent on key behaviors. "If you get up by 6:30 A.M., you can have the phone right away when you wake up. If you can't do that but are still able to sit down for breakfast at 7 A.M., you can bring your phone to the table. If you miss those goals but are on the bus by 7:30, you can get your phone when leaving the house and take it to school with you. If you miss the bus, you can still earn your phone for the afternoon if you let me drive you to school. If you allow me to drive you to school by 10:00, you can pick up your phone from the counselor at lunchtime. If you've had a rough morning and only get to school by noon, you can have your phone after school. If you stay home, you do not get to use your phone that day."

It will likely take a bit of brainstorming and trial and error to find the right increment and schedule for the reward (all rewards must be individualized). But there are several advantages to the above schedule and incremental reward structure. First, it is not all or nothing; rather, it gives the youth multiple opportunities to succeed even after initial failure. Thus, if the teen fails to get on the bus by 7:30 A.M., they could still earn access to the phone if they arrive at school by 10. If the teen passes that deadline but makes it in by noon, they can still use the phone for the evening. In traditional reward plans, the youth would have one shot to earn a reward for the day: "If you go to school today, you get your phone." This type of plan does not specify any time requirements and provides the same amount of reward for varying successes (the youth can get to school at any time during the day). The daily renewable reward aims to provide adjustable increments of reward for proportionate success. The youth is given multiple chances to succeed and earn a reward throughout the day—thus, there continues to be an incentive even after initial failure.

The second advantage of this plan rests in its *renewable* aspect. One trap that caregivers fall into is inadvertently turning a reward plan into a punishment plan by offering an initial reward but then stripping it away after the youth first fails. A parent might set up an initial (nonincremental) incentive plan such that a teen can access their phone if they get to school by 8 A.M. Once the teen passes the 8 A.M. deadline, they would no longer have any chance to access their phone. In this plan, the parent is left without any incentives to motivate their child's attendance that day. As a consequence, the parent often resorts to threatening punishment: "If you don't get to school now, you'll lose the phone tomorrow, too." In this scenario, the teen already lost the incentive to go to school on the current day and now has lost any incentive to attend school the following day. At this point, the youth is *working out of debt* and there is no obvious way to earn the phone back. Working out of debt is the quick and certain way to lose motivation! Instead, a renewable reward should be something that resets each day, effectively starting at zero. If the youth does not earn the reward one day, they do not get the privilege that day. The next day, the teen has the same ability to earn phone usage under the same rules as before.

Using a renewable scheduling system gives the teen continuous incentives to try. We recognize these plans may be daunting for caregivers. As such, initial planning may require identifying barriers to their implementation, role-playing the script with parents, and troubleshooting when the youth identifies potential loopholes (and they always find them if there is one!). The initial implementation may also require that therapists and parents stay in greater between-session communication to optimize success.

WORKSHEET 10. Daily Renewable Rewards Chart

Brainstorm step-by-step goals and rewards to go with each level. Then track success!

Theme: *School Attendance*

Goals (incremental levels)	Reward (incremental levels)	Sun	Mon	Tue	Wed	Thu	Fri	Sat	# of Days Achieved
Get up by 6:30 A.M.	*Get phone to play music in bathroom.*	—	N	N	N	N	✓	—	*1*
Get to breakfast by 7:00 A.M.	*Get phone at breakfast table.*	—	N	N	N	N	✓	—	*1*
Get on bus by 7:30 A.M.	*Get phone when leaving the house. Keep all day.*	—	N	N	N	✓	✓	—	*2*
Mom/Dad drive to school by 10:00 A.M.	*Pick up your phone at counselor's at lunchtime.*	—	N	✓	N	—	—	—	*1*
Get to school by lunchtime (noon).	*Get your phone when you arrive home after last school period.*	—	✓	—	N	—	—	—	*1*
Don't get to school at all.	*No phone.*	—	—	—	✓	—	—	—	*1*

FIGURE 5.5. Daily renewable rewards example.

97

Step 3: Observe Carefully (catch them being good)

This step (also called "catching the positive") can be surprisingly challenging as parents often require consistent practice in tracking and reinforcing the behaviors they hope to see. This step is consistent with the parenting skill of specific labeled praise in that it requires the caregiver to notice when the youth is performing a behavior as desired or achieving a goal, and then to label it appropriately: "I noticed you did your homework within the time limit!" Therapists should take note of the times when caregivers break the deal by adding additional requirements to the original agreement they made. This will often appear in the form of a "yes, but" statement ("I saw them do their homework, but they made a lot of mistakes"). If making mistakes was not part of the original goal, then it has no place in the decision to reward or not. Instead, caregivers must simply execute the agreed-upon plan each week, understanding that reward plans can be tweaked or renegotiated each week.

Step 4: Reward on Time and Consistently

Rewards should be delivered as close in time to the successful behavior as possible. In cases where the youth is earning points, stickers, or check marks on a chart, note those right away. Caregivers and youth should agree on where the chart or tracking sheet will be centrally located. For older youth, keeping track on an online spreadsheet may be an option. For rewards that cannot be given in the moment (e.g., going with friends to a movie), caregivers should acknowledge the teen's success immediately and work toward delivering the reward at the nearest feasible time. Therapists may need to work with families on the organizational aspects of reward administration based on early data and observation of the caregiver's ability to follow through consistently. Therapists will also want to validate that timely and consistent follow-up can initially feel overwhelming for parents!

Keeping track of success (Figure 5.5) helps caregivers and therapists monitor progress even when success seems variable and inconsistent. Change rarely happens in linear fashion, and caregivers may frequently arrive at a session exasperated by the latest experience. Asking caregivers to daily track progress helps provide objective data to evaluate patterns. It also helps the youth see the results of their own efforts and helps them keep their caregivers honest about keeping promises on rewards.

Extinguishing Disruptive Behaviors

In the context of anxiety and depression, CM programs rightfully focus more attention on encouraging pro-active and pro-social goals and behaviors. However, an effective CM program can also include specific, timely, and focused consequences for misbehavior. Depressed mood can manifest as irritability, and anxious avoidance can devolve into resistance and defiance when youth are pushed to scary places. Staunch refusal to participate in expected routines (e.g., school, family events) and defiance at completing important tasks (e.g., homework, chores) can escalate into conflict quickly. In these cases, both minor house rules (with regard to task refusal, arguments, name calling) and major house rules (with regard to breaking property, physical aggression) can be broken. In such instances, put in place clearly defined rules and specific and limited consequences. However, remember that CM plans do not need to be created for every imaginable undesirable behavior. Extinction plans should be reserved for serious household violations. When in doubt, try to devise a pro-active reward plan first and see if positive behaviors can be encouraged first before trying to extinguish undesirable behaviors. The following steps can be used to establish a CM policy designed to keep individuals safe and extinguish disruptive behaviors.

Step 1: Establish House Rules

House rules tend to focus on behaviors that do not fall under a reward plan. House rules vary from family to family, but it is common for most families to establish zero tolerance policies for physical aggression (hurting oneself or others), destruction of property, or significant self-endangerment or rule breaking (e.g., serious curfew breaks, running away, taking the car without permission). Demonstrating disrespect (e.g., cursing at family members) can also be targeted in CM plans. As with reward goals, establish house rules that are clear, concrete, and observable. "Not answering your phone three consecutive times" is more specific than "being available when I call you." "Throwing any household object" is more specific and observable than "destroying anything."

Step 2: Define Consequences

Clearly describe the consequences that will be levied if house rules are broken. Most typically for teens this entails removal of privileges. Help parents be specific. Restricting access to preferred objects (e.g., phones), activities (screen time, games, driving), and events (social activities, parties) is a common consequence of breaking rules. Time outs are a specified amount of time when the child is separated from other activities and people, thus removing attention. They are typical for younger children and used less frequently for teens; however, sometimes unofficial time outs are helpful to deescalate tempers during intense conflict (e.g., "Go to your corner").

When choosing consequences, advise parents to avoid taking away agreed-upon privileges from any rewards plan. If access to a mobile phone is being used to encourage the fulfillment of a goal (e.g., improved school attendance), avoid taking away the phone as a consequence for breaking some unrelated house rule. The risk to blurring rewards and consequences is that it can strip away the caregiver's ability to offer an important incentive when it is needed. If a parent removes their teen's phone because they broke curfew, then the parent will not be able to use the phone to motivate the teen later on. Mixing rewards and consequences can also confuse and breed resentment that triggers cycles of parent–youth conflict. Keep rewards and consequences separate.

Step 3: Be Consistent, Specific, and Punctual

Consequences should be imposed as soon as a house rule is broken, or as soon as is feasible. The consequence should conform to the pre-agreed-upon rules and not be overextended. It can be tempting to add additional consequences if the teen reacts angrily to their caregiver's feedback or refuses to accept the consequence; however, it is essential to deliver consequences in accordance with the original agreement. This establishes a consistency to the plan that will benefit the caregiver in the future. It is also essential to levy consequences in the same way each time so that the teen knows there is limited room for negotiations. Consistency across caregivers is also essential to prevent pitting adults against each other.

Therapists can work with caregivers to avoid emotionally reactive responses to their child and to practice maintaining neutral language and tone. Although frustration should be expected, using critical, shame-based, or coercive language only reduces the effectiveness of a calmly designed CM program. Yelling increases physiological arousal. For example, screaming, "Why do you disrespect me like this?!" only confuses the situation and likely prompts an undesired screamed-back response. The goal is to help the teen learn that the more each member sticks to the CM plan, the greater the chance for the teen and caregivers to reach goals together. We acknowledge that these parameters are much easier to discuss in the office than in the midst of an incident at home; with practice, however, it is possible for the caregiver and their teen to negotiate smoothly and more effectively at home.

COMBINING EMPATHIZE AND ENCOURAGE WITH CM

As caregivers become proficient at using empathize and encourage statements consistently and more instinctually, they can add one additional intervention—for the caregiver to remind the youth of rewards and contingencies. Ultimately, it is the effective use of CM that will encourage increased attendance to school. That exchange would sound something like this:

MOTHER: You've been spending a lot of time at home. Why don't you go meet up with some friends?

ABBY-LYNN: Nah, no one's around. Besides I'm beat.

MOTHER: It's tough getting out when you're tired [empathize]; spending time with friends can energize you [encourage]. Remember, every time you push yourself to get out of the house, you accumulate points that you can trade in for TV time by yourself—no brother [CM reminder]!

ABBY-LYNN: I don't care! I'm not a kid!

MOTHER: It's hard to get over that initial hump [empathize], and I know you can take some steps [encourage]. I really want you to get some private relaxing time [CM reminder].

ABBY-LYNN: Mom! You're not listening!

MOTHER: I see how hard it is to get going [empathize]. Try some of the skills you've been learning in therapy [encourage].

ABBY-LYNN: (stops talking)

(Mother gets up from the bedside and walks out of the room.)

In this scenario, the mother uses empathize and encourage to send an approach message to the youth. Because getting started is difficult, the mother also reminds the youth about the incentives on which they have agreed. The mother uses a nonblaming, noncritical stance when sending these reminders so that the rewards are not being dangled over Abby-Lynn. Rather, the mother is setting a tone of understanding and encouragement while also recognizing that it's up to her daughter to make the first move. The success of this approach does depend on the salience and value of the reward. If the incentives are not encouraging approach behavior, you will want to problem-solve and brainstorm revised incentives to promote action.

SUMMARY AND KEY POINTS

Parents and caregivers are influential family members in a youth's life. A number of parenting styles and practices have been linked to the development and maintenance of anxiety and depression in youth. The therapist will want to assess for potential patterns of interaction that might impact the youth's recovery and provide support where needed. This can include teaching active listening and positive communication skills, reward planning, and CM. Key points to remember:

- Caregiver control, rejection, and interparental conflict are impactful factors in maintaining youth anxiety and depression.
- The therapist can engage caregivers as partners or as agents of change based on the needs of the case.
- Caregivers often need psychoeducation to normalize the experience their teen is feeling.
- Important caregiver–youth interaction patterns are accommodation, passivity–discouragement, and aggressive–coercive spirals.
- Positive communication includes specific labeled praise, active listening, and the empathize and encourage intervention.
- CM includes efforts to reward new desired behavior and systems to set limits for the youth.

CHAPTER 6

Depression

Major depressive disorder (MDD) is an official disorder listed in the *Diagnostic and Statistical Manual of Mental Disorders* (DSM-5; American Psychiatric Association, 2013). It is one of the most common psychological conditions among youth in the United States (Merikangas et al., 2010) and can have a significant impact on a teen's academic, social, and emotional well-being. Depression affects relatively few children under the age of 13 (Costello, Copeland, & Angold, 2011; Costello, Erkanli, & Angold, 2006), but rates spike dramatically in adolescence (Kessler et al., 2012; Merikangas et al., 2010). Twelve-month prevalence of MDD among teens (13- to 17-year-olds) has been documented at 8.2%, and lifetime prevalence of any occurrence during adolescence at 11.7%. Beginning around age 13, girls become twice as likely as boys to experience depression, and this gender gap persists throughout adulthood (Hankin & Abramson, 2001; Merikangas et al., 2010). Most cases of MDD come with significant comorbidity and are associated with severe role impairment that includes interference in functioning, such as with school, work, family, and social roles (Avenevoli, Swendsen, He, Burstein, & Merikangas, 2015). Nearly 30% of teens with MDD reported some form of suicidality in the past year, and 11% reported a suicide attempt (Avenevoli et al., 2015). About 60% of teens reported obtaining some form of treatment, but the minority (34%) received depression-specific treatment or treatment from a mental health specialist. Thus, substantial work needs to be done to help identify those youth who are experiencing depression and to get them the services they need.

BIOPSYCHOSOCIAL AND INTERPERSONAL CORRELATES OF DEPRESSION

Evidence exists for a biopsychosocial model in the development and maintenance of depression with correlates evident beginning in childhood. Having familiarity with the various factors that influence the development and presentation of depression can help a clinician assess accurately, conceptualize comprehensively, and treat accordingly.

Genetic and Familial Factors

Depression in adulthood is familial and heritable, particularly recurrent forms of depression (Rice, Harold, & Thapar, 2002). Twin and adoption studies assessing depression in adults provide evidence that genetic factors account for 31–42% of the variance in the transmission of depression (Sullivan,

Neale, & Kendler, 2000). Genetic association studies have implicated particular gene variations (e.g., a serotonin transporter gene) that may interact with negative environmental factors to influence the expression of depression (Brown & Harris, 2008), likely via effects on stress response (Levinson, 2006). However, twin and adoption studies investigating the heritability of clinical depression in children and adolescents produce more modest results (Rice et al., 2002). Twin studies show that normal variation in depressive symptoms is genetically influenced, but heritability estimates tend to be low in adoption studies. Alternatively, caregiver parenting styles and practices provide a more direct pathway for influencing change. Substantial evidence suggests that intergenerational transmission of depressed mood and behaviors is related to caregiver control, rejection, and interparental hostility (McLeod et al., 2007; Yap et al., 2014). CBT therapists will want to assess for family history of depression, caregiver practices, and level of hostility and conflict in the home (see Chapter 5). Family data can inform conceptualization and provide avenues for intervention.

Cognitive Vulnerability Factors

Cognitive processes play an important role in the development and maintenance of depression (Kertz, Petersen, & Stevens, 2019; Lakdawalla, Hankin, & Mermelstein, 2007; Rood, Roelofs, Bögels, Nolen-Hoeksema, & Schouten, 2009). Substantial evidence suggests that *attentional deficits* exist in children, teens, and young adults with depression, particularly in the context of negative information (Kertz et al., 2019). Diminished attentional control, reflected in poor inhibition and shifting, can result in the failure to prevent or disrupt negative elaborative processing (i.e., rumination). Depression has been associated with poorer sustained attention, and attentional bias has been found in youth 5 to 21 years old demonstrating an attentional bias toward sad stimuli (Kertz et al., 2019).

Negative *cognitive style* is also typical of depressed teens (Lakdawalla et al., 2007). The depressed youth tends to have negative thoughts and attitudes (e.g., "I stink"), hopeless causal inferences and inferred consequences (e.g., "Nothing will get better"), and tends to respond with ruminative styles rather than with problem solving or distraction. *Rumination*, typified by continuous self-reflective thought in the absence of constructive problem solving, has been found to be consistently associated with concurrent and future depression (Rood et al., 2009). As youth confront challenges, rumination has a negative impact on mood, hinders active problem solving, and prevents the individual from accessing pleasant reinforcers. Attending to rumination may be particularly relevant for teenage girls who demonstrate significantly greater levels of rumination than boys. Thus, depressed youth may experience deficits in attentional control that make it more difficult to sustain effort, direct attention away from negative stimuli, and contribute to rumination. Furthermore, once confronted with ambiguous information, depressed teens are more likely to infer negative causes and predict negative consequences. Thus, effective CBT will want to address the negative content of thoughts through thought tracking and cognitive restructuring and train the teen to replace dysfunctional rumination with behavioral activation and mindfulness.

Maladaptive Behavioral Processes

The symptom profile of depression highlights both the stark *lack* of behaviors during a depressive episode and disrupted behavioral patterns from the youth's normal functioning, including social withdrawal, isolation, and reduction of pleasant and challenging activities. Inactivity may be related to a deprivation of available reinforcers in the environment or an inability in accessing or appreciating reinforcers (Dimidjian, Barrera, Martell, Muñoz, & Lewinsohn, 2011). Earlier research documented findings to this effect, demonstrating that depression and depressed mood were frequently associated with decreased pleasant activities, increased unpleasant activities, and decreased ability to experience pleasure in preferred activities (Hopko, Armento, Cantu, Chambers, & Lejuez, 2003; Wierzbicki & Sayler, 1991). More recently, a diversity of studies have shown that rates of depression and suicidal behaviors increased as active behaviors (e.g., in-person interactions, sports/exercise, community work) decreased and passive activities (social media use, TV time) increased (Liu, Wu, & Yao, 2016; Twenge, Joiner, Rogers, & Martin, 2018). Furthermore, longitudinal studies have shown that increased depressive symptoms lead to youth and young adults choosing increasingly passive activities over time (Heffer, Good, Daly, MacDonell, & Willoughby, 2019), creating a downward spiral of inactivity and depressed mood.

Avoidance is highly typical of depressed youth as the effort to overcome challenges increases. In a negatively reinforcing loop, teens may choose to procrastinate or quit tasks that raise their subjective distress. Escaping the task reduces stress and provides a temporary relief from the demand (Chu et al., 2014; Manos, Kanter, & Busch, 2010). Research shows that depressed youth have more difficulty than nondepressed youth in generating personal approach goals (e.g., "In the future it will be important for me to . . .") and fewer concrete plans to accomplish goals (Dickson & MacLeod, 2004). Instead, depressed youth tend to generate plans that serve to avoid their goals ("How can I avoid this?"). Thus, the primary goal of behavior-based treatment is to increase engagement in activities that are personally reinforcing.

Interpersonal Processes

Isolation, avoidance, and poor social networks create a negative feedback loop in teens with depression. Interpersonal stressors constitute a salient context for teens, particularly for girls, as stressful interpersonal events often precede a depressive episode (Grant et al., 2006; Rudolph & Hammen, 1999; Rudolph et al., 2000), and social support from peers, parents, and family can serve as essential buffering agents against the onset and duration of depression (Gariepy, Honkaniemi, & Quesnel-Vallee, 2016; Rueger, Malecki, Pyun, Aycock, & Coyle, 2016). At the same time, depression tends to affect the youths' interpersonal style, contributing to a diffident, negative, and reassurance-seeking demeanor that can disrupt otherwise supportive relationships (Rudolph, Flynn, & Abaied, 2008; Sheeber & Sorensen, 1998). In this context, help-seeking attempts may be met by rejection from peers (Gazelle & Ladd, 2003). Cognitive biases and negative attributional styles that are on guard for threats and disappointment make it harder for the depressed teen to recover from slights and rejection (Platt, Kadosh, & Lau, 2013). These factors can lead a teen into a downward spiral of interpersonal negativity, social exclusion, and depressive affect (Bukowski, Laursen, & Hoza, 2010). Treatments that provide opportunities to build positive social relations and help to build social skills can optimize the youth's access to instrumental and emotional support.

CBT MODEL OF DEPRESSION

The CBT model highlights the role that cognitive, behavioral, emotional, and interpersonal processes play in maintaining depression for an individual youth (see Chapter 2). It assumes that each factor can play important roles in explaining a youth's reaction to stressful challenges, and CBT provides interventions that can fortify relative weaknesses. A therapist identifies situations, people, external events, and internal events (e.g., thoughts, feelings, memories) that prompt the cascade of thoughts, feelings, and actions that comprise depressed mood. Deconstructing the physical, behavioral, and cognitive components of an emotion (e.g., sadness) with the cognitive-behavioral triangle (see Figure 1.1) helps the youth and therapist see where the teen has strengths and where supports are needed. For example, teens who experience sadness after receiving a bad grade may report that they can "tell [themselves] that it's not the end of the world," but the intensity of their shame and disappointment leads them to hide in the bedroom for the rest of the night refusing to talk to friends and family. Clarifying the teen's experience lets the therapist know to teach fortifying skills to help the youth manage intense feelings (e.g., through mindfulness, relaxation, or distraction). Likewise, the therapist can capitalize on the youth's strong reframing skills by having the teen repeat the coping thought ("It's just one test") and connect with other strategies. The therapist can ask, "If you truly believed it was only one test, how would you have acted differently that day? Would you have reached out to friends?" The therapist bases this formulation on the initial assessment and then continues to revisit it as new information becomes available. It thus serves as a roadmap for planning phases of treatment and selecting specific interventions and strategies to try.

CASE VIGNETTE: ABBY-LYNN

The following case (introduced in the last chapter) is a fictionalized composite of multiple real-life clients; it demonstrates how cognitive-behavioral assessment and interventions can be applied to cases where major depression is the primary referral.

Abby-Lynn is a 15-year-old White cisgender girl who is in the ninth grade. When her grades and class participation started to slide, and she began to arrive late for school (six times over the past 2 weeks), her teachers took note. Her basketball coach also noticed her diminishing attendance at practice, where she had formerly been a core member of the team. In class, Abby-Lynn could often be found resting her head on her desk, reluctant to respond to questions and prompts to participate, and failing to turn in almost half of her homework. Her basketball coach was calling Abby-Lynn out in practice for missing plays and looking distracted. Just prior to her first contact with the outpatient therapist, the coach had benched Abby-Lynn for the first time in the season; after this, she began missing practices altogether (on four occasions over the prior 2 weeks), leading to further discipline (running laps in front of her teammates) and benching. After the coach and teachers approached Abby-Lynn's school counselor, he held a meeting with the teen and her mother to recommend she seek outpatient mental health therapy.

At the initial intake, the mother noted Abby-Lynn's increased depressed mood, withdrawal, and disengagement at home. She reported that Abby-Lynn typically invited one or two girls from the team to do homework after school and then hang out, but this had not been happening of late. Abby-Lynn had also once been active on social media (especially Snapchat and Instagram), but she had recently stopped posting updates. When her mother returned from work around 7 P.M. each night, she would often find Abby-Lynn napping in her bedroom with the door closed. Abby-Lynn was generally a good student, earning mostly B's with an occasional A or C. She was regarded as a consistent community member at school and in her church youth group, even if others saw her as someone "on the quiet side." Abby-Lynn typically focused on getting her work done and leading by example, and she did have several good friends both at school and in the neighborhood.

Abby-Lynn lives with her mother and younger sister and brother (5 and 10 years old) in a small rented home in a working-class town. Her biological father lives several hours away, is divorced from her mother, and is only able to provide financial assistance intermittently. Mom works as a full-time nurse at a local hospital and takes many extra shifts to manage financially. Abby-Lynn's brother, diagnosed with mild autism spectrum disorder (ASD), frequently needs specialized attention and has intermittent emotional and behavioral outbursts. Abby-Lynn is often asked to babysit her siblings, although the mother at times hires babysitters to give Abby-Lynn some freedom. Abby-Lynn has also assumed the role of primary coach for her brother's occupational therapy to address his learning and behavioral issues. The mother acknowledges that she relies on Abby-Lynn more than she would like to, due to her own work schedule, and does not know how her oldest daughter "handles all of the pressure to do her schoolwork, practice basketball, and help with the kids."

ASSESSMENT OF MAJOR DEPRESSION

Diagnosis, Symptoms, Impairment, and Target Problems

At intake, the therapist completed separate Kiddie Schedule for Affective Disorders and Schizophrenia (K-SADS; Kaufman et al., 2016) interviews with Abby-Lynn and her mother. Abby-Lynn met the criteria for MDD and generalized anxiety disorder (GAD).

Abby-Lynn did not experience herself as having a "depressed mood" (sad, down, blue), but endorsed having less interest in things than she used to (anhedonia). She also admitted to feeling tired and fatigued most of the day and sleeping through most afternoons after school. She reported disrupted sleep where she was waking at least three to four times a night for at minimum 30 minutes, which then made it difficult for her to get up in the mornings. Consistent with this, it was difficult for her to concentrate on schoolwork or to even do fun things (e.g., basketball, respond to friends' posts on Instagram). She confessed that it took so much energy to participate in conversations that she preferred spending time alone rather than connecting with friends. She reported feeling constant shame and guilt for distancing herself from friends, letting down the basketball team, and failing to attend to her brother's therapy as much as she wanted. Abby-Lynn's mother noticed many of these same symptoms and also described that Abby-Lynn seemed down and sad, too. In addition, she had heard Abby-Lynn complain of having headaches, stomach cramps, and muscle tension in her shoulders. Both Abby-Lynn and her mother denied that the teen engaged in any self-harm or had any intentions or plans to hurt or kill herself. Abby-Lynn did acknowledge that things were getting tougher and she sometimes wondered, "if it would be easier if I just disappeared." If Abby-Lynn had endorsed any self-harm or suicidal ideation, the therapist would have assessed further with the Columbia-Suicide Severity Rating Scale (C-SSRS), consistent with the approach used in the treatment of suicidal behaviors and self-injury (see Chapter 7).

The depression diagnostic clarification checklist in Figure 6.1 outlines common conditions that could be masked by depression and require careful differential diagnosis. You can use a standardized clinical interview (e.g., K-SADS) to detect the presence of manic or hypomanic episodes,

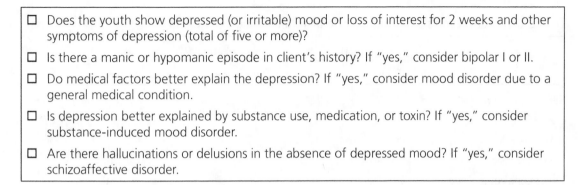

☐ Does the youth show depressed (or irritable) mood or loss of interest for 2 weeks and other symptoms of depression (total of five or more)?

☐ Is there a manic or hypomanic episode in client's history? If "yes," consider bipolar I or II.

☐ Do medical factors better explain the depression? If "yes," consider mood disorder due to a general medical condition.

☐ Is depression better explained by substance use, medication, or toxin? If "yes," consider substance-induced mood disorder.

☐ Are there hallucinations or delusions in the absence of depressed mood? If "yes," consider schizoaffective disorder.

FIGURE 6.1. Diagnostic clarification checklist for MDD.

underlying medical conditions, or substance abuse. The presence of hallucinations or delusions might suggest a more concerning schizoaffective disorder.

The diagnosis of GAD is characterized by pervasive and uncontrollable worries across multiple life domains (see Chapter 10 for diagnostic details). In addition to her anhedonia and withdrawal, Abby-Lynn described significant distress and tension related to constant worries about performance (school, sports), responsibilities (family, friends), and the future (whether things would get better for her mother). Once Abby-Lynn starts to worry, she has difficulty putting these thoughts out of her mind and only controls them by "phasing out" through napping or doing something passive like watching TV. Although many of Abby-Lynn's stresses stem from realistic demands in her life, her worries are characterized by unrealistic or exaggerated assumptions about her personal responsibility to ensure the well-being of her family, friends, or basketball team. What distinguishes these worries from her ruminative self-critical depressive thoughts is their future orientation. She quickly becomes overwhelmed thinking about messing up plays at her next practice or worrying about getting a job to help her mom out with finances. Abby-Lynn's mother and teammates have reassured her that they value her current contributions, but she nonetheless continues to worry. As such, Abby-Lynn's worries are persistent (present more days than not) and enduring (present for at least 6 months), and contribute to significant impairment in school, family, friendships, and self-care. She also reports a number of physical symptoms, such as muscle tension, difficulty concentrating, and restless sleep.

Objective measures were also helpful in diagnosing Abby-Lynn's mood and anxiety problems. Abby-Lynn and her mother completed the Revised Children's Anxiety and Depression Scale (RCADS; Chorpita, Yim, Moffitt, Umemoto, & Francis, 2000; Chorpita, Moffitt, & Gray, 2005), and their responses reinforced the results of the semi-structured interview, showing T-scores in the clinical range for MDD and GAD (see Table 6.1).

In summary, semi-structured interviewing and evidence-based parent and youth questionnaires support a diagnostic picture that includes MDD and GAD as primary targets for treatment. Research shows that these two disorders often co-occur, particularly in teens (see Cummings, Caporino, & Kendall, 2014), and are conceptually related around the diffuse distress and persistent negative thinking styles that characterize them (Barlow, Allen, & Choate, 2004; Watson, 2005). The practicing clinician will want to be prepared for this common copresentation of psychological disorders.

TABLE 6.1. Abby-Lynn's Symptom Profile at Intake Using the RCADS

	Mother		Father		Youth	
	Raw score	T scores	Raw scores	T scores	Raw scores	T scores
Separation anxiety	4	58	–	–	2	48
Generalized anxiety	8	65*	–	–	13	67*
Panic disorder	0	41	–	–	0	36
Social anxiety	13	59	–	–	14	53
Obsessions/compulsions	2	50	–	–	0	35
Depression	18	80**	–	–	19	81**
Total anxiety	27	57	–	–	29	49
Total anxiety and depression	45	66*	–	–	48	57

*T scores higher than 65 indicate borderline clinical threshold. **Scores of 70 or higher indicate scores above clinical threshold. T scores are normalized based on youth's age and gender.

Goal Setting and Defining Target Problems

To set treatment goals, the therapist reviews his assessment with Abby-Lynn and her mother and leads a collaborative discussion to identify concrete treatment objectives. When trying to address depression, youth and parents can struggle to develop concrete goals. The most pressing problem often appears to be diffuse emotional states (e.g., sadness, depression, feeling overwhelmed, feeling worthless). Helping clients realize these broad emotional states is the first step toward achievable goals. The therapist helps Abby-Lynn and her mother visualize what kind of day-to-day change they would like to see in meaningful life domains (school, peers, family, health). How would they know if Abby-Lynn was feeling less sad? Less overwhelmed? The lists of parent, youth, and therapist goals below show a mixture of diffuse emotional goals ("improve sad mood," "enjoy life more"), as well as more concrete, achievable goals ("spend more time with friends"). The key point is to formulate the youth's treatment goals around specific changes that the client and family want to see in the youth's life.

Parent's Goals for Abby-Lynn

- Improve sad mood; enjoy life more.
- Decrease isolation (hanging out in room all day, napping).
- Improve sleep.
- Better handle responsibilities like grades and basketball practice.

Teen's Goals

- Spend more time with friends.
- Re-engage with things that she doesn't do any more; enjoy them more.
- Not feel so overwhelmed by everything (school, family obligations).

Therapist's Goals for Abby-Lynn

- Re-engage with things that she used to enjoy; increase enjoyment.
- Increase sense of control over demands and decrease self-criticism.
- Increase social contact and social supports.
- Improve sleep hygiene and regulate sleep cycle.

To help monitor progress, the therapist converts treatment goals into an idiographic outcome measure (see Figure 6.2; a blank version is available as Worksheet 11 in Appendix A). Personalized measures are a helpful and feasible way to track progress, giving both the therapist and client feedback about whether treatment is progressing as expected (Hoffman & Chu, 2019; Weisz et al., 2011). The more specific and concrete the desired outcomes, the easier it will be to track change, as well as provide the client with any additional concrete treatment goals to pursue. However, observing flexibility in defining outcomes (such as frequency of events, dimensional ratings of distress) can help bridge common and distinct goals across family members or the therapist.

As discussed in Chapter 1, feedback monitoring systems provide quantifiable data to the clinician that can be used to correct any family discouragement of slow progress. In this case, Abby-Lynn and her mother had several similar goals, including increasing social engagement and improving mood (sadness, feeling overwhelmed). The mother also was concerned about Abby-Lynn improving her sleep habits and accomplishing concrete tasks like completing homework assignments and making it to basketball practice. Abby-Lynn was focused on enjoying activities more fully. The therapist integrated both of their goals on the tracker form, giving him a framework around which to conceptualize Abby-Lynn's depression and anxiety and to plan treatment. After creating individualized goals and outcomes, the therapist can have the youth and caregivers rate progress on treatment goals on a weekly basis. Using an assessment (e.g., RCADS, CESD) weekly, biweekly, or monthly can also help provide a standardized way to balance idiographic measures.

CASE CONCEPTUALIZATION

CBT Model for Abby–Lynn

Abby-Lynn's depression and anxiety are characterized by diffuse distress (negative affect); anhedonia and avolition; social withdrawal; and functional impairments to her sleep, attention, and perseverance. Furthermore, her thought process is characterized by self-focused, negative ruminations and future-oriented worries about her family, basketball team, and eventual prospects. When confronted with demands that overwhelm her, Abby-Lynn tends to avoid the situation (e.g., taking naps, withdrawing from friends), which leaves the problem unsolved and perpetuates her feelings of helplessness. To make sense of this disparate collection of symptoms and impairments, the therapist diagrams a case conceptualization using the CBT model to identify how Abby-Lynn reacts cognitively, behaviorally, and physically to potent triggers (see Figure 6.3).

During the initial assessment, Abby-Lynn described her reactions to being singled out by her basketball coach when she became distracted during a play. Her first thought was "I really messed that up," which triggered facial flushing and pressure in her forehead, and then led to her freezing

WORKSHEET 11. Goals Tracker

Work with your therapist to brainstorm possible specific, meaningful, and achieveable goals. Think out what outcomes you expect to see. And then, keep track of how your child does each week.

Parent Goals:	Desired Outcomes	Week 1	Week 2	Week 3	Week 4	Week 5
Improve sad mood; enjoy life more.	Rate sad mood (0–10). Rate weekly enjoyment (0–10).	Sad: 9 Joy: 0	Sad: 9 Joy: 0	Sad: 7 Joy: 0	Sad: 6 Joy: 3	Sad: 5 Joy: 3
Decrease isolation (hanging out in room all day, napping).	Frequency of hang-outs with friends (inside and outside house)	0	0	1	2	1
Improve sleep.	Number of times she wakes up at night	3	4	2	1	0
Handle responsibilities like grades and basketball.	Handing in homework (%) Practices attended (%)	HW: 25% Practice: 50%	HW: 40% Practice: 50%	HW: 70% Practice: 95%	HW: 80% Practice: 100%	HW: 80% practice: 100%

Youth Goals:	Desired Outcomes	Week 1	Week 2	Week 3	Week 4	Week 5
Spend more time with friends.	Frequency of hang-outs with friends (inside and outside house)	0	0	1	2	1
Re-engage with things that she doesn't do any more; enjoy them more.	Frequency of fun activities; rate enjoyment (0–10).	# activities: 1 Joy: 0	# activities: 0 Joy: 0	# activities: 1 Joy: 1	# activities: 4 Joy: 5	# activities: 2 Joy: 4
Not feel so overwhelmed by everything (school, family obligations).	Rate how overwhelmed you feel (0–10).	10	10	8	6	6

FIGURE 6.2. Completed Goals Tracker worksheet for Abby-Lynn.

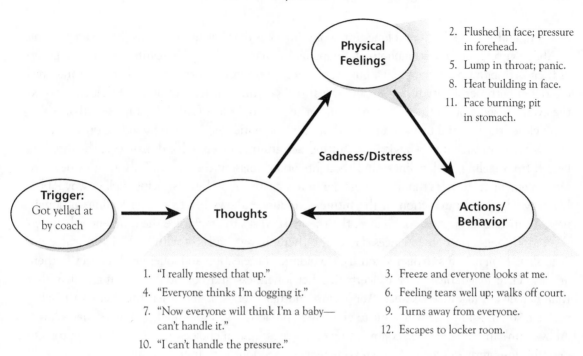

Physical Feelings

2. Flushed in face; pressure in forehead.
5. Lump in throat; panic.
8. Heat building in face.
11. Face burning; pit in stomach.

Sadness/Distress

Trigger: Got yelled at by coach

Thoughts

Actions/ Behavior

1. "I really messed that up."
4. "Everyone thinks I'm dogging it."
7. "Now everyone will think I'm a baby— can't handle it."
10. "I can't handle the pressure."

3. Freeze and everyone looks at me.
6. Feeling tears well up; walks off court.
9. Turns away from everyone.
12. Escapes to locker room.

FIGURE 6.3. Individualized CBT conceptualization for Abby-Lynn. Her thoughts, feelings, and behavior cycle continuously in a downward spiral (follow the numbers in order: 1, 2, 3, etc., to see how the thought–feeling–action cycle flows into another).

on the court. This initial sequence cascades in a downward spiral, leading to increasingly negative thought–feeling–action cycles. Without intervention, one negative cycle begets another until Abby-Lynn escapes the scene, which confirms her final thought: "She can't handle the pressure." Figure 6.3 illustrates how thoughts, feelings, and behavior cycle continuously in a downward spiral.

The therapist also provides Handout 12 (a reproducible version is available in Appendix A) to help Abby-Lynn understand how others experience the same patterns. Spelling out this case conceptualization helps demystify an overwhelming scenario for the parent and youth, illustrates where depressive episodes begin (i.e., identifies the trigger), and provides hints for fruitful targets for intervention. Here, her naturalistic reactions to this stressful scenario provide ample evidence that Abby-Lynn could benefit from techniques designed to identify and challenge negative thinking, strategies that address anxious tension, and behavioral activation that counters avoidance instincts.

Functional Assessment

A second method in case formulation is to conduct a functional assessment. A functional assessment helps identify behavioral chains that follow daily stressors and the specific contingencies that maintain the youth's avoidant and maladaptive reactions. Figure 6.4 (a blank version is available as Worksheet 1 in Appendix A) shows the results of a functional assessment that outlines Abby-Lynn's reactions to common stressors. As discussed in Chapter 1, the therapist will want to pay close attention to (1) the youth's immediate emotional response, (2) the initial behavioral reaction, and (3) the short- and long-term consequences of the youth's actions. For example, one of Abby-Lynn's friends posts a photo on Snapchat of an event that Abby-Lynn missed. The group of friends respond with comments, but Abby-Lynn's response illustrates how her avoidance has interfered with her ability to forge friendships. Abby-Lynn feels left out and sad that she missed the event. Instead of posting her own comment (e.g., "Looks like fun! Sorry I missed it!"), Abby-Lynn closes the app and turns to unrelated isolating activities (e.g., searching videos on YouTube).

What motivates this behavior? By shifting her attention to unrelated activities, she distracts herself from feelings of loneliness and thoughts about missing the event. This form of negative reinforcement (behaviors that permit escape from negative mood states) helps explain why Abby-Lynn avoids social interaction in the future: avoidance allows her to escape feelings of loneliness. To invoke motivation for change, the therapist works to emphasize the differences between short- and long-term consequences. Here, the therapist sympathizes with Abby-Lynn: there are clear *short-term* benefits to distraction (i.e., avoidance of rejection and loneliness). However, there are also clear *long-term* effects: exacerbating her loneliness and potentially creating real (rather than perceived) distance between Abby-Lynn and her friends. Later, when the therapist teaches problem-solving skills, he will want to emphasize proactive, goal-oriented responses that address Abby-Lynn's initial fears (e.g., commenting on the post). Such choices are more likely to promote desirable long-term outcomes (e.g., creating real connections with friends) than avoidance, even if they require effort in the short term.

The first two examples in Figure 6.4 demonstrate negative reinforcement chains (avoidance of distress perpetuates harmful patterns). The third trigger shows how positive reinforcement can promote helpful patterns. In this case, Abby-Lynn feels compelled to help her brother learn his occupational therapy skills even though she is not in the mood. She pushes herself through it and experiences positive feelings as a result. Her responses illustrate how choosing proactive, goal-oriented actions (being productive despite her mood) can produce both short-term outcomes (feeling helpful) and long-term consequences (regular helping) even when her initial instinct might have been to shut down and avoid making the effort.

TREATMENT PLANNING

Armed with a diagnosis, case conceptualization, and list of target problems, the therapist can then plan interventions to address the youth's concerns. Tables 6.2 and 6.3 are designed to help in writing managed care treatment plans and reports. Table 6.2 lists broad treatment goals and appropriate interventions that match Abby-Lynn's case. Table 6.3 shows a delineated sequence of interventions for a 22-session course of treatment for depression, specific to Abby-Lynn (18 weekly sessions, 4 biweekly) with an agreement to check in with the family after Session 10 to review her progress and determine if therapy continues to be an appropriate fit. There is limited research to suggest the order in which interventions should be presented. Some research suggests that social skills and problem-solving interventions are among the most potent for depressed adolescents (Kennard et al., 2009) even as behavioral activation and cognitive restructuring remain key strategies in treatment (Oud et al., 2019). Thus, it makes sense to present these skills early in treatment when possible. These interventions also match Abby-Lynn's particular profile as she is presenting with limited activation, significant anhedonia, and social inhibition. Behavioral activation and pleasant events can expose Abby-Lynn to reinforcing and stimulating environments that might

WORKSHEET 1. Trigger and Response

Tell us about your triggers and how you reacted. Describe your feelings, what you did (action), what happened right away (immediate outcome), and then what happened later (long-term outcome).

```
┌──────────────┐        ┌──────────────────────┐        ┌──────────────┐
│  Antecedent  │ ─────► │   Behavioral and     │ ─────► │ Consequences │
│              │        │  Emotional Response  │        │              │
└──────────────┘        └──────────────────────┘        └──────────────┘
```

Trigger	Feeling (emotional response)	Action (behavioral response)	Immediate Results (What keeps it going?)	Long-Term Results (What gets you in trouble?)
My friends share a Snapchat	Sadness (feeling left out)	Close out app. Watch YouTube.	Phased out, distracted	Feeling lonely, isolated. Avoid friends.
Getting benched on team	Embarrassed, guilty	Skip next practice.	Avoid coach and embarrassing scene.	Harder to return to practice.
Have to coach Bobby (brother) in skills	Tired, bored	Do it because I have to.	Felt good about helping him.	Do it pretty regularly because he seems to like it.

FIGURE 6.4. Individualized functional assessment of Abby-Lynn's depressed mood and avoidant behavior.

113

TABLE 6.2. Abby–Lynn's Broad Treatment Plan for Depression

Treatment goals	Interventions
Improve sad mood; enjoy life more	Psychoeducation about depression, thought–action–mood tracking, progress monitoring
Re-engage activities that the youth used to enjoy; increase enjoyment of activities	Behavioral activation, reward charts, problem solving, mindfulness, cognitive restructuring
Increase sense of control over demands and decrease self-criticism	Cognitive restructuring, problem solving, graded exposures to challenges/demands
Increase social contact and social supports	Behavioral activation to social situations, graded exposure to support seeking
Improve sleep hygiene and regulate sleep cycle	Sleep hygiene, relaxation, mindfulness, reward charts

instill hopefulness for the future. As Abby-Lynn becomes more active and experiences naturally reinforcing responses from her friends, her self-esteem may, in turn, improve and her self-criticism abate. However, it is helpful to institute formal thought monitoring and cognitive restructuring midway through treatment to help internalize lessons. Active exposure exercises and behavioral challenges are implemented to help Abby-Lynn practice her skills in increasingly challenging situations to generalize her skills and solidify her gains.

In keeping with the current evidence base, the treatment approach outlined hereafter describes some of the common interventions and steps to address depression for teens. Specific cognitive and behavioral interventions are based on a thorough assessment of presenting problems, diagnoses, and treatment goals. Abby-Lynn's treatment plan reflects interventions designed to address each of these individual problems: depression, anxiety disorder, social problems, and skills deficits (Cummings et al., 2014; Hammen, 2009; King & Merchant, 2008; Segrin, 2000). The focus here will be on psychoeducation about depression, self-monitoring of mood, behavioral activation, problem solving, cognitive restructuring, mindfulness, active exposure exercises, and behavioral challenges. Additional work to educate the youth in proper sleep hygiene and relaxation to improve sleep regulation may also be beneficial.

INTERVENTION COMPONENTS AND PROCESSES

Psychoeducation

In the process of developing a joint case conceptualization and treatment plan with the youth and parents, the therapist provides introductory education on the nature of depression in the youth, its impact on the teen and family functioning, and outlines appropriate treatments. To help summarize, the therapist can provide Handout 7 to the parent and Handout 13 to the youth to provide facts about the symptoms, impairments, and effective treatments for depression (reproducible versions of both handouts are available in Appendix A). The therapist can also direct the family to reliable online resources (e.g., the Association for Behavioral and Cognitive Therapies, Society for Clinical Child and Adolescent Psychology) as listed in Appendix B. The therapist highlights

TABLE 6.3. Abby–Lynn's Detailed Treatment Plan for Depression

Sessions 1–2

Assessment

- Assess presenting problems.
- Conduct diagnostic assessment with a focus on impairment (real-life functioning).
- Administer symptom profile measures (e.g., RCADS).
- Assess target problems and treatment goals, focusing on improving daily functioning.
- Assess past attempts (including past treatment) to address problem.
- Assess parent–child interactions.
- Conduct collateral assessments as needed with the youth's school (e.g., counselor, teacher, school nurse); retrieve past psychological assessments (e.g., academic/learning assessments); request parents' complete release of information to speak to school contact(s).
- Evaluate co-occurring medical conditions; consult with pediatrician or specialist (e.g., gastroenterologist) as indicated.
- Assess need for medication and psychiatric referral.

Psychoeducation

- Review assessment and generate target problems with youth and parents.
- Create idiographic target problems tracker.
- Collaborate on case conceptualization: CBT model and functional assessment.
- Provide parents and youth with information handouts on depression and cognitive-behavioral therapy.
- Educate parents about potential for medication.

Home practice

- Monitor depression triggers over the week: CBT model and functional assessment.
- Have the youth track their reactions to distress and short- and long-term outcomes (functional assessment) in relation to school routines.
- Have parents track parent–youth interactions around depressed mood/irritability episodes.

Sessions 3–4

Assessment

- Evaluate and discuss home practice.
- Complete the target problems tracker.
- Every fourth session, complete the symptom tracker (e.g., RCADS).

Interventions

- Implement in-session incentive plan (reward chart) for home practice completion.
- Review and refine individual functional assessments. Conduct motivational interviewing to highlight the trade-off between short-term gains and long-term consequences.
- Introduce activity monitoring, focusing on the connection between events, activities, and mood.
- Introduce behavioral activation, focusing on the connection among triggers, emotional response, and avoidant behaviors. Use functional assessment to highlight how avoidant behaviors are interfering with long-term goals.
- Assign pleasant activities and brainstorm proactive, goal-oriented activities.
- Describe self-reward and contingency management, focusing on assigning rewards for actions that are naturally difficult.

(continued)

TABLE 6.3. *(continued)*

Home practice
- Monitor the activity mood tracker.
- Monitor functional assessments, helping youth to distinguish short- and long-term consequences.
- Monitor the youth's completion of pleasant and goal-oriented activities.
- Monitor reward programs.

Sessions 5–6

Assessment
- As in Sessions 3–4

Interventions
- Continue behavioral activation assignments and review completion.
- Introduce problem solving.
- Connect problem solving with behavioral activation, focusing on helping the youth choose the solutions that achieve their own long-term goals.
- Connect reward plan to efforts to problem-solve and attempt proactive solutions.

Home practice
- Practice problem solving.
- Monitor behavioral activation and pleasant activities.
- Monitor reward plan.

Sessions 7–8

Assessment
- As in Sessions 3–4

Interventions
- Provide psychoeducation around good sleep hygiene, emphasizing routine regulation. Discuss developmental expectations around sleep routines.
- Teach relaxation exercises to use at sleep time.
- Obtain update in any medication treatment the youth is receiving; consult with presiding psychiatrist.
- Obtain updates from collateral systems (e.g., school, extracurricular leaders). Assess the youth's functioning across home/family, school/work, peer, and recreation domains.

Home practice
- Monitor sleep changes.
- Monitor use of relaxation exercises.

Sessions 9–10

Assessment
- As in Sessions 3–4

Interventions
- Monitor self-talk: teach the youth about the link between thoughts and depression/distress.
- Cognitive restructuring: teach the youth to identify thinking traps and challenge unrealistically negative thoughts with more realistic coping thoughts.

(continued)

TABLE 6.3. *(continued)*

Home practice
- Monitor the thoughts–action–feelings tracker.
- Monitor the thinking traps tracker.

Sessions 11–12

Assessment
- As in Sessions 3–4
- Review symptom report forms and progress on target goals. Discuss with the youth and their caregivers interest in and fit for continuing therapy.

Interventions
- Exposures and behavioral challenges: build challenge hierarchy or hierarchies, focusing on core youth goals. Situations will help the youth practice skills to overcome barriers they normally face.
- Practice first steps of hierarchy in session.

Home practice
- Youth refines steps of challenge hierarchy.
- Youth attempts first steps of hierarchy outside of session. Monitor reward chart for successful completion of challenges.

Sessions 13–14

Assessment
- As in Sessions 3–4

Interventions
- Exposures and behavioral challenges: continue practicing mild to moderate steps of challenge hierarchy, focusing on the youth's core goals and barriers.
- Include caregiver in behavioral experiments as necessary to address miscommunication and family problem solving.

Home practice
- Youth continues practicing hierarchy challenges outside of session.
- Monitor use of coping skills and self-reward for successful attempts at challenges.

Sessions 15–16

Assessment
- As in Sessions 3–4
- Review symptom report forms and progress on target goals. Discuss continued progress with the youth and their caregivers. Consider transition to maintenance or termination phase.

Interventions
- Exposures and behavioral challenges: continue practicing moderately challenging steps of challenge hierarchy, focusing on the youth's core goals and barriers.
- Include caregiver in behavioral experiments as necessary to address miscommunication and family problem solving.

(continued)

TABLE 6.3. *(continued)*

Home practice
- Youth continues practicing hierarchy challenges outside of session.
- Monitor use of coping skills and self-reward for successful attempts at challenges.

Sessions 17–18

Assessment
- As in Sessions 3–4

Interventions
- Exposures and behavioral challenges: practice increasingly/difficult challenging steps of challenge hierarchy, focusing on the youth's core goals and barriers.
- Include the caregiver in behavioral experiments as necessary to address miscommunication and family problem solving.
- Discuss transition to biweekly maintenance sessions.

Home practice
- Youth continues practicing hierarchy challenges outside of session.
- Monitor use of coping skills and self-reward for successful attempts at challenges.

Sessions 19–22 (biweekly for maintenance)

Assessment
- As in Sessions 3–4

Psychoeducation
- Introduction to relapse prevention phase.
- Discuss termination.

Interventions
- Exposures and behavioral challenges: Practice increasingly/difficult challenging steps of challenge hierarchy, focusing on youth's core goals and barriers.

Home practice
- Youth continues practicing hierarchy challenges outside of session.
- Monitor use of coping skills and self-reward for successful attempts at challenges.

several key points, including the facts that depression is distinctive from normative sad moods by its persistence and intensity, and is pervasive in terms of the symptoms and impairment seen in the youth. Depressed mood or loss of interest is observed consistently across at least 2 weeks and marks a distinctive change from prior functioning. Significant changes in sleeping, eating, and daily routines (activities, hygiene) and socialization may also be evident, and early intervention is crucial for effective treatment.

By reviewing this information with Abby-Lynn and her mother, the therapist provides a common set of knowledge, normalizes Abby-Lynn's experience, and rallies the family around this established condition. When presenting the handouts enumerating facts on depression (Handouts 7 and 13), the therapist is careful to attend to any questions the family has and to present information in a nonstigmatizing way: depression is a real and impactful condition, it does not reflect a person's personality or lack of willpower, and psychological interventions can help the youth build on their strengths and return to baseline functioning.

Motivational Interviewing

Avolition (limited motivation) and anhedonia (disinterest in previously desired activities) are two symptoms of depression that can compromise a youth's natural inclination to work toward goal-directed behavior, including therapy participation and therapy-related goals. Having collected an assessment of functional impairment and identified specific behavioral traps (via functional assessment), the therapist leads Abby-Lynn through the Change Plan worksheet (Figure 2.1) to identify goals she cares about, steps she is willing to take to reach those goals, and barriers that will challenge her success. Broaching these topics early in therapy can help identify certain obstacles right away and engender a positive working alliance by aligning the therapist and youth around common goals. When discussing specific goals (e.g., returning to basketball practice after an embarrassing exchange with the coach), the therapist brainstorms the pros and cons of pursuing and not pursuing the goal (Figure 2.2). A decisional matrix can be used at any time in therapy; however, it may prove particularly useful when the youth is stuck and questioning whether they are committed to a particular goal. The decision matrix clarifies the youth's own reasoning and values in pursuing a goal.

Activity Monitoring and Behavioral Activation

Teens experiencing depression suffer from deprived environments and activities because they isolate themselves, withdraw from social contacts, and refuse activities that used to bring them joy. Even when they do engage in activities, many depressed teens report they don't enjoy those activities as much as they formerly did (anhedonia). The goals of behavioral activation are to (1) increase physical activity, (2) increase pleasant or mastery activities, and (3) enhance the youth's appreciation of those activities. The goal is to expose the youth to settings with natural rewards and reinforcers. However, even when exposed to natural rewards, some youth will have difficulty appreciating them or experiencing the same joy. Thus, a goal is to enhance the youth's ability to appreciate those reinforcers.

The first step of behavioral activation is activity monitoring. As described in Chapter 2, we review activity trackers looking for automatic behaviors, triggering events, fluctuations, and patterns. The therapist has Abby-Lynn complete the activity tracker in Figure 6.5 (a blank version is available as Worksheet 12 in Appendix A) and reviews the following patterns:

1. **Automatic behaviors.** Several patterns emerged that had not been obvious to Abby-Lynn before. First, it was clear that staying up on the phone late into the night (on Monday and Wednesday) was disruptive to her sleep and contributed to difficulties waking the next day. The isolative behavior (searching YouTube for clips) contributed to a poor mood while she was doing it and then made it difficult for her to fall asleep. The behavior was problematic for several reasons: she chose activities that were isolating (she searched YouTube rather than engaging friends on social media) and she was only involved in the activity half-heartedly, noting that she really wasn't searching for anything in particular; she was just bored. Noticing these kinds of automatic patterns gives some direction about places for intervention.

WORKSHEET 12. Activity Tracker

Sometimes we don't even know when we're getting stuck. Over the next week, track your activities, mood, and important events that happen each day! Then rate your mood from 0 to 10:

0 = "The worst mood I've ever felt."   **5** = "I'm feeling OK but not great."   **10** = "The best I've ever felt."

Example:

| Looked after my little sister. | 10 |

	Monday	Tuesday	Wednesday	Thursday	Friday	Saturday	Sunday
Morning	Couldn't get out of bed. Felt so tired; thought about miserable week. **2**	Woke up late; didn't eat breakfast. Forced myself to school. **3**	Got up late, but ate breakfast. Got to school on time. Talked to Jenn in Math. **5**	Late to school; ignored friends in class. **1**	Got to school on time. Finished math homework in class. **5**	Slept in. **4**	Watched tv. **4**
Lunch	Pushed myself to get to school by lunch. **3**	Sat with girls from team. Felt phased out. **3**	Sat with Jenn and Cara; talked about team. Motivated to go to practice. **6**	Was going to skip lunch; girls made me sit with them. Jenn had funny stories. **5**	Sat with girls, talking about weekend plans. **6**	Mom gave me a hard time about sleeping and not doing anything. **3**	Did some homework. Ate lunch. **5**
Afternoon	Felt so tired in class; barely paid attention. **3**	Covered new stuff in history; felt behind. **4**	Teacher was funny in class. **6**	Got a bad grade back on Science homework. **4**	Still struggling in Science. **4**	Helped brother with OT; he was a pain the whole time. **5**	Practiced ball handling in driveway. **6**
After school/late afternoon	Went straight home. Crashed in room, b/c I was tired. **3**	Went home. Tried to do homework, but too tired. Took nap. **3**	Friend dragged me to basketball prac-tice. Coach chewed me out. **1**	Skipped basketball; went home and did homework. **2**	Went to basket-ball practice. Felt normal. **6**	Texted with Jenn; looked at posts on Snapchat. **7**	Texted with friends. **7**
Evening	Stayed in room all night; YouTubed random clips; up most of night. **2**	Mom made me help brother with OT. **6**	Crashed; skipped dinner. On phone (web) all night. **0**	Emailed coach, said I was having a tough time. She said to come back. **4**	Got pizza with some of the girls; did homework. **7**	Went to movies with Jenn and Alex. **8**	Worried about upcoming week; getting anxious. **4**

FIGURE 6.5. Completed Activity Tracker worksheet for Abby-Lynn.

2. **Mood antecedents (triggers).** Events that appear most linked to poor moods seem to be associated with *isolative behaviors* (e.g., searching YouTube at night; ignoring friends in class; crashing in bed after school), *disengagement* during activities (e.g., being disconnected during lunch with friends; not participating in class), and *performance* (e.g., being chewed out by a coach; getting bad grade). In contrast, social interactions (actively engaging friends at lunch; getting pizza or texting with friends) and competence-enhancing activities (e.g., emailing coach; going to practice; helping brother) seem linked to positive moods.

3. **Fluctuations and patterns.** When working with Abby-Lynn, it would be important to see how social and engaging activities might tend to prompt improvement in her moods, even after she starts the day in a bad mood. For example, on Thursday, she reported a low mood after ignoring her friends in class, but it improved when her friends made her sit with them at lunch. Likewise, she started Saturday in a bad mood after her mother, in her view, criticized her, but the day improved as she helped her brother and engaged friends. In contrast, her mood can slip when she chooses to avoid and disengage. On Thursday, Abby-Lynn felt good at lunch after sitting with her friends, but then became increasingly disengaged after she received a bad grade in science. She faded out during class and skipped basketball practice, leading to a declining mood. Once she did something proactive (i.e., emailed her coach to explain her situation), her mood started to improve and potentially helped her get to school the next day. These observations further lend support to ongoing challenging global or all-or-nothing attributions (e.g., "I had a bad day," as in the whole day was bad) and supporting self-efficacy (e.g., "Even though the morning started out bumpy, I was able to do something to turn it around").

Behavioral activation then works to encourage physically active and pleasant/mastery activities to encourage approach-oriented activation. In Abby-Lynn's case, the therapist starts by identifying the triggers and circumstances that prompt Abby-Lynn to withdraw and avoid. These might include: having a bad day and crashing in bed, searching YouTube instead of using social media, ignoring friends in class even when she's been invited to join them, getting criticized by a coach, or receiving a bad grade.

The therapist then brainstorms options that help prevent withdrawal and inactivity. Proactive responses should be personalized, context-specific, and designed to prompt problem solving or pleasant/mastery choices rather than avoidance. These are not just arbitrary fun activities, but are designed to energize Abby-Lynn's strengths and target her particular vulnerabilities. When Abby-Lynn feels depressed after a bad day, her natural inclination is to crash in bed and sleep through the evening. Her choice to stay in bed makes good emotional sense in that doing this helps Abby-Lynn avoid the persistent rumination about the day's failures and limits her emotional dismay. However, such a solution is short-lived. She rarely feels rested when she awakes, and her concerns remain (her homework is no closer to being completed; she still feels isolated from friends). Alternative proactive solutions could include a number of activities that are freely available, inexpensive, and under the youth's control. They can promote any of the following:

1. **Physical activation:** practicing basketball in the driveway or at the gym, going for a run or other conditioning exercises
2. **Pleasant activities:** walking her dog around the block, texting/calling friends, posting on social media, commenting on YouTube, listening to music, going to the movies with a friend, eating her favorite dessert after dinner

3. **Mastery exercises:** helping her brother in OT, attempting some homework, helping prepare dinner for family, finishing a homework exercise, organizing an outing with friends on the basketball team

4. **Attempts to problem-solve:** texting friends or posting on social media to resolve feelings of loneliness

These options may be combined to potentially maximize effects, for example, texting a friend to go for a run together or shoot hoops. The therapist then matches the proactive activities with the triggers that call for them the most, as shown in Figure 6.6 (a blank version is available as Worksheet 13 in Appendix A).

Any of the proactive responses may come with struggles or frustrations, but they serve several vital functions. First, the physical activities tend to have mood-elevating properties. Second, Abby-Lynn may actually directly address (problem-solve) some of the concerns that led to her bad mood. And third, behavioral activation's greatest gift may be how it can lead to a *pleasant surprise.* This refers to the fact that it is impossible to predict what outcomes may happen by any action we take; unknown positive results can occur. For example, by texting her friend, Abby-Lynn may

WORKSHEET 13. Getting Active and Building Mastery

We all feel down and stuck sometimes. When you feel stuck, bored, disengaged, or depressed, think up active, pleasant, or mastery activities to get you un-stuck.

- Physical activation: Try physical or mental exercise or exertion
- Pleasant activities: Try anything that you find fun and pleasant
- Mastery exercises: Try something that helps you build a skill
- Problem-solve: Brainstorm solutions to solve the problem, using problem-solving STEPS.

List Situations That Get You Stuck (lead to avoidance, withdrawal, procrastination, quitting, isolation)	Proactive Physical, Pleasant, Mastery or Problem-Solving Options
1. Crashing in bed after a bad day	Practice basketball in driveway; help brother in OT; do some homework; text friends; post on social media
2. Searching YouTube	Text friends or post on social media; call friends
3. Ignoring friends in class	Talk to friend; ask other classmate questions; ask teacher question; raise hand in class
4. Getting criticized by coach	Go to coach and ask for feedback or explain situation; get support from teammate
5. Receiving a bad grade	Ask teacher for help and explain situation; go to friend for support

FIGURE 6.6. Brainstorming active responses to Abby-Lynn's avoidant behaviors.

learn about events she had not been aware of and earn an invite. By responding to one friend's post on social media, she may become aware of another classmate's common interests. This may lead to connecting with this other classmate and forging a new friendship. It is true that taking action can bring both "good" and "bad" outcomes, but on average the unexpected good outcomes, the pleasant surprises, tend to outweigh the bad. The therapist can counter youth resistance by noting that no matter what happens, making an attempt to do something has a greater chance of success than the teen's original choice (lying in bed) and that most undesirable outcomes that may result from trying are hardly worse than the outcomes that arise from the original choice (remaining fatigued and lonely).

Self-Reward and Reward Charts

Self-reward and rewards from others are critical to help foster proactive movement. Depressed youth tend to have lost intrinsic motivation and appreciation for activities. External rewards help promote antidepressant behaviors by (1) recognizing the effort it takes to initiate action (i.e., a focus on efforts to cope!) and (2) helping reinforce continued activity until the youth begins to appreciate them again. It's helpful for therapists to brainstorm with youth about rewards they can give themselves and those that may require some help from their parents or others. The key elements of CM plans are that the rewards are available and, in fact, rewarding! The criteria by which teens evaluate themselves should also be attainable. Ideally, goals should be clearly defined, easy to monitor, and broken into small steps. Then rewards should be readily available and easy to give to the youth (whether it's a self-reward or other reward) as soon after goal accomplishment as possible.

Figure 6.7 (a blank version of Worksheet 14 is available in Appendix A) provides examples of goals and rewards for Abby-Lynn. Notice that Abby-Lynn's reward chart is divided into goals that she feels comfortable monitoring and rewarding herself for and other goals that enlist the help of her mother. The self-monitored rewards help emphasize to Abby-Lynn that she deserves rewards for accomplishing these goals and that she should be looking to self-reward as immediately after success as possible. The mother's assistance is also enlisted so that Abby-Lynn knows her mother is aware of her daughter's success in accomplishing goals. Abby-Lynn begins to see that others are becoming interested in her growth and achievement of goals. Involving the mother also ensures that Abby-Lynn will receive some kind of reward even when she does not believe she deserves one.

Problem Solving

Problem solving was particularly useful for Abby-Lynn because she often took a defeatist attitude toward problems and had difficulty seeing the available options. Below is an example where the therapist helped Abby-Lynn build her problem-solving skills (Chorpita & Weisz, 2009) with regard to a situation where she felt helpless. The therapist uses the problem-solving approach called STEPS (say, think, examine, pick, see; refer to Chapter 2). Abby-Lynn came to session distressed that the situation on the basketball team was deteriorating quickly. After several practices during which Abby-Lynn became distracted, her coach benched her while the first-string team practiced. After one noticeable mistake (she passed the ball to the opposing team), the coach made Abby-Lynn run laps around the gym. Abby-Lynn's anxiety had been building over the past week, and the day after running laps (Wednesday), she skipped practice (Thursday). Abby-Lynn came to session distraught, fearing that she would never be able to resume playing on the first-string team and

WORKHEET 14. Goals and Rewards Chart

Whenever we're trying new skills, we should reward ourselves for making the effort. First, brainstorm achievable, meaningful foals. Then decide how you would reward yourself for each accomplishment.

Goals I Can Match Myself	Reward	M	T	W	TR	F	Sat	Sun	# of Days Achieved
Respond to texts from friends right away (within 10 min).	1 pt per response; at 10 points, get to watch favorite TV by self.	Y	N	Y	Y	N	Y	Y	5
Go for a run when I get home from school.	Get to take a shower before doing any HW or chores.	Y	N	N	Y	Y	Y	Y	5
Help brother do a practice exercise.	Take 30 min for myself (ex: crafts, surfing YouTube).	Y	–	–	Y	–	N	–	2

Goals My Mom Can Reward Me For	Reward	M	T	W	TR	F	Sat	Sun	# of Days Achieved
Finish one class assignment before dinner.	At least 4 successes, gets to borrow car on weekend.	Y	N	N	Y	Y	–	–	3
Get to school on time.	Gets 1 hr of free time (no one bothers her) after dinner.	N	Y	Y	N	Y	–	–	3

FIGURE 6.7. Goals and rewards chart for Abby-Lynn.

expressed a desire to quit. After listening to Abby-Lynn's concerns and normalizing her distress, the therapist wondered aloud if there was anything Abby-Lynn could do to repair the situation before she made such a rash decision.

> THERAPIST: I can hear how upset you are about your coach and being embarrassed in front of the team. Is there anything that can be done about this?
>
> ABBY-LYNN: No! The coach is so unforgiving. Once she makes a judgment, she writes you off forever. I might as well just quit now.
>
> THERAPIST: Well, I'd hate to see you make that decision when you're so upset, especially knowing how important basketball is to you. Would you be willing to brainstorm some options to see if we can improve the situation?
>
> ABBY-LYNN: I guess we can try.

S: Say What the Problem Is

> THERAPIST: OK, the first trick to solving any problem is getting clear on what the problem is.
>
> ABBY-LYNN: Well, my coach hates me.
>
> THERAPIST: So, it seems like she's upset with you, and you want her not to be upset with you.
>
> ABBY-LYNN: I guess.
>
> THERAPIST: Sometimes I find it's difficult to get other people to change their feelings. What else is a problem here?
>
> ABBY-LYNN: I'm not getting any playing time.
>
> THERAPIST: OK, you're not getting any playing time, and you'd want more.
>
> ABBY-LYNN: I also want the coach to get off my back. She doesn't know what pressure I'm under.
>
> THERAPIST: OK, so maybe another problem is that your coach doesn't understand why you're struggling.
>
> ABBY-LYNN: Yeah.
>
> THERAPIST: If we were to just focus on one problem first, which is more important to you?
>
> ABBY-LYNN: I guess getting the coach off my back.

Notice that the therapist is trying to achieve several things: She is helping Abby-Lynn choose which problem is most important to her and she is helping to clarify what the specific problem is. Next the therapist will transform the problem into a goal. It is always easier brainstorming solutions when you know what the goal is.

> THERAPIST: OK, can we turn this into a goal? What would you want most in this situation?
>
> ABBY-LYNN: To get the coach off my back. Have her understand why I'm so distracted and messing up.
>
> THERAPIST: OK, that sounds like a start: Helping the coach understand what you're going through.

T: Think of Solutions

Next the therapist helps Abby-Lynn brainstorm solutions in nonevaluative ways.

> THERAPIST: OK, the first step to problem-solving is to brainstorm as many solutions as possible—without prejudging them! They can be rationale or implausible—let's just get them on paper.

The therapist and Abby-Lynn brainstorm a number of solutions as seen in Figure 6.8 (a blank version is available as Worksheet 15 in Appendix A). Note that the pros and cons are not discussed until after all solutions have been offered. (See Chapter 2 for review of problem-solving steps.) When necessary, the therapist helps prompt more creative and outlandish solutions (e.g., skywriting a message to the coach!). The goal is to truly consider the whole range of possibilities. This helps the youth feel less trapped into a designated set of commonsense solutions. One will notice that even one of the later solutions ("Get there early and put in extra work") seems promising to Abby-Lynn, but it might never have surfaced if she and her therapist started evaluating prematurely.

E: Examine Each Solution

Once Abby-Lynn and the therapist finish brainstorming, the therapist then helps the teen consider the pros and cons of each solution. The critical lesson here is that each solution, no matter how promising on its face, has both pros and cons. This examination reveals that no one solution is expected to solve a problem on its first try, and that a person should expect to have to try several solutions to resolve any problem.

P: Pick One Solution and Try It

After considering the pros and cons of each solution, the therapist prompts Abby-Lynn to rank-order (or rate on a scale) which solutions seem most promising. Again, the aim is to emphasize that multiple solutions may be needed before a satisfying one is found. This process prepares the youth to think of problem solving as a continuous process.

S: See If It Worked

After rank-ordering the solutions, Abby-Lynn is ready to try one of them. After a discussion with her therapist, Abby-Lynn prioritizes emailing her coach as her first choice. She likes the idea of being able to spell out her thoughts ahead of time, even though she can't be certain when the coach will read the message. This solution also stays focused on the primary goal of communicating to the coach how much pressure she is under, not necessarily asking the coach to give her playing time. Abby-Lynn composes the email in session and sends it off to the coach. To her surprise, the coach writes back the same evening, showing concern (the coach had wondered if something was wrong) and encouraging Abby-Lynn to return to practice the next day. This interaction brings relief to Abby-Lynn. It also challenges certain expectancies and assumptions she may have

WORKSHEET 15. Problem-Solving STEPS

To solve problems, take these steps: say what the problem is, think of solutions, examine each solution, pick one solution and try it, and see if it worked!

Say What the Problem Is: *Getting the coach to understand what I'm going through*

Think of Solutions	Examine Each Solution		Rank
	Pros	**Cons**	
1. Go up to coach after practice to tell her I'm having trouble.	I can tell her what's going on.	She might still be mad at me at practice. I might be too emotional.	4
2. Go up to coach <u>before</u> practice to talk to her.	I can tell her what's going on.	Better than after practice, but I might still be too emotional to tell her.	3
3. Have my friends talk to coach for me.	I don't have to face my coach.	Might not be as believable. Friends might say the wrong thing.	5
4. Email coach to explain my situation.	I get to spell out my words.	Won't know if/when the coach reads it. Sometimes emails are misread.	1
5. Don't tell her anything and just focus more in practice.	Actions speak louder than words.	I might still mess up and then make things worse.	6
6. Get there early and put in extra work.	Will show her I'm sorry and help get me back on the team.	Doesn't really tell coach about everything going on in my life right now.	2
7. Quit the team.	Easiest thing to do.	Sad to not play basketball.	7
8. Talk about the coach on Instagram.	Get out my anger. Maybe she'll know how hurt she made me feel.	Will make me feel bad. And probably make things worse.	9
9. Send her flowers to apologize.	Will show I'm sorry.	Kind of corny. Doesn't really tell her what's going on.	8
10.			

Pick One Solution and Try It: *Email coach to explain my situation.*

FIGURE 6.8. Brainstorming problem solving for Abby-Lynn.

(see below). Though the exchange does not solve the overall problems of her mood, distractibility, and aimlessness, it helps to know that the coach is going to give her some leeway to figure things out. This is enough to help Abby-Lynn sleep better that night and motivate her to go to school the next day.

Sleep Hygiene, Relaxation

Sleep hygiene is the next target the therapist will address (Sessions 7–8). Sleep disruptions are a frequent and significant symptom in many depressed youth (Brand, Hatzinger, Beck, & Holsboer-Trachsler, 2009; Rao, Hammen, & Poland, 2009). Depressed youth often shift their sleep cycle such that they end up going to sleep later, experience disrupted and restless sleep, have difficulty rising, and feel unrested. As a result, depressed youth will nap and sleep at various points of the day. That leads to a number of functional impairments, including poorer cognitive functioning and school attendance.

Like other depressed youth, Abby-Lynn had a disrupted sleep cycle: she had difficulty falling asleep because she did not feel tired at her desired bedtime (10 P.M.), would then lie in bed thinking about the day for 1–2 hours before dozing off, only to wake spontaneously at various points during the night. When her alarm clock rang at 6:00 A.M., Abby-Lynn felt groggy, sick, and "like she ran a 5-mile race." No amount of prompts by her mother could wake her. About half the week, Abby-Lynn would wake up after 9:00 A.M. and rush off to school, missing her first two periods. Upon returning home, she would crash for 1–2 hours before her mother awakened her to do homework and help prepare dinner. To address Abby-Lynn's dysregulated sleep cycle, the therapist conducted a module of therapy that included psychoeducation (including the use of Handout 4, which is available in Appendix A) that emphasized the importance of healthy sleep hygiene. The therapist analyzed Abby-Lynn's sleep routine, taught her relaxation exercises, and reviewed cognitive restructuring to identify the anxious and negative thoughts contributing to her restless sleep.

In conducting an analysis of Abby-Lynn's sleep cycle, it became apparent that she would wait until an hour before bedtime to review her planner to see if she had completed all her homework. When she realized she missed an assignment, she would either rush to complete it then, or give up and try to go to sleep but lie awake worrying about the missed assignment. In addition, sometimes she would make coffee or consume an energy drink to improve alertness to complete her homework. After this, she would lie awake until 4–5 A.M. recycling thoughts of her failure. This cycle led her to feel fatigued throughout the day and compelled her to crash when she came home, leading her to not feel tired at bedtime many a night.

The therapist first provided education about good sleep hygiene using Handout 4, correcting Abby-Lynn's misperceptions about how to create a conducive sleep environment. The therapist helped her construct a plan where they agreed on an official "cutoff time" of 7 P.M. for homework and secured her mother's support of this plan. This was relieving to Abby-Lynn both because it prevented her from looking at her planner at bedtime, and it also gave a finite deadline by which she could quit homework each night. Paradoxically, having this concrete deadline contributed to greater completion of homework because Abby-Lynn procrastinated less after school. In line with this, Abby-Lynn agreed to not drink any caffeinated drinks after 5 P.M. and focused on pleasure reading and talking to friends in the evening. She also agreed to not watch YouTube or go onto Instagram after 9 P.M., which tended to activate her anxious or negative thoughts. To help feel awake in the mornings, Abby-Lynn agreed to place her alarm across the room and to do 10 jumping jacks on her way to shutting it off. The therapist and Abby-Lynn also worked on preemptively identifying thoughts and urges to quit the plan likely to surface in the morning when she was more vulnerable and sleepy (e.g., "Ugh this is stupid" or "I'll hit snooze" or "I just need a few more minutes"). They also worked on self-coaching statements Abby-Lynn would practice instead (e.g., "This is not stupid but important for my health" or "My depression wants me to hit snooze but that leads to me feeling worse" or "I *want* 5 more minutes but do not *need* 5 more minutes"). Engaging in physical exercise was something Abby-Lynn conceptually valued, so the therapist asked her to walk around the block first thing after waking. Abby-Lynn tried this and even turned this ritual into a short jog around her neighborhood. In the first 2 weeks of the trial, this jog led to Abby-Lynn being late for school. The therapist got her mother and school to permit this lateness for a while, to help Abby-Lynn prioritize activation to reset her sleep–wake cycle. Even when late, Abby-Lynn arrived at school more alert and activated, prompting positive reports from her teachers. With this early success, Abby-Lynn became motivated to wake earlier and complete her running routine in time for her to reach school by first period most days.

Identifying Thinking Traps and Cognitive Restructuring

At this point in therapy (Sessions 9–10), the therapist had prioritized behaviorally oriented interventions as a way to initiate socioemotional activation, provide a sense of self-efficacy, and teach problem-solving skills that could help Abby-Lynn gain control over the challenges and hassles of daily life. As a result, Abby-Lynn had developed a better sense of which events and interactions triggered negative mood states and how she fell into behavioral traps. She began to problem-solve her way out of these traps by looking for more proactive strategies to engage the activities that were meaningful to her (e.g., basketball, taking care of her brother) and to reward herself accordingly (e.g., self-care, borrowing the car). Seeing Abby-Lynn's initial success at implementing these skills, the therapist thought it was the appropriate time to conduct thought tracking and cognitive restructuring. This was consistent with the therapist's conceptualization that self-critical and discouraged thoughts contribute to avoidant, negative cycles that lead to increased isolation and depression. To help identify Abby-Lynn's thinking traps and to challenge unrealistic thinking, the therapist followed the steps below (see Chapter 2 for an extended discussion of these same guidelines):

Step 1: Track Events, Thoughts, and Mood

To help Abby-Lynn identify *automatic thoughts* that lead to a depressed mood, the therapist recalled that Abby-Lynn often commented that some of her toughest self-criticism came in the form of "hearing" her mother's or coach's voice criticizing her or pushing her harder. The therapist noted that the thoughts in our head can often sound as loud as real voices and that it can be easy to internalize their commands with little questioning. However, the thoughts Abby-Lynn was attributing to her coach or mother really reflected her own self-doubts and criticism. Using Handout 2 and Worksheet 5 (reproducible versions of both are available in Appendix A), the therapist encouraged her to start tracking such automatic thoughts to see what events trigger them, and what mood and actions follow (see Figure 6.9).

THERAPIST: So, how was going to practice yesterday after emailing your coach?

ABBY-LYNN: I almost didn't go. I was nervous that everyone would be looking at me for how I stormed out the other day.

THERAPIST: OK, so it sounds like this is an example of having other "voices" in your head. I wonder if those are your own thoughts.

ABBY-LYNN: Yeah, I know. I guess I just imagine the worst thing they could be thinking of me, and assume it's true.

THERAPIST: Well, that's what we're going to be looking into today. When you do notice those thoughts, like one of your teammates thinking, "What's she doing back? She's a quitter." How does that make you feel?

ABBY-LYNN: Embarrassed. Disgusted with myself.

THERAPIST: And what's the first thought you notice coming into your head?

ABBY-LYNN: They all think I'm a loser; I shouldn't be there.

THERAPIST: And what's your instinct to do?

ABBY-LYNN: Get out of there.

THERAPIST: OK, well let's spell out that link here.

The therapist and Abby-Lynn use the Thinking Traps Tracker in Figure 6.9 to start spelling out the link between events, thoughts, mood, and action. Upon seeing her automatic thoughts laid out, Abby-Lynn begins to see how certain events (performance situations, interpersonal expectations) triggered routinely negative thoughts. "I guess I knew I had these thoughts, but I didn't realize how many times I had them." Over the week that follows, the therapist assigns Abby-Lynn to track her thoughts in reaction to any events that lead to a negative mood and to return to the next session with the tracker. Even though the tracker includes a space for "Thinking Trap," the therapist tells Abby-Lynn to leave that column blank; they will review that concept the following week.

Step 2: Identify Unrealistic Assumptions and Label Thinking Traps

When Abby-Lynn returns the following week with a completed thought tracker, the therapist reviews the trends and notices the same pattern that Abby-Lynn had. Abby-Lynn seems to be most routinely upset when there is an expectation to perform or when there are ambiguous social cues that suggest others want something from her. The therapist then introduces the concept of "thinking traps," the common ways in which individuals make false assumptions or draw unrealistic conclusions based on ambiguous information.

THERAPIST: OK, I'm noticing there are some common themes in your thinking patterns. You seem to be most sensitive when you have to perform, or when you think others want something from you.

ABBY-LYNN: Yeah, I just keep thinking that I'm failing. Or, that I'm not living up to people's expectations.

THERAPIST: Those thoughts can really be strong that way. And yet, does that really reflect what's going on?

WORKSHEET 5. Thinking Traps Tracker

What thinking traps do you fall into when feeling sad, anxious, or distressed? For each situation, describe and rate how you feel. Describe your automatic thought (the first thought that comes into your head). What thinking trap might you be falling into? How does that make you feel (the result)?

Trigger	Feeling (Rate 0–10: "not at all" to "excruciating")	Thought	Thinking Trap	Result?
Walk into practice, think teammates are thinking I'm a loser.	Embarrassed (7) Disgusted (7)	"They think I'm a loser." "They don't want me there."	Mind reading	Disgusted with myself (9) Wanted to leave the gym (10)
Missed a pass during practice. Other team stole it for a point.	Frustrated (8) Embarrassed (6)	"I suck at this." "I've lost my touch."	Catastrophizing	Frustrated (9) Angry at myself (8)
Didn't help my brother out with his OT.	Sad (6) Frustrated (5)	"My mother hates me." "I can't get anything done."	Mind reading, looking for the negatives	Sad (8)

FIGURE 6.9. Completed Thinking Traps Tracker worksheet for Abby-Lynn.

131

ABBY-LYNN: Yeah, everyone's been hating me because of my flakiness and messing up. I threw the ball to the wrong team last week!

THERAPIST: OK, so you made some mistakes, but how do you know your teammates thought you were flaky, or that they hated you?

ABBY-LYNN: I don't know. . . . They seem to be treating me differently.

THERAPIST: Like how?

ABBY-LYNN: They're ghosting me.

THERAPIST: Are they avoiding you, or are you avoiding them?

ABBY-LYNN: I don't know.

THERAPIST: Because you seem like you've been avoiding them a lot lately, like, you haven't been texting back and when you go into the locker room, you kind of go right to your locker.

ABBY-LYNN: I guess . . .

THERAPIST: Is it possible that you're making some assumptions based on how awkward you feel?

ABBY-LYNN: Maybe.

THERAPIST: When people are depressed, they often make assumptions that don't reflect what's fully going on. They draw the most negative conclusion without really having the cause. Could this be happening to you? Let me share with you a list of common thinking traps that people can often fall into. There are a number of different kinds, each reflecting different assumptions or false conclusions we make. Let's go through them and see if any apply to this situation.

The therapist and Abby-Lynn review the thinking traps list in Table 2.2 (a reproducible version is available as Handout 2 in Appendix A) and start to apply various traps to assumptions Abby-Lynn has been making. They identify that Abby-Lynn is falling prey to a number of consistent traps, including mind reading, catastrophizing, and looking for the negatives. For example, when she walked into the locker room, she assumed that her teammates' tentative actions resulted because they were judging her past performance. A review of the evidence suggests that several teammates came up to her and asked how she was doing. This provides an example of mind reading whereby the client assumes they know what another person is thinking without asking them. Likewise, when Abby-Lynn missed one pass, she criticized herself harshly, thinking, "I've lost my touch." She was making unreasonable assumptions about the impact of this single pass, so she may have been falling prey to the catastrophizing trap (thinking the worst possible outcome). It also could have been an example of looking for the negatives (Walking with Blinders On, only looking at the situation a certain way), because she neglected to count the dozens of other successful passes she made during the day. The therapist helps Abby-Lynn consider whether adequate evidence exists for her conclusions, and where her assumptions are getting the better of her. Using a formal thinking trap label makes it easier to identify them in the moment, rather than having to do a sophisticated analysis each time a negative emotion strikes.

Step 3: Generate More Positive, Realistic Coping Thoughts

The therapist next helps the youth develop more realistic and adaptive coping thoughts by taking into account the full reality of their situation. Ideal coping thoughts directly address the specific thinking trap the youth may be falling into. When Abby-Lynn resorts to mind reading when assuming that her teammates think she is a loser, the therapist helps her build a coping thought around some of the facts they have uncovered (see Figure 6.10; a blank version is available as Worksheet 16 in Appendix A).

THERAPIST: So, when you were standing by your locker, did anyone say anything to you?

ABBY-LYNN: Yeah, Jazmin came over and asked how I'd been.

THERAPIST: That doesn't sound like they didn't want you there, at least for Jazmin.

ABBY-LYNN: I guess I was assuming she'd be mad at me.

THERAPIST: Is there a more realistic thought that can help you cope with the mind reading you're doing?

ABBY-LYNN: What do you mean?

THERAPIST: I'm looking for a slogan that would respond to the negative assumption that your teammates are mad at you.

ABBY-LYNN: I guess that they do care. They asked if I was OK.

THERAPIST: OK, would that help remind you that your friends are there for you? Would it help counter that niggling thought that everyone's mad at you?

ABBY-LYNN: I guess.

THERAPIST: OK, so the trick of this is to recite that coping thought any time your negative thinking gets triggered. So, the next time you enter the locker room, say to yourself, "They're just concerned." Now there may be similar situations, like walking into a class or lunchroom, where you're also not sure what people are thinking. Is there another coping thought that could cover these types of situations where you're not sure what people are thinking?

ABBY-LYNN: I don't know . . . maybe "I don't know what people are thinking" or "Friends are more supportive than I give them credit for"?

THERAPIST: OK, I like those. Now we can test those out for specific situations. But for now, I do believe that if you entered friend situations thinking those things, you'd be more open for good things to come than if you entered assuming they were mad at you.

ABBY-LYNN: That's probably true.

As discussed in Chapter 2, avoid forming coping thoughts that are *unrealistically positive* as well. The goal is not to sell the youth on false platitudes or superficial pleasantries. Adopting the coping thought "People like me no matter what I do" would have been hardly believable and less effective than citing specific evidence that Abby-Lynn's friends were concerned about her. In truth, not everyone may like us just as we may not be expected to like everyone we encounter. Thus, the goal of devising coping thoughts is to open the youth to the possibility that things could

WORKSHEET 16. Coping Thoughts Tracker

Brainstorm coping thoughts that could respond to your thinking trap! Try and come up with coping statements that are more realistic and ask, "How am I not seeing the whole picture?"

Trigger	Thought	Thinking Trap	Coping Thought	Result?
Walk into practice, think teammates are thinking I'm a loser.	"They think I'm a loser." "They don't want me there."	Mind reading	"They showed concern; asked if I was OK."	Felt calmer; went into practice with clearer head.
Missed a pass during practice. Other team stole it for a point.	"I suck at this." "I've lost my touch."	Catastrophizing	"I made a dozen other passes."	Felt calmer; more confident; kept going.
Didn't help my brother out with his OT.	"My mother hates me." "I can't get anything done."	Mind reading,		
Looking for the negatives	"I can only do what I can, and I'm doing a lot."	Felt less sad; played with my brother later.		

FIGURE 6.10. Completed Coping Thoughts Tracker worksheet for Abby-Lynn.

be more positive (or at least less negative) than they are assuming. Being open to that possibility, the youth may have the confidence to activate and approach when they normally might have withdrawn.

Behavioral Challenges and *In Vivo* Exposures

Building Challenge Hierarchies for Mood Problems

The therapist moved to integrating *in vivo* behavioral challenges in Session 11 to help Abby-Lynn practice her developing coping skills. Based on Abby-Lynn and her mother's goals and the therapist's case conceptualization, the therapist generated (with the family) several challenge hierarchies focused on *life re-engagement, building Abby-Lynn's social network, balancing responsibilities and stress,* and improving her *sleep hygiene and sleep.* Even though Abby-Lynn's mother had listed "improve sad mood" as an initial goal, the therapist communicated that mood is sometimes a difficult thing to address directly; instead, the therapist built consensus around the notion that if they made progress on some of the social, behavioral, and cognitive goals, an improved mood would follow. Abby-Lynn and her mother agreed that focusing on enhancing her activity level and outlook on life would lead to increased positivity.

Challenge hierarchies for depression tend to include two forms of experiments. As discussed in Chapter 2, they are most typically referred to as behavioral experiments in the sense that challenges are created wherein concrete goals are identified and the therapist coaches the youth to achieve those goals. For example, one useful experiment might be to direct Abby-Lynn to phone a friend, have a 5-minute conversation, and then invite the friend to hang out. Accomplishing the specific goals (calling the friend, maintaining a conversation, extending the invitation) can have a meaningful impact on Abby-Lynn's life—such as in building a social network, or simply appreciating the friend's conversation. Within this context, experiments can be used to test out faulty cognitions and challenge negative assumptions and thinking traps. So, as Abby-Lynn is talking to her friend, she may notice self-critical thoughts ("She's wondering why I'm calling—she must think I'm a loser") that fall into her characteristic thinking traps (mind reading). Behavioral experiments help obtain evidence to counter unrealistically negative assumptions Abby-Lynn is making. During, or following, the experiment, the therapist can ask, "Did your friend say she was bored?" "Was there any evidence that she liked your call?" Conducting behavioral experiments in real time with the youth during session (such as Abby-Lynn sending her coach an email) allows the therapist to be a real-life observer and challenge the youth's negative cognitive filters.

A second kind of experiment can take on the form and function of classic *in vivo* exposures. Exposures typically refer to confronting an anxious youth with a feared stimulus and having the youth habituate to the stimulus or learn to tolerate the distress that results from the stressful situation. These types of exposures help challenge the youth's notion that they will become incapacitated by the feared stimulus or that catastrophic outcomes will occur. Depressed youth can likewise become incapacitated by mood. Youth prone to depression come into contact with task demands or opportunities to get more active, and instead of engaging, they often decline, withdraw, or isolate. For Abby-Lynn, homework time was always a stressor. Even though she liked language arts, the notion of sitting down, thinking about what to write, and then composing connected sentences and thoughts felt overwhelming. Her typical response was to push her books away and crash on her bed. The demand for *sustained effort* was its own trigger. When her friends would text, Abby-Lynn would put her phone down because she could foresee the effort it would take to text back, maintain the back-and-forth conversation, and then maybe plan some outing. While she acknowledged that she liked her friends, she rarely felt the reward (connecting with friend) was worth the effort (texting, planning) it required. The therapist can share Handout 14 (a reproducible version is available in Appendix A) to help convey these concepts to the youth.

In these cases, *in vivo* exposures can be used to expose the youth to the feeling of sustained effort and to help them complete a task. Dimidjian and colleagues (2011) use a similar technique when helping adult clients respond to rumination. They ask their clients to practice identifying instances where rumination or passivity leads to disengaging life; they instruct clients to notice whenever they have ruminated for longer than 5 minutes and to use that as a "cue for activation." In the case of exposures, the therapist is there to create a situation that calls for "effortful action" (Chu et al., 2014), to help the youth recognize the temptation to quit, and to push past that feeling, similar to tolerating distress in traditional exposures for anxiety. In Abby-Lynn's case, the therapist might request that she bring in homework, watch her initiate composition of an essay, and then help Abby-Lynn become aware of the moment when her perception of "effort" calls to her to quit. The therapist then coaches Abby-Lynn through that moment using any number of coping skills taught earlier in therapy. The goal is to show Abby-Lynn that (1) she can overcome the urge to quit and (2) the rewards are worth sustaining effort.

Several hierarchies are generated that give options for the therapist and Abby-Lynn to practice skills during session or afterward at home. Each challenge falls within one of the general themes from treatment goals, but they are not necessarily hierarchical. Each challenge taps into different dimensions of the particular goal. The first hierarchy below references the goal to engage activities that used to be fun for Abby-Lynn. This challenge and many of the others also make use of the "effortful action" form of exposure described above.

*Challenge Hierarchy A: Re-engaging with Former Activities
and Pushing Through with Sustained Effort*

1. Practice dribbling.
2. Practice free-throws.
3. Play basketball one-on-one with a teammate.
4. Practice drills with a teammate.
5. Post images on Instagram.
6. Comment on other people's Instagram accounts.
7. Film myself doing basketball drills.
8. Post a basketball video on YouTube.
9. Text friends.
10. Make plans with friends.
11. Do writing homework.
12. Help my brother with his OT.

As the therapist helped Abby-Lynn begin to activate and learn to appreciate the positive results of activation, she wanted to make sure that Abby-Lynn was building a real support network that would help maintain her activity once Abby-Lynn started to reach out. To this end, the therapist and Abby-Lynn brainstormed a number of challenges that would help give her practice in reaching out to others and planning activities. Some were doable in session, and some had to be completed as home practice outside of session. The goals of each activity differed depending on the particular skill they wanted the teen to practice most that week. When making plans with a friend, Abby-Lynn expressed numerous negative assumptions. The behavioral experiment helped to identify her thinking traps and challenge them with evidence.

Challenge Hierarchy B: Increasing Social Contact and Social Supports
1. Comment on a friend's Instagram.
2. Post on my Facebook or Instagram account.
3. Text a friend.
4. Make plans with friends.
5. Hang out with friends.
6. Sit with friends at lunchtime.
7. Talk with a friend during class.
8. Call a classmate after school about homework.
9. Ask a teacher for help after class.
10. Talk to the basketball coach about having a hard time.

At the same time, the therapist wanted to help Abby-Lynn practice concrete problem solving to help manage real-life stressors and daily *hassles*. The therapist planned a series of family problem-solving exercises where Abby-Lynn could practice her assertiveness skills and Abby-Lynn and her mom might collaboratively manage her responsibilities.

Challenge Hierarchy C: Managing Responsibilities while Balancing Stress
1. Engage in family problem solving with my mother.
2. Practice assertiveness skills while asking for breaks.
3. Plan breaks and rewards in between chores and schoolwork.
4. Problem-solve realistic expectations.

Abby-Lynn had reported significant sleep disruption when she first entered treatment. The therapist provided education on sleep hygiene, taught relaxation and mindfulness skills, and introduced cognitive restructuring to help the teen create a conducive sleep routine. Some of the steps focused on problem solving these routines. Others gave Abby-Lynn and the therapist a chance to practice skills in session. For example, the therapist would simulate bedtime in session and lead Abby-Lynn through relaxation and mindfulness exercises, identifying and challenging anxious thoughts that would keep Abby-Lynn awake.

Challenge Hierarchy D: Improving Sleep Hygiene and Regulating the Sleep Cycle
1. Practice relaxation and mindfulness exercises to use before sleep.
2. Practice coping thoughts for easing anxious fears before sleep.
3. Plan out a sleep routine.
4. Plan rewards for waking at a consistent time.
5. Plan rewards for staying awake during the day.

Performing Behavioral Experiments and Exposures in Session

Before conducting each exposure, the therapist and youth identified the goals, challenges, and coping efforts that would be required. Chapter 2 provides an overview of exposure preparation and execution. Here, we provide two case examples of a behavioral experiment. These were designed to help Abby-Lynn challenge negative assumptions when building social networks. The second also exposed her to sustained effort (effortful action) when trying to complete homework.

BEHAVIORAL EXPERIMENT: BUILDING A SOCIAL NETWORK

Figure 6.11 is an exposure worksheet as completed by Abby-Lynn (a blank version is available as Worksheet 6 in Appendix A) that illustrates a social exposure related to the goals of establishing a broad social network and challenging her negative assumptions. In collaboratively choosing with her therapist an exposure to conduct in session, Abby-Lynn mentions talking with a girl at lunch with whom she used to be closer but has had less contact with in recent months. Abby-Lynn agrees to text Kelly and attempt to make plans with her (see items 3 and 4 in Challenge Hierarchy B), hoping to challenge her own fears that Kelly would not want to hear from her. In preparing for the behavioral experiment, the therapist assists Abby-Lynn in identifying her feelings (anxious, sad), her distress rating (85), and negative thoughts related to the challenge. All of these are noted on the worksheet. In talking through her fears, the therapist helps Abby-Lynn notice that she is falling prey to *mind reading* ("She'll think it's weird I'm texting her out of the blue") and *taking things too personally* (playing the Self-Critic; "I must be so desperate to do this"). The therapist challenges Abby-Lynn to identify evidence for and against each negative thought. Abby-Lynn acknowledges that Kelly had always responded to her texts in the past. She then generates a relevant coping thought ("Kelly might be excited to hear from me") to counter her anxious thought. She also reasons that being proactive is not an act of desperation, but a move to help herself. The therapist helps her identify examples of people who have struggled with challenges and have had to ask for supports or take small steps to reestablish themselves (as an athlete, Abby-Lynn is receptive to examples of pro basketball players who overcame long stints in rehab). She decides to then use this coping response: "It's proactive to do something to help yourself."

Having identified the negative thoughts and fears that could potentially interfere with Abby-Lynn accomplishing her goal, the therapist and Abby-Lynn generate achievable behavioral goals to focus their efforts. These goals are intentionally designed to be small, achievable, and incrementally advance Abby-Lynn toward a larger functional goal (establishing contact with a potential friend). Rewards are then identified that will help acknowledge her accomplishment of each goal. These rewards do not have to be elaborate; their primary function is to recognize the effort she will have to make to attempt something that remains very difficult. The final reward ("Search the Web for frozen yogurt and other places to visit") is designed to both acknowledge and capitalize on the success of Abby-Lynn's efforts. Successful attempts to reach out to friends will next trigger the planning of what fun activity to do.

After sketching the outlines of the experiment, the therapist initiates the process by recording Abby-Lynn's beginning distress rating, which elevates to 90 as the start of the experiment approaches. The therapist then prompts Abby-Lynn to text Kelly. The teen initially protests, revealing that her anxious thoughts are still salient and emotionally interfering. "She's going to think I'm so weird. This is so stupid. Why do I have to do this? No one else has to do experi-

WORKSHEET 6. *In Vivo* Exposure/Behavioral Experiment

> Complete this worksheet with the youth as you are preparing for a behavioral experiment.

1. Situation (What's the situation?):

Text Kelly to see what she's doing; maybe make plans.

2. Feelings: **Distress Rating:** _85_

Anxious, sad

3. Anxious/Negative Thoughts: | **Thinking Traps (See list below.)**

"We haven't talked in so long; she'll think it's weird I'm texting her out of the blue."

"I must be so desperate to do this. I'm such a loser to not have friends."

Mind reading

Taking things too personally; overgeneralizing

Thinking Traps: mind reading, fortune-telling, catastrophizing, jumping to conclusions, what if's, discounting the positives, looking for the negatives, overgeneralizing, all-or-nothing thinking, should statements, taking things too personally, blaming.

4. Coping Thoughts (How do you respond to your anxious thoughts?):

Mind reading: "She might be excited to hear from me." "She's always responded before."
Taking things too personally: "Doing things to help yourself is not desperate, it's proactive."
"Everyone has something they're working on."

Challenge Questions: Do I know for certain that _____? Am I 100% sure that _____? What evidence do I have that _____? What is the worst that could happen? How bad is that? Do I have a crystal ball?

5. Achievable Behavioral Goals (What do you want to accomplish?):

Goal	Accomplished?
a. Text Kelly. Make comment about class today.	
b. Talk about last time we hung out.	
c. Suggest getting fro-yo after school tomorrow.	

6. Rewards:

Reward	Earned?
a. High five, self-praise "Go me!"	
b. Accept praise from therapist.	
c. Search Web for fro-yo places and other places to stop off.	

FIGURE 6.11. Completed behavioral experiment worksheet to help client broaden social network.

ments!" The therapist reminds Abby-Lynn of her thinking traps and prompts her to recall her coping thoughts: "I guess she's always answered before." "Sheryl Swoopes had to relearn how to jump after her knee injury." The therapist also reminds Abby-Lynn that she does not have to text Kelly; but she is choosing to lift her mood and try this step to see what happens. After recalling her coping thoughts and taking a deep breath, Abby-Lynn initiates the first step of texting Kelly. After finishing her text ("Did Mr. Whitmore make any sense to you today???"), Abby-Lynn lets out a huge exhalation but quickly becomes anxious: "What a loser! I can't believe I said that! She'll never respond!" The therapist prompts Abby-Lynn to again recall her relevant coping thought ("She's always responded before") and identifies the teen's distress rating at 95. As Abby-Lynn and the therapist are preparing for the next step, Kelly texts back: "fr—so clueless." Relieved and suddenly emboldened, Abby-Lynn immediately texts, "lol save me." And, "It's been too long. Hang out?" To which Kelly responds, "I know! I was thinking the same thing" and "Need an Abby-Lynn dose!" Capitalizing on the momentum, Abby-Lynn replies, "Fro-yo??" Kelly enthused, "Definitely!"

After the final text, Abby-Lynn rates her distress a 0 and acknowledges, "I was so nervous, but it went so quickly," which the therapist emphasizes as a helpful "take-home message." We often build up stressful situations in our mind, due to our thinking traps, but once we engage in them, we find that they are easier than expected. Consistent with the behavioral experiment model, the therapist asks Abby-Lynn if any of her feared outcomes occurred. Abby-Lynn could not identify any. Indeed, Abby-Lynn accomplished each of her behavioral goals. The therapist takes the time to review each step with Abby-Lynn, identifies any challenges she encountered, and reinforces the coping skills she used to persist. Most importantly, the therapist prompts the youth to receive her reward. Here, the therapist lavishes specific praise on Abby-Lynn's ability to push through a stressful moment and to recall her coping thoughts. She also prompts Abby-Lynn to praise herself and asks her to list what specific skills she was most proud of using. Together, they took the next 5 minutes of therapy "off" to search for the closest frozen yogurt places near Abby-Lynn's school.

Behavioral experiments do not always go according to plan, and in fact, ambiguous outcomes are as, if not more, valuable in helping test out coping skills as clearly successful outcomes. In this case, Kelly might not have responded immediately for any number of reasons. These reasons may not have had anything to do with her interest in talking or hanging out with Abby-Lynn, but absent or ambiguous text responses would understandably arouse fears and anxious thoughts. In those moments, remind the youth of their coping thoughts and proceed with planned goals as appropriate. In this situation, Abby-Lynn could have completed a series of texts without having even gotten a response from Kelly. It would not have been entirely socially inappropriate to write three separate texts: "What was Mr. Whitmore talking about today???" "It's been too long, let's hang out." "Fro-yo?" Each would have served as an opportunity to practice coping in the face of ambiguous outcomes and each would have deserved praise. Recall, we cannot control the outcomes of life; we can only do our part to bring about the desired results.

IN VIVO EXPOSURE TO SUSTAINED EFFORT: COMPLETING WRITTEN ASSIGNMENTS

Figure 6.12 is an exposure worksheet as completed by Abby-Lynn (again, a blank version is available as Worksheet 6 in Appendix A) that illustrates a challenge designed to give the teen practice at pushing through situations that call for sustained effort and to help her appreciate the benefits of perseverance. Abby-Lynn has noted that she often quits and withdraws (crashes on bed, watches YouTube) when it is time to do homework, especially when completing writing assign-

WORKSHEET 6. *In Vivo* Exposure/Behavioral Experiment

> Complete this worksheet with the youth as you are preparing for a behavioral experiment.

1. Situation (What's the situation?):

Have to write a bio of a historical figure—I don't care and it'll take forever

2. Feelings: **Distress Rating:** _80_

Frustrated, unmotivated

3. Anxious/Negative Thoughts:	**Thinking Traps (See list below.)**

3. Anxious/Negative Thoughts:

"Why bother? This is a stupid assignment."
"This is going to take so long; I just don't have it in me."

Thinking Traps (See list below.)

Looking for the negatives; discounting the positives
Catastrophizing; discounting the positives

Thinking Traps: mind reading, fortune-telling, catastrophizing, jumping to conclusions, what if's, discounting the positives, looking for the negatives, overgeneralizing, all-or-nothing thinking, should statements, taking things too personally, blaming.

4. Coping Thoughts (How do you respond to your anxious thoughts?):

Focusing on the negative: "You have to do it, so make the best of it."
Catastrophizing: "Work for the break." "Every step is one step further than I took yesterday."

Challenge Questions: Do I know for certain that _____? Am I 100% sure that _____? What evidence do I have that _____? What is the worst that could happen? How bad is that? Do I have a crystal ball?

5. Achievable Behavioral Goals (What do you want to accomplish?):

Goal	Accomplished?
a. Turn on the computer.	
b. Read assignment.	
c. Bullet-point thoughts about first paragraph.	
d. Write one sentence.	

6. Rewards:

Reward	Earned?
a. Praise self; repeat coping thought: "Every step is one step further...."	
b. Get to sip favorite coffee drink.	
c. 5-min break with jumping jacks and stretching.	
d. Watch 5 min of YouTube.	

FIGURE 6.12. Completed behavioral experiment worksheet to help client sustain effort.

ments. To give Abby-Lynn practice at pushing through the urge to quit, she agreed to bring in a writing assignment and work on it in session (see item 11 in Challenge Hierarchy A). As with behavioral experiments, it is helpful to identify the negative assumptions the youth is making in confronting such a challenge. Here, Abby-Lynn presumes the effort it will take to complete the task is insurmountable and painful. Relatedly (or as a result of her negative attitudes), she finds the assignment boring and unrelated to her interests. These thoughts demonstrate mild catastrophizing ("This is going to take so long"), but they mostly reflect the fact that the required effort will be unpleasant. This is an example of emotional reasoning, where the youth assumes a task is unachievable because of the distress they feel about it. In these cases, validate the youth's feelings ("I know writing is a struggle for you" "It can feel impossible to know where to start") and provide encouraging statements that orient them to generating proactive coping statements (empathize and encourage). Here, Abby-Lynn comes up with coping thoughts ("I might as well make the most of it" "Work for the break") that remind her this challenge is within her capacity. She recalls how her basketball coach would treat the team when they were drilling. "Whenever we would do two-a-days, she would always break the drills up and then push us to earn the water breaks." Thus, Abby-Lynn uses the experience of pushing herself physically to take a similar approach to mental/academic exercises. "If I think of them as brief drills, I think I can get through these assignments."

Goals are established that mimic brief outcome-focused drills. Each step (e.g., turning on the computer, finding the assignment, initiating any form of writing) had derailed Abby-Lynn in the past because she felt that every step unlocked further steps in an unending series of tasks. She had experienced frustration after completing tasks, instead of accomplishment, because she saw no end in sight. The act of outlining her required tasks for this exposure gives her a sense of concrete finality, and instituting breaks in between each step gives her something to look forward to ("Work for the break"). The therapist also encourages a realistic, self-nurturing approach by reminding Abby-Lynn that she doesn't have to complete all components of the challenge—they are merely goals. She reserves the right to stop at any time. In this way, completing each task brings her a sense of meaningful accomplishment. Completing more tasks would be even more awesome, but stopping at any point does not detract from earlier achievements. With that encouragement, Abby-Lynn and the therapist also derive this key coping thought, "Every step I take is one step further than I took yesterday." Accordingly, the rewards are designed to fit naturally into Abby-Lynn's writing workflow (i.e., could serve as natural stopping points, but not distract her from returning to the writing task). The final reward (watching 5 minutes of YouTube) reflects one of Abby-Lynn's behavioral traps (withdrawing with YouTube). While the therapist at first hesitated, not wanting to reinforce the notion of YouTube as Abby-Lynn's ultimate reward, she agreed in keeping with the mantra of "Work for the break." To motivate short bursts of activation, truly gratifying rewards are needed.

Conducting a sustained effort exposure is similar to other distress tolerance exposures in that the goal is to present the youth with a challenging task, to get them to notice when "quitting" feelings (apathy, boredom, frustration, unease) surface, and to help them bear those feelings as they get over the hump (push through) and continue with the task. Typically, one "hump" is a series of multiple humps to be navigated. Reminding the youth to recall coping statements can help them ride the emotional waves. The therapist can also elect to solicit distress ratings at regular intervals to track distress and demonstrate afterward that distress ebbs and flows over the course of a challenge. In this exposure, the therapist prompts Abby-Lynn to initiate the first step (turn on the computer), after which Abby-Lynn nonchalantly responds, "No big deal. See this isn't going to be like when I'm at home." Abby-Lynn turns on the computer and the therapist insists that she praise herself and repeat her coping thought ("Every step I take is one step further than I took yesterday"). When the therapist nudges her to find and read the assignment, Abby-Lynn starts to protest:

ABBY-LYNN: This just isn't like it is at home. When I have someone to watch me, I can do it.

THERAPIST: That's OK if it's easier. Just like in basketball, you practice your drills in low-pressure situations to prepare for game time.

ABBY-LYNN: I just don't see the point.

THERAPIST: I wonder if this is one of your behavioral traps? What is your distress rating thinking about opening your assignment?

ABBY-LYNN: No . . . oh, I guess 75. I just don't want to do it.

THERAPIST: We seem to be climbing up the challenge hump. What coping thought can we use here?

ABBY-LYNN: No . . . uh, Work for the break.

THERAPIST: So, let's push over the hump so we get to the next break.

ABBY-LYNN: Aaargh! I hate this. (*Abby-Lynn searches through her laptop to find her assignment. She opens a document.*) There, I found it. Happy?

THERAPIST: What was your goal for this drill?

ABBY-LYNN: To finish a paragraph.

THERAPIST: No, just this step.

ABBY-LYNN: To read the assignment.

THERAPIST: OK, read the assignment. Distress rating?

ABBY-LYNN: Ugggh. 80. [*Abby-Lynn reads out loud the assignment: to write an essay on a historical figure.*]

THERAPIST: Nice!!! That's awesome. There were some rocky moments there, but you really pushed yourself over the reading hump. How does it feel?

ABBY-LYNN: Relieved. I just want to stop.

THERAPIST: Well, first reward yourself with a drink of your caramel macchiato! If that's not working for the break, I don't know what is?!

ABBY-LYNN: I can't believe I'm doing this.

The exposure continues in this way, wherein the therapist acts as a coach pushing her athlete through her drills while also continually assessing where the youth gets stuck: Where are her natural behavioral traps, where does she escape or avoid, and when does frustration take over? Throughout, Abby-Lynn's tone reflects a mixed sense of disbelief ("Why am I doing this?") and surprise ("I can't believe I finished this step"). We take that iterative process as an index of a successful exposure—sufficiently activating to cause hesitation and protest, but achievable enough for the youth to accomplish goals.

Evidence suggests that learning can be enhanced in exposures when individuals are held at a high level of challenge throughout the exposure (Craske et al., 2014). The goal is to demonstrate that the individual can survive high levels of distress and that feared consequences do not occur even when distressed. While no concrete criterion has been set for optimal distress to target in an exposure, we aim to maintain our clients in the 70–85 range out of a 100-point distress scale (or 7–8 out of 10). This activation level ensures sufficient stimulation of fear and distress structures while keeping the client in the exposure. If a client escapes or becomes dissociated, learning is also defeated. If a therapist senses that an exposure is too easy for a client, the therapist can use imagery or spontaneous challenges to raise the challenge level. For example, in Abby-Lynn's homework exposure, the therapist could have prompted Abby-Lynn to envision her bedroom, to recall past homework failures, or offered criticism that she received from her mother or teacher. The therapist evokes these memories not to discourage Abby-Lynn, but to arouse the same level of emotional intensity that she feels in real-life circumstances. Likewise, the therapist can add challenges that intensify the emotional valence of each task. When bullet-pointing her thoughts about the first paragraph of the essay, the therapist could prompt Abby-Lynn to add additional subpoints or to justify each point with a conversation. After completing all four tasks, the therapist can also continue the challenge by moving on to subsequent paragraphs. If the therapist chooses this approach, they must first celebrate the accomplishment of the initial four goals. Next the therapist can suggest that Abby-Lynn continue the same process with as much of the essay that she will tolerate. In the end, if writing in front of the therapist is easy, then Abby-Lynn will still come away with the experience of having completed a task that had previously remained incomplete, thus achieving a meaningful functional outcome!

WORKING WITH FAMILIES: COMMUNICATION AND PROBLEM SOLVING

At various points in therapy, it became apparent that conflict and misunderstandings between Abby-Lynn and her mother contributed to Abby-Lynn's negative mood and inhibited her from using her skills fully. For example, one weekend, Abby-Lynn turned down an outing with friends because her mother had lectured her a few days prior about getting more homework done. Another time, Abby-Lynn skipped basketball practice because her mother had asked her to lead an OT session with her younger brother. In each situation, Abby-Lynn could point to a reason as to why she was turning down friends or missing practice, contributing to her social isolation, withdrawal, and inactivity. What was unclear is if Abby-Lynn's mother was also aware of the consequences of these choices, or if alternative solutions could have worked in each situation. How much of each situation was due to immutable circumstances, how much was related to Abby-Lynn's defeatist and discouraged stance, and what kinds of creative solutions could be pursued with direct problem solving and open communication? When the therapist noticed these conflicts, she arranged for joint sessions with Abby-Lynn and her mother.

In one session, the therapist supported Abby-Lynn by inviting the mother to attend the session and problem-solve the teen's difficulty in completing homework. Importantly, the therapist and Abby-Lynn discussed the agenda and goals for this session ahead of time. The therapist helped the family identify a common problem (improving homework) while acknowledging other interests (maintaining social connections), brainstorming solutions, and trying them out. While attempting to orient Abby-Lynn and her mother around the first part of STEPS (say what the problem is), the therapist used a form of *communication analysis* (e.g., Young, Mufson, & Benas, 2014) to help each person acknowledge what the other person was saying and to align around common goals. Here's how this looked:

THERAPIST: We've been working on helping Abby-Lynn improve her consistency in completing her homework, and we've come to see how hard it is for her. Mom, I can understand how concerned you are about her grades, but I think we also want to make sure Abby-Lynn's getting out and seeing friends. If she has these social contacts, there will be more incentive to doing her work and having a reason to finish her work.

MOM: I get that, and I didn't know she had turned down hanging out with her friends because of our argument.

ABBY-LYNN: How could you not know that? You yelled at me the day before telling me I was going to be a failure if I didn't get my grades up!

MOM: I didn't say you were going to be a failure, Abby-Lynn. But you can't not do your homework and pass your classes.

ABBY-LYNN: I'm passing my classes! I'm getting C's and B's in all my classes.

MOM: But you've wanted to go to State since you were a little kid. You need better grades than that.

[*Silence.*]

THERAPIST: So, can we do a little experiment? Can you each summarize what the other person is saying?

ABBY-LYNN: She wants me to get good grades.

THERAPIST: Mom, is that what you're trying to say?

MOM: Well, I don't care about grades just for grades sake. I thought that's what Abby-Lynn wanted.

THERAPIST: Abby-Lynn, what do you hear when your mom says that?

ABBY-LYNN: I don't know. I guess she wants me to do the best that I can. . . .

THERAPIST: Or, maybe she's wanting to help you on your goals? Mom, what do you hear?

MOM: She thinks I think she's a failure, but I don't.

THERAPIST: Abby-Lynn, what do you hear? Do you think your mom thinks you're a failure?

ABBY-LYNN: No . . . It's just a lot of pressure. And I don't want to fail either.

THERAPIST: So, it sounds like you both kind of agree that we just want Abby-Lynn to do as best she can, but it can be hard.

MOM/ABBY-LYNN: I guess so.

From this, the therapist helps Abby-Lynn and her mother narrow down to a specific goal of increasing the amount of homework she completes in the next week (moving from half to 75%), with the expectation that Friday nights are kept free for her friends' weekly get-together. To assist in the brainstorming step (thinking of solutions), the therapist has Abby-Lynn and her mother list as many solutions as each can think of on separate pieces of paper, following this approach so that they will not interfere with each other's creative solutions. Occasionally, the therapist throws out a prompt suggesting a creative but far-fetched solution (e.g., pay someone else to do it; move to a pull-out classroom where homework is easier). Once Abby-Lynn and her mother have generated a range of solutions, the therapist asks the pair to list them all collectively on a whiteboard and then identify the strengths and weaknesses of each (examining each solution). The solutions that seemed to have the best ratio of pros to cons focused on breaking assignments into small increments, taking breaks, and rewarding completion. Examples include the following:

1. Post for 5 minutes on Instagram after every 15 minutes of completed homework.
2. Walk around the block after completing an assignment.
3. Ask the babysitter to watch Abby-Lynn's younger brother on an afternoon when she wants to do homework.

Abby-Lynn and her mother select these three options to try out and also institute a rewards plan that includes daily rewards (Abby-Lynn will get out of washing the dinner dishes if she completes 75% of her homework that day) and weekly rewards (Mom will pay for Abby-Lynn's movie ticket on Friday if Abby-Lynn hits 75% for 3 out of 5 days) to give acknowledgment to incremental and sustained efforts.

By involving the parent at key moments, the therapist serves several goals, including helping to improve communication between Abby-Lynn and her mother to reduce conflicts around misunderstandings. The therapist aims also to improve and strengthen their relationship to bolster Abby-Lynn's social support network. Furthermore, through joint problem solving, Abby-Lynn practices proactive assertiveness and problem solving that will help her counter the negative assumption that her mother might be unmoved by her concerns. In addition, the therapist is able to shape the mother's parenting behaviors to become more clear in her communications with Abby-Lynn; this increases active listening and empathizing statements, and supports Abby-Lynn's efforts and incremental successes with praise and rewards.

PROGRESS MONITORING

After 16 weeks of therapy, Abby-Lynn had demonstrated improvement across a number of primary goals and symptom profiles. The therapist assessed the progress of her therapy goals every week because they required simple, single-item endorsement. In addition, every 4 weeks, the therapist asked Abby-Lynn and her mother to complete the RCADS so there would be a standardized assessment of anxiety and depression symptoms over time. This enabled the therapist to compare Abby-Lynn's generalized anxiety and depression symptoms to representative norms monthly while tracking individual goals more frequently.

A review of Abby-Lynn's RCADS scores over the 16 weeks shows how change occurred during the course of treatment (see Figure 6.13). Depressive symptoms as reported by Abby-Lynn and her mother seemed to change first, suggesting that the initial behavioral activation and problem solving matched with Abby-Lynn's need to feel less stuck. Increasing her pleasant activities and giving her a way to approach challenges provided an immediate boost to her confidence and helped overcome discouragement. By Week 8, Abby-Lynn had obtained the majority of the relief she would experience with regard to depression; the second half of therapy saw mostly stable

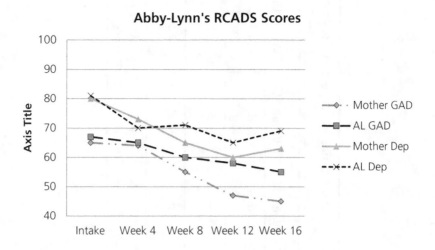

FIGURE 6.13. Ratings of Abby-Lynn's anxiety and depression symptoms as reported by the teen and her mother.

depressive symptoms that hovered just below the clinical threshold. This early response in treatment is not uncommon among clients receiving CBT for depression, and this kind of early gain can signal a good overall prognosis (Renaud et al., 1998; Tang & DeRubeis, 1999). Abby-Lynn's generalized anxiety symptoms took a slower and more gradual trajectory from intake to termination. This may reflect the greater chronicity of worry and anxiety that Abby-Lynn had experienced long before her depressed mood set in. Recovery from anxiety may have benefited from engaging in more positive experiences and then challenging deeply held beliefs about her abilities and how others viewed her. The behavioral experiments allowed Abby-Lynn to formally test and challenge her worry beliefs.

Reviewing the goal trackers as completed by Abby-Lynn and her mother also provided a personalized way for the therapist to monitor progress and discuss change with the teen (see Figure 6.14; a blank version is available as Worksheet 11 in Appendix A). Each week, the therapist assessed Abby-Lynn's progress on desired outcomes to set priorities and identify problem areas. The therapist and Abby-Lynn collaboratively agreed to attempt behavioral goals first because they seemed more concrete, easier to initiate, and simpler to monitor for success. Early on, Abby-Lynn increased her number of social engagements and enjoyable activities (e.g., basketball, social media), which may have contributed to early mood alleviation. Abby-Lynn's mother also reported that her daughter had completed a greater proportion of her homework in the first few weeks, potentially contributing to an improved sense of accomplishment and, pragmatically, freeing time up to spend with friends. Abby-Lynn's feelings of being overwhelmed changed on a slower course as she reported, and this is consistent with her RCADS scores. Thus, as therapy progressed, the therapist could see that their work was having a positive effect on behavioral goals early on, which would increase the teen's joy and open up reinforcing opportunities. The therapist could also observe that distressed feelings were improving at a slower rate and deserved greater attention in the second half of therapy. In this way, progress monitoring provided an ongoing check that the dyad was headed in the right direction. It could also be used to give Abby-Lynn explicit feedback if she were to become discouraged at any point. Frequently depressed youth will minimize success and express negative hopes for future change. Using individualized and standard assessments

WORKSHEET 11. Goals Tracker

Work with your therapist to brainstorm possible specific, meaningful, and achievable goals. Think out what outcomes you expect to see. And then, keep track of how your child does each week.

Parent Goals	Desired Outcomes	Week x	Week 14	Week 15	Week 16
Improve sad mood; enjoy life more.	Rate sad mood (0–10) Rate weekly enjoyment (0–10).	…	Sad: 4 Joy: 6	Sad: 3 Joy: 7	Sad: 2 Joy: 8
Decrease isolation (hanging out in room all day, napping).	Frequency of hang-outs with friends (inside and outside house)	…	4	3	3
Improve sleep.	Number of times she wakes up at night	…	2	1	0
Handle responsibilities like grades and basketball.	Handing in homework (%) Practices attended (%)	…	HW: 90% Practice: 95%	HW: 95% Practice: 100%	HW: 95% Practice: 100%

FIGURE 6.14. Abby-Lynn's Goals Tracker worksheet at the conclusion of treatment.

gives the therapist concrete data to discuss with their client when they have made progress and to indicate where they may still need to do continued work.

TERMINATION AND RELAPSE PREVENTION

Given research that suggests effective treatments can have a meaningful impact within 8 to 12 weeks (Brent et al., 2008; March et al., 2004), the therapist initially proposed a therapy plan consisting of about 10 meetings before reevaluation. At Week 10, the family had seen noticeable change in depression and anxiety symptoms and improvement in the personal goals Abby-Lynn had set. The teen had completed several behavioral experiments by this time and was feeling more confident, but both she and her mother decided continued practice would help consolidate her gains and generalize her skills across settings. For example, Abby-Lynn had become comfortable asking her basketball teammates to hang out after practice, but she still had difficulty talking to new people and initiating friendships. As a result, the family agreed to continue for another six to eight sessions to practice building Abby-Lynn's social network and to keep her rhythm going with schoolwork.

At Session 16, the family reconvened to discuss therapy progress and future plans. Since the last check-in, Abby-Lynn had initiated a new friendship with a classmate in her math class with whom she could study. Abby-Lynn also spent fewer Friday nights at home. Along the way, the therapist had led family sessions to address misunderstandings in communication. Abby-Lynn's sleep hygiene was also addressed. Given the continued progress and Abby-Lynn's growing confidence, the therapist suggested that this acute phase of therapy might be coming to an end. The therapist suggested that occasional booster sessions could be helpful (Clarke, Rohde, Lewinsohn, Hops, & Seely, 1999; Gearing et al., 2013), but that ending weekly sessions would allow Abby-Lynn to practice skills on her own. Abby-Lynn and her mother agreed to attend two more weekly sessions (Sessions 17–18) and to then return to biweekly meetings (Sessions 19–22) after that to conduct check-in's and reinforce growth.

As therapy came to an end (Sessions 21–22), the therapist reviewed the lessons that Abby-Lynn had learned and highlighted the unique accomplishments she had made in the prior months. These included establishing concrete friendships, strengthening communication with her mother, and becoming more adept at structuring homework time. The therapist provided copies of Abby-Lynn's progress-monitoring graphs (symptoms and target goals) to illustrate her improvement. The therapist also listened to Abby-Lynn's worries and doubts about ending therapy and maintaining her success without supports. The therapist reminded her of the natural supports Abby-Lynn had developed as a function of her good work (friends, family, teachers) and reviewed how to access these supports when needed. The therapist reviewed the concepts of "lapse," "relapse," and "collapse" (see Chapter 3) to set realistic expectations. Abby-Lynn felt reassured by the therapist's confidence in her and also looked forward to updating the therapist on her progress at monthly check-ins.

SUMMARY AND KEY POINTS

Abby-Lynn came to therapy in a state of significant discouragement and worry with regard to her place at school and with friends and family. Her self-doubt was perpetuating a downward spiral that prevented her from accessing her strengths and moving toward her personal goals. Through a course of CBT, her therapist helped build a strong working alliance with Abby-Lynn, one focused on common goals, and then tailored interventions that would supplement Abby-Lynn's strengths and fortify her limitations. Below are key points from this successful collaboration that can be applied with other clients:

- Build a strong working alliance with your client through active listening; comprehensive, holistic assessment; and matching interventions to their needs and strengths.
- Assessments that include diagnosis, symptoms, and personal goals can help you develop a holistic picture of the youth's social context, daily functioning, concerns, strengths and limits. Compare past to present functioning.
- Conduct targeted functional assessments when there are sticking points. Where does the youth get stuck? What emotions do they feel? How does the youth respond? What keeps them stuck in that cycle?
- Active engagement and pleasant and mastery experiences can provide an initial push and early relief when sad feelings and inertia are problematic.
- Reward programs (from self and others) can help reinforce efforts to move and cope.
- Problem solving and cognitive restructuring can help youth learn active coping strategies to change a situation when possible and to adapt to the situation when they have less control.
- Behavioral challenges and exposures consolidate skills and produce new learning opportunities that talking cannot replicate.
- Monitoring progress and providing feedback throughout therapy help keep you on track and can provide valuable feedback to the youth.

CHAPTER 7

Suicidal Behaviors
and Nonsuicidal Self-Injury

Suicidal ideation (SI) and behaviors, including nonsuicidal self-injury (NSSI), are common in depressed and anxious youth. Clients and caregivers may identify SI and NSSI as part of the initial presenting problems, or they may surface at any point in therapy. Despite their common presence, SI and NSSI can be challenging and frightening to manage, even for the experienced clinician (Dexter-Mazza & Freeman, 2003; Feldman & Freedenthal, 2006). This chapter provides guidelines for how therapists can conduct risk assessments, devise a risk designation, create safety plans, and address suicidal phenomena and NSSI as part of ongoing treatment.

PREVALENCE AND IMPACT OF SUICIDAL IDEATION
AND SUICIDE ATTEMPT

In the general population, thoughts about death, dying, and killing oneself (SI) are relatively common, identifiable in nearly 10% of adults (Nock et al., 2008). In adolescents, nearly 3% report SI at any one time, and upward of 19% of teens report a lifetime history of ideation (Lewinsohn, Rohde, & Seeley, 1996). Rates of SI are even more common among clinical samples, in which nearly 30% of youth meeting criteria for major depression report some form of suicidality during the past year and over 10% report a suicide attempt (SA) (Avenevoli et al., 2015).

The risks of attempting or completing a suicide are real. Recent figures by the Centers for Disease Control and Prevention (CDC, 2022; *www.cdc.gov/vitalsigns/suicide*) show an increase in suicides by Americans of 36% from 2000 to 2018. In the Youth Risk Behavior Surveillance System, which monitors various health risk behaviors, 18% of teens reported having seriously considered suicide, 15% of teens reported having made a plan for an attempted suicide, 9% had reported having made one or more attempts over the previous year, and 3% described having made an attempt that required them to get medical attention (Kann et al., 2016). Physical harm to oneself where there is at least some intent to kill oneself (SA) has been identified in an alarming number of high school students, with 9% reporting a suicide attempt in the past 12 months CDC, 2022). Accordingly, suicide has become the second leading cause of death in young people 10–24 years old, accounting for over 5,000 deaths in a year (Sullivan et al., 2015). An estimated 804,000 lives were lost to suicide worldwide in 2012 (World Health Organization [WHO], 2014). The methods by which people kill themselves are commonly available in American homes. In the general population, death by firearm is the most common method for suicide, followed by suffocation and poisoning (Jack et al., 2018). For adolescents, hanging has been identified as the most frequent method for attempting suicide (Kolves & De Leo, 2017; Sullivan, Annest, Simon, Luo, & Dahlberg, 2015). Furthermore, over half of people who died by suicide over the last decade-and-a-half did not have a known mental health condition (CDC, 2022). Thus, clinical disorders like depression call for particular alertness, but the risk of suicidal ideation and behaviors come with any client who seeks care.

PREVALENCE AND IMPACT OF NSSI

NSSI is distinguished from suicidal behaviors by the absence of any observable intent to die. NSSI includes multiple forms of self-injury, including cutting, carving, burning, scratching, hitting oneself, and it occurs in an alarming proportion of youth (Nock, 2010). In general community samples, 13–45% of teens report having engaged in self-injury at some point in their lifetime (Lloyd-Richardson. Perrine, Dierker, & Kelley, 2007; Plener, Schumacher, Munz, & Groschwitz, 2015; Ross & Heath, 2002). In clinical samples of adolescents, 40–60% report prior self-injury, as NSSI often precipitates treatment referrals (Asarnow et al., 2011). The frequency of self-harm varies widely among those who engage in NSSI, from only a few times (< 10 lifetime episodes) to highly frequent among inpatient populations > 50 times) (Nock, 2010). While the wish to end one's life is not a principal directive in NSSI, the risk of unintentionally killing oneself or causing other serious bodily injury is high. Furthermore, NSSI is a robust predictor of SAs, particularly among adolescents with more severe and frequent NSSI (Asarnow et al., 2011; Hamza, Stewart, & Willoughby, 2012). Nock and colleagues (2006) reported that 70% of adolescents engaging in NSSI reported a lifetime SA and 55% of youth reported multiple attempts. A longer history of NSSI, use of a greater number of methods, and absence of physical pain during NSSI increase the likelihood of an SA. Even in the absence of eventual SAs, NSSI is correlated with significant psychological pain, bodily harm, and interpersonal/family distress and conflict (Nock, 2010).

RISK FACTORS AND PREDICTORS OF SUICIDAL AND NONSUICIDAL BEHAVIORS

The strongest predictor of future SAs is the occurrence of recent attempted suicide and self-injury. Heightened attention is required shortly after any crisis as the risk for repeated suicidal behavior is highest in the first 3 to 6 months after an attempt (Stanley et al., 2009). Comprehensive reviews provide evidence for multiple social and interpersonal factors that predict adolescent suicidality (King & Merchant, 2008; Auerbach, Stewart, & Johnson, 2016). Common circumstances that add to the risk of suicide and NSSI among individuals with or without a history of mental health issues include relationship problems/loss, life stressors, recent/impending crises, harmful use of alcohol, hopelessness, chronic pain, among other factors (Kiekens et al., 2017; Stone et al., 2018; WHO, 2014). Systemic and community factors also contribute to suicide risk, including barriers to health care access, access to means, inappropriate media reporting, stigma associated with seeking help, discrimination, and trauma/abuse, to name a few (WHO, 2014). Public policy matters too, as states with same-sex marriage legislations evidenced reductions in reported suicide by high school students (Raifman, Moscoe, Austin, & McConnell, 2017), and explicit and inclusive anti-bullying protections for sexual minority youth are associated with a reduction in SAs (Hatzenbuehler &

Keyes, 2013). Variations in youth demographics (age, sex, race, and ethnicity), gender identity and sexual orientation, pathology, and educational abilities may also help predict vulnerability to suicidal behaviors and self-harm.

Age, Sex, Race, and Ethnicity

Suicidal behavior and NSSI show similar developmental trajectories. Both are relatively rare before the ages of 11–12 and rise dramatically during adolescence (Nock et al., 2013). SI is more common in young females than males, with twice as many adolescent girls reporting lifetime SI than boys (Lewinsohn et al., 1996). However, boys account for nearly 2 to 4 times the completed suicides in America due to the more lethal methods they choose (CDC, 2018; Sullivan et al., 2015). A firearm was the leading mechanism of suicide for males, and suffocation was the leading cause for females. Sex differences extend to NSSI in both community and clinical samples (DiCorcia, Arango, Horwitz, & King, 2017; Sornberger, Heath, Toste, & McLouth, 2012). In an examination of teens presenting to a psychiatric emergency room (DiCorcia et al., 2017), adolescent girls reported about 50% more lifetime engagement in NSSI than boys (79% vs. 50%, respectively). Girls also endorsed using the methods of cutting, carving, burning, scraping skin, picking at wounds, and pulling out hair than boys, but no difference in hitting, punching, biting, inserting objects into skin and nails, or swallowing dangerous substances. Adolescent females also endorsed using NSSI to stop or numb bad feelings more than boys. Engaging in NSSI to communicate to others or stop suicidal urges was equally endorsed between girls and boys.

Little research has been conducted to specifically isolate the impact of race/ethnicity and culture on suicidal behaviors or NSSI (King & Merchant, 2008). However, national trends do show significant increases in rates of suicide across all racial/ethnic groups (White, Black, Asian, Native American, Hispanic, and non-Hispanic) of young people (ages 10–24) from 1994 to 2012 (Sullivan et al., 2015). In addition, certain racial and ethnic minority statuses (e.g., Black, Asian, Native American) are associated with reduced treatment seeking, particularly when symptoms are less severe (Nestor, Cheek, & Liu, 2016). Thus, early detection and intervention may be particularly challenging in minority communities.

Sexual Minorities

Membership in a sexual minority group is significantly associated with an increased risk for SI, SA, and NSSI (Batejan, Jarvi, & Swenson, 2015; Marshal et al., 2011). Identifying as lesbian, gay, or bisexual (LGB) conveys almost 3 times the risk for suicidality, with average estimates ranging from 15 to 49% of youth participating in some kind of suicidal behavior. Individuals identifying as transgender or gender nonconforming have an even higher rate of SI and SA, in which nearly half of trans men and women report a lifetime SA (Haas, Rodgers, & Herman, 2014). The escalated rates of suicidal ideation and behavior may result from the increased discrimination and peer victimization associated with being a sexual minority (Liu & Mustanski, 2012; Mueller, James, Abrutyn, & Levin, 2015). Special care is required in assessing risk in these vulnerable individuals.

Psychopathology, Developmental Disabilities, and Coping

Psychopathology and socioemotional distress are common in youth who report NSSI. In psychiatric inpatient populations (Nock et al., 2006), as many as 88% of adolescents engaging in

NSSI met the criteria for a DSM-IV Axis I diagnosis, including externalizing (63%), internalizing (52%), and substance use (60%) disorders. The majority (67%) also met the criteria for an Axis II personality disorder. In broader community samples, nearly 30% of youth with major depression reported some form of suicidality in the past year and 11% reported a SA. Youth with disabilities have higher levels of suicide than youth without them. In large community samples, elevated rates of SA were found in youth with autism spectrum disorder (ASD), sensory impairments, physical mobility disabilities, speech/language disabilities, and chronic health conditions (Moses, 2018). Coping styles that tend to be associated with pathology also predict SI in teens. For example, disengagement coping styles (use of avoidant and passive strategies to manage distress) are a strong predictor of SI among teens and young adults (Horwitz, Czyz, Berona, & King, 2018).

Reasons for and Functions of SI and NSSI

Evidence suggests a number of identifiable functions that NSSI serves for distressed youth. Youth who eventually attempt suicide tend to have a longer history of NSSI, using a greater number of methods. Thus, NSSI may serve as an early warning sign of later SAs.

Nock and colleagues (Nock, 2010; Nock & Prinstein, 2004) have provided support for a four-factor model describing the functions of NSSI that can help to identify and clarify intervention. Two factors describe NSSI functions in *intrapersonal* domains: one reflects a positive reinforcement function—"To feel something even if it is pain"—and the other reflects a negative reinforcement function—"To stop bad feelings." Two factors describe NSSI functions in *interpersonal* domains: one reflecting a positive—"To get a reaction out of someone" "To let others know I'm unhappy"—and the other reflecting a negative reinforcement function—"To avoid punishment from others" "To avoid something unpleasant." Through these four functions, NSSI serves as both a means of regulating one's emotional and cognitive experiences and way of communicating with or influencing others. Accordingly, the risk of NSSI is increased by the presence of distal risk factors (e.g., childhood abuse) that contribute to problems with affect regulation and interpersonal communication. Social influences (e.g., peer modeling) can escalate risk even further (Nock, 2010).

To understand risk in greater depth, research has explored the contextual features in which NSSI occurs. Youth self-reported data suggest that NSSI is typically performed impulsively (the youth contemplates it for a few minutes or less), without the use of alcohol or drugs, and experienced without pain (Nock & Prinstein, 2005). Reported greater pain was associated with a longer contemplation time. The number of friends who engage in NSSI is also correlated with endorsement of the positive social function of one's own NSSI, suggesting evidence for social modeling and social approval functions. Using an ecological momentary assessment (EMA; electronic diary) approach, research has also been able to identify more proximal contextual factors that precede self-harm behaviors (Nock, Prinstein, & Sterba, 2009). For example, NSSI and suicidal thoughts most typically began when a youth was socializing, resting, or listening to music. At the same time, youth most often indicated they were either alone or with a friend when NSSI or SI occurred. Drugs and alcohol were used minimally, and youth reported that worry, a bad memory, and feeling pressure most frequently led to the thought. In a small percentage of youth, NSSI followed encouragement by others. The odds of engaging in NSSI significantly increased when a youth was feeling rejected, angry toward themselves, self-hatred, numb, nothing, and anger toward another. Daily diaries also gave some suggestions for coping strategies that could help. Youth self-reported that changing thoughts, talking to others, doing homework, and going out were useful strategies to distract from NSSI. It is apparent that NSSI and SI can follow many individual triggers. Thus, it is incumbent on the clinician to conduct thorough idiographic functional assessment so that treatment can then be tailored to address the youth's needs and offer alternatives to self-harm.

SUICIDAL INCEPTION AND GROUP CONTAGION: WHAT ARE THE REAL RISKS?

Clinicians are sometimes reluctant to raise issues about suicide out of fear they will inadvertently create a risk that was not already there. Compelling data demonstrate that suicide risk screening and assessment do not increase the risk of distress or SI (e.g., Gould et al., 2005). Instead, assessment and safety planning can maintain, and even enhance, rapport through skilled assessment of thoughts and behaviors (Pettit, Buitron, & Green, 2018). A large experimental trial by Gould and colleagues (2005) randomly assigned high school students to receive a health care survey either with or without questions assessing suicidal ideation and behavior. There were no differences between the experimental and control group in distress, depressive feelings, or SI either immediately after the survey or 2 days later. High-risk students who had been identified with depressive symptoms, substance use problems, or SAs did not report any more distress or suicidality in either survey condition. On the contrary, depressed students and those with previous SAs appeared less distressed and suicidal after receiving the survey with suicide items, compared to the high-risk control students. Similar research has also been conducted for NSSI. Across three studies that exposed adolescents to repeated images or words of self-injurious thoughts and behaviors as part of an implicit attitude experiment, teens did not show any reliable increase in their desire to self-injure or desire to die (Cha et al., 2016). There was a moderate mood decline for females only, and only in response to images compared to words. These findings were consistent regardless of NSSI history. Given the evidence, clinicians can comfortably conduct risk assessments and inquire about suicidal thoughts and behaviors without fear of inserting suicidality where none existed (inception). Rather, it is imperative that the therapist conduct responsible, thorough, and sensitive assessment to determine the presence of any real risks (Pettit et al., 2018).

Effect of Personal Role Models and Media Exposure

In contrast to unrealistic fears of inception, therapists should be alerted to the occurrence of suicide clustering (contagion) and modeling. Evidence suggests a temporal relation between public suicide accounts (e.g., celebrities) and national and local suicide rates (Gould & Kramer, 2001; Stack, 2003, 2005). Geographic and temporal clustering of suicides has been identified in local regions (Baller & Richardson, 2002; Gould, Wallenstein, Kleinman, O'Carroll, & Mercy, 1990). One meta-analysis estimated that about one-third of suicide cases in the United States involve suicidal behavior following dissemination of a suicidal model in the media (Stack, 2005). Models can be real (e.g., celebrities, local individuals) or fictional (e.g., novels, TV shows), and one analysis suggested that youth are particularly at risk of suicide suggestion via fictional suicides (Stack, 2009). The duration of risk is relatively brief, such that greatest risk escalates rapidly after a salient suicide and gradually weakens over 2 to 4 weeks (Abrutyn & Mueller, 2014; Brent et al., 1989; Phillips, 1974; Stack, 1987).

There are factors that increase the risk of suicide contagion. The closeness that a youth feels toward the individual who committed suicide can be influential. Research suggests that suicides by personal role models (e.g., friends, family) trigger new suicidal thoughts (Abrutyn & Mueller, 2014). Girls tend to be more vulnerable than boys, and role models who are friends tend to be more influential than role models who are family members. At the same time, these effects fade over time, so the immediate period following a completed suicide is a time to watch closely. A therapist will want to be on heightened alert when a client's friend has attempted or completed suicide. The closer the friend, the greater the potential risk.

How the youth receives the news may also be important. Availability of vivid, detailed information about completed suicides in the media has been associated with increased risk (CDC, 2018; Gould, Kleinman, Lake, Forman, & Midle, 2014; WHO, 2014). As a result, suicide prevention organizations have offered guidelines for responsible reporting methods (http://reportingonsuicide.org). These guidelines emphasize the need to deglamorize coverage of SAs and to limit the amount of salacious details about suicide method. Risk of additional suicides (suicide contagion, copycat suicides) increases when a youth is exposed to media stories that explicitly describe the suicide method, use dramatic, graphic headlines or images, and when repeated coverage sensationalizes or glamorizes a death. When working with an at-risk teen, be aware of highly publicized suicides (both locally and globally) and assess the youth's proximity to the death or exposure to media coverage. You will want to assess for misperceptions and falsely optimistic views of suicide (e.g., "It seemed to work for him") or evidence that the youth is habituating to the consequences of suicide (e.g., "If she can do it, why shouldn't I?"). Therapists can also recommend that parents limit their child's exposure to media coverage of the suicide and coach parents in having open-ended conversations with their teen. Advise parents to start by asking what the youth has heard and then to insert fact-based education to normalize anxiety and sadness and to dispel misperceptions. In summary, responsible discussion of suicides in the community or in popular media should entail deglamorized fact-based presentation, limited exposure, and provision of supports and resources during discussion.

EFFECTIVE TREATMENTS FOR SI/NSSI

Although common, SI/NSSI will not ameliorate on its own. CBT has support for reducing SI and NSSI and reducing the distress surrounding suicidal behaviors, particularly for adults, though evidence is building for adolescent formats as well (Shaffer & Pfeffer, 2001; Brausch & Girresch, 2012). The typical length of stand-alone SI/NSSI treatments lasts 11 sessions but can range from 2 to 104 weeks. Formats and components most associated with successful CBT include individual, family-based, and school-based group formats (Paschall & Bersamin, 2018; Wolff et al., 2017; Stanley et al., 2009; Wasserman et al., 2015). Effective components include intensive early intervention with safety planning, chain analysis (functional assessment), and standard CBT skills (e.g., behavioral activation, problem solving, cognitive restructuring, parent education/training) (Wolff et al., 2017; Stanley et al., 2009). Dialectical behavior therapy (DBT) has also received support in reducing NSSI and suicide risk for adults, particularly as they occur in the context of borderline personality disorder (Hunnicutt Hollenbaugh, & Lenz, 2018). Because SI/NSSI commonly co-occurs in the presence of other mental health distress, this chapter presents strategies consistent with an initial detection (first session at which SI/NSSI is reported) and showcases a four-session treatment plan for conducting initial assessment, safety planning, and integration with other treatment goals (see Table 7.1).

TABLE 7.1. Modular Treatment Plan for Addressing Suicidal and Nonsuicidal Thoughts and Behaviors

First Session at Which SI/NSSI Is Detected

Assessment
- Suicidal and nonsuicidal ideation and actions (SI/NSSI) or suicidal attempts (SA) can occur at an initial intake or at any point in therapy. This first session refers to the initial point at which SI/NSSI or SA is detected. The assessment, psychoeducation, and intervention activities suggested in this first session are comprehensive and likely take longer than the traditional 50-minute session. However, the assessment, safety plan, and check-in system are necessary to ensure the youth's safety prior to allowing the youth to depart from the clinician's office.
- Assess the presence and severity of SI/NSSI with the Columbia-Suicide Severity Rating Scale (C-SSRS), Self-Injurious Thoughts and Behaviors Interview (SITBI), or diagnostic interview (e.g., ADIS, K-SADS).
- Organize scope of problem using the SHIP framework/worksheet: severity, history, intent, plan.
- Determine the acuity of risk using Pettit et al.'s (2018) algorithm for assessing acute suicide risk.

Psychoeducation
- Review the assessment and risk designation with the youth and their caregivers.
- Review key information using the SI/NSSI fact sheet.

Interventions
- Develop a safety plan (Stanley & Brown, 2012), identifying key risk factors, supports, and internal/external coping strategies.
- Create an SI intensity thermometer to provide common language between the caregiver and youth.
- Develop a check-in system to reduce the barriers that might prevent a youth from disclosing SI to caregivers. Frequency is based on the severity of SI/NSSI, and the nature of check-in is fit to family context.

Home practice
- Family implements a check-in system at the agreed-upon frequency and enacts appropriate elements of a safety plan as necessary.

Second Session after Which SI/NSSI Is Detected

Assessment
- Assess the presence of continued SI/NSSI with C-SSRS.
- Administer a depression symptom measure (e.g., Beck Depression Inventory [BDI]).

Interventions
- Assess if the caregivers or youth have new or continuing questions about SI/NSSI.
- Assess the family's reliability and fidelity in implementing a check-in system and safety plan as intended. Problem-solve adherence issues.
- Conduct chain analysis to determine the triggers and sequelae of SI/NSSI.

Home practice
- Family implements a revised check-in system and safety plan.
- Youth and/or caregivers complete a chain analysis of SI/NSSI.

(continued)

TABLE 7.1. *(continued)*

Third Session after Which SI/NSSI Is Detected

Assessment
- Assess the presence of continued SI/NSSI with C-SSRS.
- Review the depression symptom measure (e.g., BDI); readminister it weekly.

Interventions
- Problem-solve adherence issues with a check-in system and safety plan as needed.
- Review chain analysis of the youth's triggers and sequelae of SI/NSSI.
- Reconcile data on youth's SI/NSSI with other treatment goals (e.g., depression, anxiety, social isolation). In what ways are the treatment goals for SI/NSSI compatible with other treatment goals? In what ways will they require a unique focus?

Home practice
- Family implements a revised check-in system and safety plan.
- Youth and/or caregivers complete a chain analysis of SI/NSSI.

Fourth Session after Which SI/NSSI Is Detected

Assessment
- Assess the presence of continued SI/NSSI with C-SSRS.
- Review the depression symptom measure (e.g., BDI); readminister it weekly.

Interventions
- Review chain analysis of the youth's triggers and sequelae of SI/NSSI. Identify new triggers and greater insights into reinforcing functions.
- Integrate SI/NSSI focus into existing treatment plan, making use of CBT strategies that are being implemented for other treatment goals (e.g., behavioral activation, problem solving, cognitive restructuring).

Home practice
- Make use of home practice exercises consistent with relevant CBT strategies (as recommended in depression and anxiety chapters).

CASE VIGNETTE: LUZ

The case study that follows illustrates a CBT approach to (1) conducting risk assessments and introducing safety plans, (2) assessing the function of SI/NSSI, and (3) implementing SA/NSSI prevention strategies. All three components are commonly implemented at the beginning of any treatment course where SI/NSSI has been detected, often following a comprehensive assessment battery that indicates past or current SI/NSSI, and certainly when any past or recent SA has been reported. After a history or current risk of suicidal behavior has been detected, you will want to conduct ongoing monitoring of SI/NSSI regularly, depending on its severity, and revise the safety plan as needed. In the current case, we describe a targeted focus on the youth's suicidal ideation and behavior due to their severity and recency of SA.

Luz, a 16-year-old Latina cisgender female, was referred to an outpatient office as a step-down referral after having completed a 1-week inpatient stay and an 8-week intensive outpatient program (IOP) following her first SA. The SA consisted of Luz taking multiple (< 4) Xanax pills that she had gotten from a friend, sharing a bottle of wine, and making 3–4 horizontal cuts across her wrists using a razor blade. Her father found Luz conscious, but disoriented and intoxicated, crying in her bedroom holding a towel over her wrists. The father brought Luz by car to the emergency room, where she received a psychiatric assessment and was admitted to the adolescent inpatient unit. During her stay on the inpatient unit, Luz began taking an antidepressant medication (Lexapro) and a mood stabilizer (Seroquel). In the IOP, Luz participated in group process meetings and skills-building groups that provided introductions to distress tolerance and emotion regulation skills. Her father became involved in family sessions at the IOP and served as her primary caregiver. At discharge from the IOP, Luz's dose on Lexapro was stabilized and maintained, but the psychiatrist on staff discontinued the Seroquel. Luz was referred to outpatient treatment to prevent future SA and NSSI and reinforce her coping skills to regulate stressors.

Upon outpatient intake, the father reported that he first saw Luz's mood start to decline about 3 years prior, when the parents' conflict intensified and they ultimately decided to divorce. The mother remarried shortly thereafter and moved out of state with her new husband. Luz's younger sister (10 years old) moved with her mother, but it was decided that Luz should remain with her father, to maintain stability as she entered high school. Luz agreed with her father's assessment: that her parent's divorce, the splitting up of the family, and her mother's decision to "leave me behind" contributed to her self-doubt, depressed mood, and social withdrawal. At age 14 (in the ninth grade), she felt socially isolated and was spending less time with her established friends and gravitating to a new group of schoolmates whom she described as "moody" and "kind of outsiders." Luz reported that her first instance of NSSI (scratching herself with a nail clipper) occurred at the end of ninth grade after she heard her friends talking about doing it. It was also a stressful period as her grades were declining and Luz had withdrawn from most activities at school.

Luz's NSSI occurred sporadically but frequently during intense episodes (e.g., multiple times per day over 2–3 weeks), and the method and harm intensified with time. Prior to her admission to the hospital, her most severe NSSI consisted of exacting 4- to 5-inch cuts in her thighs or torso with a razor blade and watching them bleed for minutes before blotting the cuts with a towel. She usually cut herself during stressful times, such as when she failed to keep up with schoolwork or experienced social rejection or victimization. Luz was open about her NSSI with her friends. Her father noticed cuts on three or four occasions and demanded that Luz stop but he rarely followed up. In the tenth grade (when she was 15), the father sought outpatient treatment for Luz. She attended about 12 sessions, did not find them helpful, and so terminated treatment.

At the current therapy's intake, Luz reported that peer rejection and bullying played a significant role in her NSSI and recent SA. Luz disclosed that she was attracted to both males and females and had pursued sexual activity with both sexes. She did not feel comfortable with labeling her sexual orientation as "bisexual," but instead preferred to describe herself as "questioning" and "unsure." Other times she sounded more self-assured and described herself as "queer" and "liking both." Prior to her SA, Luz had begun a discreet relationship with another girl in her grade at school. The girl's "boyfriend" found out about their relationship and confronted Luz in the school hallway in front of other students. The boy shoved Luz against the locker, pinning her there for minutes before a teacher intervened. Parents and legal authorities became involved, and the boy was ultimately suspended. Before long, it seemed everyone at the school was aware of the incident, and the story became a major source of gossip and aggression toward Luz. Peers at the school and in the surrounding community expressed anger and disgust at Luz on social media sites, and homophobic threats against her were made through public and private venues. Supportive messages were far fewer. The school issued formal statements condemning physical aggression but insisted it could not intervene in Web-based activities. Luz's father was protective of Luz, telling her he would defend her against any physical violence, but he was also invalidating about sexual orientation that suggested Luz had contributed to the initial assault and resulting social rejection.

After several weeks of gossip and threats, Luz went to a friend's house and shared a bottle of wine with her. She also took Xanax that the friend had procured from her parents' medicine cabinet. After commiserating with her friend about the intensifying bullying, Luz went home and cut her wrists with a razor she had used previously to cut herself. She was surprised by how deep she had cut her wrists and by how long she let the wounds bleed, but she also remembered having clear thoughts about death and killing herself: "Everyone else wants me to die. I might as well just keep going." Luz eventually covered her cuts with a towel, helping to stop the bleeding (about 20–30 minutes after cutting herself), but continued to feel ambivalent about living.

Suicide Risk Assessment and Designation

Suicidal risk can occur at any point in therapy, and patients may present as being at acute risk and/or chronic, ongoing risk. Therapists can prepare themselves by having relevant resources readily available when the occasion arises. A number of assessment measures and systems are available (for a review, see Goldston & Compton, 2007; Wingate, Joiner, Walker, Rudd, & Jobes, 2004). Formal suicide screens help structure the risk assessment and can normalize the process by demonstrating that the questions included are routine. We recommend two measures that are easy to administer, publicly available, and have established reliability and validity. The Columbia-Suicide Severity Rating Scale (C-SSRS; Posner et al., 2011; *http://cssrs.columbia.edu*) is a clinician-administered measure that asks five questions about the presence and intensity of SI (e.g., wish to be dead, thoughts about killing oneself) and presence of intent and plan for both lifetime and past month time frames. If the youth has already made an attempt, detailed questions are asked about the method and lethality. The Self-Injurious Thoughts and Behaviors Interview (SITBI; Nock, Holmberg, Photos, & Michel, 2007) is a 169-item structured interview that assesses the presence, frequency, and characteristics of five types of self-injurious phenomena: SI, suicide plans, suicide gestures, SAs, and NSSI. Many structured diagnostic interviews (e.g., Anxiety Disorders Interview Schedule [ADIS], Kiddie Schedule for Affective Disorders and Schizophrenia [K-SADS]) also include questions that assess for the presence of SI and SA.

At the time of intake, the therapist was aware of Luz's SA and past NSSI behaviors. The therapist conducted the C-SSRS to determine current risk. Luz reported that she still experienced a significant degree of anxiety and tension and episodic SI, but she had no intention of making any attempts at the current time. Specifically, Luz reported chronic mild SI nearly every day but no current plan or intent. She could not guarantee that she would never make another SA; she wanted to "keep it as an option." However, she felt she was presently safe and not at acute risk.

After collecting relevant data on SI and past SAs, we recommend that the therapist organize the information in a conceptual heuristic. Much like the use of a CBT conceptualization, having an organizing framework helps the therapist conceptualize risk and lays the groundwork for safety planning. We use the acronym SHIP (severity, history, intent, plan) as a heuristic to organize our assessment of SI, SA, and NSSI and to help clinicians recall relevant data as they are assessing level of risk.

S: Severity

Severity refers to frequency, persistence (controllability, duration), and intensity (intrusiveness, subjective distress) of suicidal thoughts. Does the child experience SI monthly, weekly, or multiple times a day? Are the SI fleeting thoughts that come and go, or do they reflect persistent rumination that the youth can't shake? What is the youth's subjective experience of the SI? Is the intensity mild, equivalent to diffuse thoughts about death? Or, is the SI highly intense, intrusive, and pressing for action? The greater the intensity and frequency, the greater the severity and potential risk.

H: History

History refers to the chronicity and pattern of SI and SA. It also includes common risk factors, such as NSSI, drug and alcohol use, access to methods, availability of social models who have attempted or committed suicide, and social isolation. Is the current episode the first episode of SI? Does it reflect an ongoing pattern of dark, hopeless rumination? Does the youth have any history of NSSI or SA? Is there a history of trauma and/or stressors that tend to trigger SI and SA, and are those stressors present in the youth's current life? Does the youth have a history of acting impulsively in a dangerous way? Research has suggested that general impulsivity does not indicate greater suicide risk, but other research posits that specific NSSI and SA acts are enacted impulsively in the moment (Nock, 2010). It behooves the clinician to note past incidents where the youth hurt themself "accidentally" or their present impulsive decisions that could lead to unintentional harm (e.g., driving recklessly; alcohol and drug use; severe isolation; missing curfew).

I: Intent

Does the youth report or demonstrate an intention to carry out any plan? Is the youth describing adaptive future-oriented thinking (e.g., going to college) or able to identify reasons for living? Have they initiated any preparatory acts, such as giving away valued possessions or telling friends good-bye. How do they respond to questions like these: "Do you wish you were dead? Would you ever do anything about it? How safe can you keep yourself?"

P: Plan

Does the youth have ideas about how they would hurt or kill themself? Have they done Internet searches investigating potential means of suicide? The more specific the details of a plan, the greater the risk, but any conceptualization of a plan is concerning. Access to planned methods (e.g., sharps, medications, or firearms in the home) should also inform the level of risk and help establish how proximal the risk of any harm is.

Using SHIP, the therapist organized the data about Luz's current episode and relevant suicidal, NSSI history (see Figure 7.1; a blank version is available as Worksheet 17 in Appendix A).

WORKSHEET 17. Suicidal Risk Heuristic: Severity, History, Intent, Plan (SHIP)

Client Name: *Luz*	Date: *[xx/xx/xx]*

Severity	
Frequency and duration	*Passive SI nearly every day. Comes in clusters throughout the day, but can distract away in 1–2 minutes.*
Intensity	*Rated a 6 out of 10. Mostly passive SI, sounding like dysphoria ("Nothing's changed") and hopelessness ("The kids won't ever change" "They'll always hold a grudge against me").*
History	
Chronicity and history of SI	*Most recent episode started about 4–5 months ago coinciding with bullying/ harassment by peers. SI ("Everyone wants me to die") and hopelessness ("I might as well end it") intensified to a 9/10 and culminated in a SA about 9–10 weeks ago. Since attending inpatient and IOP programs, intensity of SI has reduced (6/10) even as SI stays relatively constant.*
NSSI history	*Youth reports history of NSSI dating back to ninth grade as a way to deal with social, family, and academic distress. Methods focus on cutting with sharp objects and razors. Mostly nonlethal with minor bleeding that can stop on its own or with light pressure.*
SA history	*Youth made SA 9–10 weeks ago with combination of wine, Xanax, and cutting wrists with razor blade. Father found her crying and alert. Admitted to inpatient. This was first attempt.*
Impulsive/risk behaviors	*Youth has minimal Hx of risk behaviors, reporting minimal experimentation with drugs and alcohol and minimal Hx of physical injury.*
Chronic stressors/ risk factors	*Family stressors (Mo/Fa divorced; estranged from Mo) and peer bullying and harassment that preceded SA.*
Intent	
Stated or inferred intent	*Since inpatient/IOP, youth has denied intent ("No, I know it doesn't solve anything") but reserves it as an option ("I know I could always do it").*
Preparatory acts	*Youth has made commitments to Fa and friends to "stick around" until I give it a try. No evidence of preparatory acts.*
Plan	
Planned methods	*In recent/only SA, used alcohol, Xanax, and razor blades. Youth has agreed to have these items locked away at home.*
Access to methods	*Fa agreed to lock away all liquor, potentially dangerous medications, and sharps (razors, small knives that can be hidden).*

FIGURE 7.1. Using the SHIP approach to SI/NSSI risk assessment.

Designation of Risk

The therapist determines acuity of risk based on the detailed SI, NSSI, and SA history. Risk assessment and designation, in turn, directly inform action steps. Pettit and colleagues (2018) have created an algorithm for designating level of risk (low, moderate, high, severe) based on past SA or NSSI and current SI, plan, intent, and access to means (see Figure 7.2; a blank version is available as Worksheet 18 in Appendix A).

In Luz's case, past NSSI and a recent SA suggest that she is at least at moderate acute risk of making another attempt. Because she also reports current SI, but no current plan or intent, it would be best to designate her as a high acute risk. High acute risk indicates the current presence of a suicidal crisis that could rapidly escalate to a SA (Pettit et al., 2018). Youth at high acute risk deserve continuous monitoring by a treatment team and immediate steps to safeguard the environment. Another tool for therapists and administrators in behavioral health clinics who need to monitor chronic risk is the Assessment of Chronic Risk in Youth (ACRY; Dackis, Eisenberg, Mowrey, & Pimentel, 2021). This is an instrument that allows for systematic tracking of risk status over time based on clinician review of empirically supported risk and protective factors in youth (see Figure 7.3; a blank version is available as Worksheet 19 in Appendix A).

INTERVENTION COMPONENTS AND PROCESS

Safety Planning

When a therapist first becomes aware of suicide risk, it is crucial to conduct safety planning to reduce the risk of the youth making further SAs. A safety plan generally consists of a review of the stressors that trigger escalation of SI and NSSI, a brainstorming of short-term coping strategies to use during acute episodes, and connecting the youth with helpful resources and supports to keep the youth safe (Pettit et al., 2018; Stanley & Brown, 2012). Stanley and Brown (2012) have also developed a single-session approach designed to be completed in 20–30 minutes in an emergency room setting, assuming that a clinician might only have a single contact with clients who come in for acute intervention. The same approach can be used in an outpatient setting and has been adapted for adolescent populations (Stanley et al., 2009).

A safety plan stands in contrast to "no-suicide contracts" in which the client makes a written or verbal agreement to refrain from suicidal behavior. No-suicide contracts traditionally do not spell out the coping skills or resources that a client is expected to use to keep themself safe. In this format, no-suicide contracts have limited if any value in preventing future suicidal behavior (Kelly & Knudson, 2000; Reid, 1998; Shaffer & Pfeffer, 2001). Instead, in the Stanley and Brown (2012) model of safety plans, the clinician collaborates with the youth to: (1) list the warning signs of increased SI and NSSI; (2) brainstorm internal coping strategies that can be used to quickly distract the youth from intense SI; (3) identify social situations and people who can help distract the youth; (4) pinpoint the individuals who will be supportive; (5) list local resources (e.g., doctors, mobile response teams, suicide hotlines) that the youth can contact in emergencies; and (6) generate a plan to limit access to dangerous objects (e.g., sharps, alcohol/drugs, guns, materials which can be used to asphyxiate) that the youth could then utilize to hurt themself. For teen clients, the therapist frequently collaborates directly with the youth, but it also often helps to involve a caregiver who can assist the youth in identifying local resources to access as well as making the

WORKSHEET 18. Acute Suicide Risk Algorithm

Circle any endorsed risk indicators to determine level of acute risk.

☐ Low: Youth may not need a safety plan.

☒ Moderate and High Risk: Youth will routinely require some elements of safety planning.

☐ Severe Risk and some High Risk: Therapist should be prepared to alert mobile response or direct youth to emergency room.

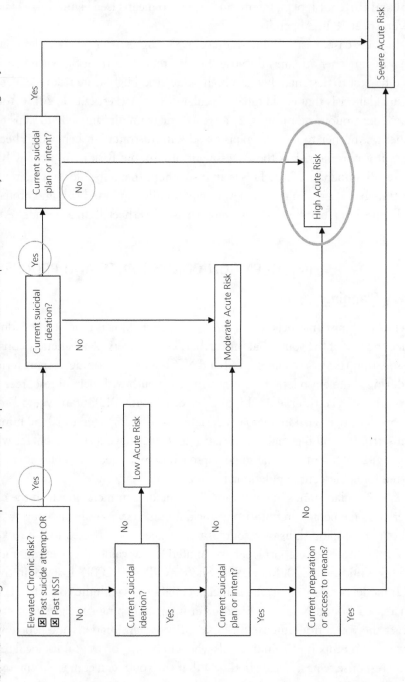

FIGURE 7.2. Algorithm for assessing acute suicide risk in Luz's case. Adapted with permission from Pettit et al. (2018).

WORKSHEET 19. Assessment of Chronic Risk in Youth (ACRY)

Patient Name: _LUZ_ Date Completed: _3/20/23_

Primary Therapist: _____ Date Reviewed: _____

Psychiatrist (Y/N): _____ ☒ Baseline (past 6 months)

Other Team Provider(s): _____ ☐ Follow-up (past 3 months)

| RISK FACTOR | Current | | Lifetime | | COMMENTS |
	YES	NO	YES	NO	
Suicide Attempt *If yes in past 2 years →* **HIGH**	Date(s): 01/06/23 #attempts: 1 Med attn: Y		Date(s): 01/06/23 #attempts: 1 Med attn: Y		*Multiple Xanax (< 4) with wine; 3–4 cuts on her wrist*
Assaultive/Violent Behavior *If yes past 2 months and caused bodily harm and led to arrest/ hospitalization →* **HIGH**		X		X	
Suicidal Ideation	Passive/Active Intent/Plan	Y	Passive/Active Intent/Plan	Y	
Suicidal Behaviors		Y		Y	
Homicidal Ideation	Passive/Active Intent/Plan	N	Passive/Active Intent/Plan	N	
Psychiatric Hospitalizations	#: 1	N	#: 1	Y	*1 week*
Psychiatric Emergency Room Visits	#: 1		#: 1		
Nonsuicidal Self-Injurious Behaviors	Y Med attn? Y		Y Med attn? Y	Y	*Cutting arm, leg, torso with a razor*
High-Risk Behaviors		N		N	

(continued)

FIGURE 7.3. Completed Assessment of Chronic Risk in Youth (ACRY) for Luz. Adapted with permission from Dackis, Eisenberg, Mowrey, & Pimentel (2021).

RISK FACTOR	Current		Lifetime		COMMENTS
	YES	NO	YES	NO	
Substance/Alcohol Use	TBD		TBD		Pt drank wine during SA
Treatment Noncompliance		N		N	
Medical Condition/ Complications		N		N	
Perceived Burden to Others	Y		Y		
Child Maltreatment/ Trauma		N		N	
Impulsivity	Low / <u>Mod</u> / High		Low / <u>Mod</u> / High		
Other	Y		Y		Paternal invalidation related to sexual orientation

PROTECTIVE FACTORS

☐ Family cohesion, connectedness	☒ Verbal, cooperative/engaged in treatment
☒ Perceived parental involvement	☐ Attendance/engagement in sports/religion
☐ Involvement of other caring adult/teacher	☐ Reasons for living
☐ School connectedness, positive feelings toward	☐ Restricted access to means
☐ School safety	☒ Self-esteem
☐ Academic achievement	
☐ Social support/positive friendships	

Designate Overall Risk

Low Risk	Moderate Risk	High Risk

FIGURE 7.3. *(continued)*

environment safe. Furthermore, in most cases, state laws require a therapist to disclose to caregivers when a minor has reported SI and SA. Thus, the caregiver can become a vital partner in implementing a safety plan at home. To aid with this, we often develop a formal "check-in plan" that schedules routine checks between a caregiver and youth. Mental health professionals must additionally be aware of mandated suicide-reporting guidelines in their respective states.

For Luz, the therapist followed the risk assessment by collaboratively generating a safety plan with the teen. Building a safety plan when SI or SA first becomes apparent helps the therapist teach the importance of open communication around SI, NSSI, and SA and ensures the therapist is aware of the youth's warning signs and range of coping skills. Following Stanley and Brown's (2012) approach, the therapist and Luz completed the safety plan shown in Figure 7.4 (a blank version is available as Worksheet 20 in Appendix A). Notice that the focus of this brief safety plan is to help the youth navigate acute episodes of SI or urges to hurt themself. Thus, the internal coping strategies focus on activities that serve the simple function of distraction and can be executed alone by the youth. They aim to disrupt the ruminative and intrusive thoughts and experiences that contribute to suicidal mood and intent.

Likewise, social support is divided into situations and people that can help distract and those who would be able to provide emotional or instrumental support. When identifying people who can help, identify *at least one adult* so that the youth is not relying solely on peers when SI arises. When identifying professional supports, the therapist and Luz identified people she could contact both inside and outside of school. It may be necessary to identify who *not* to include on this list, that is, peers who create access to means (e.g., the peer who gave her the Xanax). In addition to a general national suicide hotline, the therapist listed the contact information for the Trevor Project, which provides special guidance for sexual minority youth who are suicidal. Luz's father was also asked to be involved, to safeguard the environment by locking up razors and small knives (which Luz could hide), removing sedatives and other toxic medications and safeguarding the rest, and throwing away any alcohol in the home.

As noted above, in many situations we recommend developing a formal check-in plan between the caregiver and youth (Step 7 in the worksheet) at regular intervals (e.g., daily, 2–3 times weekly). A formal check-in plan is indicated when the caregiver was previously unaware of the youth's SI, NSSI, and SA, and the youth is isolative and caregiver–youth communication is poor. Depending on the specific state laws, age for consent, and disclosure rules for self-harm, the therapist may be obligated to disclose the presence of SI, NSSI, or SA to parents.

In addition, the evidence suggests that interpersonal connectedness and increased monitoring can reduce SI and SA (Stanley & Brown, 2012). Thus, we incorporate a daily check-in between the youth and parents so that caregivers may develop greater awareness of the presence of and changes in SI, and parents and youth are using a standardized method for assessing severity.

To create a common language and scale, we start by creating a SI Intensity Thermometer (see Figure 7.5; a blank version is available as Worksheet 21 in Appendix A) aimed at developing subjective feeling labels that fit the youth's experience for each score and identifying personalized behavioral anchors that match the youth's personal history of SI, NISS, and SA. With the caregiver and youth present, the therapist begins by normalizing the presence of SI and NSSI and notes that not all SI are created equal. Some feel more intense and intrusive. Others feel like niggling thoughts at the back of one's mind. Both are real and deserve attention, but each type reflects different levels of risk. The therapist helps the youth assign different subjective labels for each score on the scale. Here, Luz labels lower scores as "fine," "calmer," and "foggy"; medium

WORKSHEET 20. Safety Plan

> Therapist and client (and caregiver when appropriate) work together to clarify warning signs that the youth might experience elevated self-harm thoughts; then, they brainstorm coping strategies to help manage thoughts and feelings and prevent harm.

Step 1: Warning signs

1. Seeing people mention me on Snapchat

2. Kids looking at me in the hallway

3. Thinking about how things will never get better

Step 2: Internal coping strategies: things I can do to distract myself without contacting anyone

1. Draw

2. Listen to music

3. Write music lyrics

Step 3: Social situations and people who can help to distract me

1. Text my friend Zoe (phone: 000-000-0000)

2. Message Zoe, Jazmin, Sofie online

3. Go to art classroom where people hang after school

Step 4: People whom I can ask for help

1. My dad (phone: 000-000-0000)

2. Go by Zoe's place

Step 5: Professionals or agencies I can contact during a crisis

1. Therapist Name: Dr. Sandy Pimentel (Phone: 000-000-0000)

2. School Counselor: Precious Diodonet (at school)

3. Local Hospital/Mobile Response: University Mobile Response (Phone: 000-000-0000)

4. Suicide Hotline: (800) 273-TALK; Trevor Project: (866) 488-7386; www.thetrevorproject.org

Step 6: Making the environment safe

1. Dad will keep razors and small knives locked away.

2. Dad will remove sedatives and other dangerous meds.

3. Throw away alcohol.

Step 7: Regular check-in's

1. Check-In Adult: Dad

2. Frequency of Check-In's: nightly after dinner

FIGURE 7.4. Safety plan for Luz. Adapted with permission from Stanley & Brown (2012).

WORKSHEET 21. Suicidal Ideation Intensity Thermometer

When it comes to thoughts about harming ourselves, it is important that we can describe the feeling and intensity to others. Try to rate the intensity of your suicidal thoughts and feelings on a 0 to 10 scale. What words would you use to describe each rating? Can you remember a time when you've felt that way?

Suicidal Thoughts/ Feeling Intensity	What feeling you are rating:		
	How intense is it? (0 "Not at all" to 10 "the worst")	Describe the feeling (in your own words) for each level.	Describe past times you've felt this way.
	10	?	Never got here.
	9	Hopeless	My first night in the hospital, sobering up.
	8	Searing pain in my head	The day I drank and cut my wrists, thinking, "Might as well end it all."
	7	Scared for myself	When that kid pinned me against the locker choking me.
	6	Pitiful	Every time kids get all homophobic on Snapchat.
	5	Depressed	Sitting in my room wondering if things will ever make sense for me.
	4	Mad	Hanging out with Zoe, complaining about the other girls at school.
	3	Foggy, blah	Everyday level, kinda like: "Oh great, another day."
	2	Calmer	Calmer: just hanging out, doing nothing.
	1	Fine	Sleeping in.
	0	Nothing	No thoughts.

FIGURE 7.5. Suicidal Ideation Intensity Thermometer with personalized anchors in Luz's case.

169

scores as "mad," "depressed," and "pitiful." As intensity increases, the subjective labels also intensify: "scared for myself," "searing pain," and "hopeless." Notice that the score of 10 has been left blank because Luz's feelings have never reached that level and she wanted to leave room for greater intensity.

While the youth is applying affective labels, the therapist helps the youth identify times (events, actions) when they experienced each level of intensity. Personalized anchors help the youth concretely connect numeric scores with a level of true intensity. The labels also begin to detail the progressive steps that lead to greater risk for self-harm. Finally, personalized anchors provide concrete warning signs for caregivers to recognize objectively when the youth is intensifying in SI.

Once a personalized scale is created, it provides a common language for the youth and caregiver. A caregiver could ask for a youth's "intensity rating," and the youth can simply give a number, and both will immediately know the affective label and life experiences to which that number corresponds. In other words, it gives a standardized shorthand for youth and caregiver to communicate. This will be essential for implementing a robust youth–caregiver check-in plan. With a common scale in hand, the therapist collaborates with the family to create a regular SI and NSSI check-in. This helps establish a routine by which the parent can monitor the youth's mood and potential SI at the established interval.

Key Steps in a Check-In Plan

1. **Identify check-in frequency and a specific time when the caregiver can assess the youth's SI and NSSI.** The frequency of the check-in can be tailored to the severity of risk. For a youth with mild SA risk, a weekly check-in may suffice. Alternatively, the youth can be instructed to seek help or enact their safety plan when their SI Intensity rises above a certain level. For a youth with moderate or high SA risk, daily check-ins may be necessary. The selected time of day should be a time when the caregiver and youth are likely to be together. Examples include checking in after dinner, right before bedtime, or during the car ride from school to home.

2. **Identify a way in which the caregiver can conduct the check-in that is acceptable to the youth.** With the use of a personalized intensity thermometer, the check-in can be relatively quick since the family has already established a common language for mood and associated risk. A daily check-in could simply consist of the caregiver requesting the youth's SI intensity rating. If the rating appears elevated from baseline, the caregiver could follow up to check for any increased risk. The parent uses the personalized anchors from the thermometer to inquire if the youth has experienced any of the stressors typically associated with elevated SI: "I know you feel bad about yourself when the kids give you a hard time. Did anything like that happen today?"

3. **Determine a threshold for executing the safety plan.** Using the intensity thermometer, the therapist helps the youth and caregiver determine what intensity levels trigger which elements of the safety plan. For example, if Luz were to report scores of 1–3 (see Figure 7.5), her father would want to encourage her to execute Step 2 or 3 (internal coping strategies, distracting social situations) (see Figure 7.4). If Luz were to report more intense scores of 4–6, she should ask for help from people she trusts (Step 4) and from counselors or therapists (Step 5). For Luz, a score of 7 is highly intense and immediately precedes the intensity level (8) at which she made a SA. Thus, any rating of 7 would call for a consultation with a mobile response unit and possible assessment at a local emergency room. The goal is to intervene before Luz develops any intent to self-harm.

4. **Problem-solve likely challenges to the plan.** A busy household or a hectic family routine may challenge the caregiver and youth's ability to adhere to plan. Help the family problem-solve by identifying time frames for the plan (e.g., "Do this every day for 2 weeks. If there are no problems, switch to once a week"). Also identify likely interruptions. If the caregiver and youth pick a time when others might be around (e.g., right after dinner), help devise a plan to account for this; for example, have the youth give a "sign" after dinner that would draw the caregiver away and seek a private location (e.g., have the child say, "Mom, I need your help on math").

In summary, the goal of the SI intensity thermometer and check-in system is to give the caregiver a tool to help assess how serious they believe their youth's risk is and provide them with ways to monitor their youth's behavior. In the session after a check-in system is established, you should plan to reassess its use and problem-solve any challenges to consistent implementation. These tools also provide youth with a way to assess their own severity level to become more self-aware of their thoughts, feelings, and specifically SI or NSSI urges, and increase their efficacy in knowing when to implement the safety plan. Neither a check-in system nor a safety plan intervention replaces professional risk assessment when the youth is reporting serious SI and NSSI. These tools provide a method to help the caregiver and youth know when a formal risk assessment is needed.

Integration with Other Treatment Goals

As treatment progresses, the therapist will need to balance the need to secure the safety of the client while making strides toward other goals the client finds important. Intrusive SI and self-harm often appear in the context of other psychological disorders. Clients may appreciate the seriousness with which a clinician takes their suicidal thoughts and behaviors, but they may also become frustrated if their SI and NSSI are the only topics that get covered in therapy. The degree to which SI and NSSI exist at the foreground of therapy depends on the youth's risk designation and how active their SI and NSSI are. If SI and NSSI are current, then the therapist will want to conduct their own regular check-in at each session, similar to the caregiver check-in. The therapist may also want to weekly or biweekly administer a standard depression measure (e.g., the Beck Depression Inventory [BDI]; Beck, Steer, & Brown, 1996) to assess the escalation of depressed mood. If the youth has ever made a SA or has active NSSI, then review the safety plan each meeting to reinforce the strategies the youth can use when SI intensifies. Besides risk assessment, safety planning, and check-ins, how does a therapist address suicidal thoughts and behaviors in therapy? We will now turn to how therapists can use functional assessment and chain analysis to facilitate skills development and embody an educational, calm, and confident therapeutic posture.

Posture of Therapist during SI and NSSI Psychoeducation

Effective therapeutic work with SI and NSSI communicates the importance of the topic while also normalizing the experience (Pettit et al., 2018). Assuming a matter-of-fact manner can lower defenses and facilitate honest discussion. Clinicians want to communicate that any thoughts about death, desires to die, and visions of methods or plans should be attended to, and when the youth experiences them, they should be discussed. At the same time, communicate the idea that questions about living are not synonymous with wishes to be dead and that having SI does not mandate the youth will follow through with such thoughts. Many thoughts may be fleeting, even if intense, and the goal is to help the youth bare the intensity of those more difficult moments. Providing such education helps to normalize the experience and to limit any secondary guilt, shame, or hopelessness that may develop from SI. The following is an example series of statements that can help communicate these very messages:

> "Sometimes when people are feeling upset or going through a difficult time, they have thoughts about hurting themselves or wanting to die. These thoughts are important to pay attention to, and when you experience them, I want you to tell me. At the same time, just because you have these thoughts, it doesn't mean that all is lost or that you have to carry those thoughts out. As we work together, I will work to help you practice strategies to ride out those stressful moments and to remember that things can get better."

The therapist can provide Handout 15 (a reproducible version is available in Appendix A) to highlight essential information about suicide and NSSI. The youth or family can also be directed to reliable organizations, such as the Association for Behavioral and Cognitive Therapies and the Society of Clinical Child and Adolescent Psychology (see Appendix B for further details). In the case of NSSI, where the youth is actively causing bodily harm to themselves, clearly communicate that any self-harm is antithetical to the therapy process and interferes with the teen achieving personal goals (Linehan, 1993). Thus, if the youth evidences any NSSI behaviors, the therapist should pay close attention to them at each session. The rationale for this is that any issues likely to result in termination or significant disruption to therapy (e.g., through death or hospitalization) deserve to get the highest priority in treatment (Rizvi & Ritschel, 2014).

Chain Analysis and Functional Assessment

One of the first interventions therapists use to gain a greater understanding of the function of SI, NSSI, and SAs is to conduct a chain analysis (Stanley et al., 2009). A chain analysis helps identify the youth's personal risk factors by identifying the stressors and sequence of responses that result in SI, NSSI, and SAs (Rizvi & Ritschel, 2014). A chain analysis identifies any vulnerability factors (e.g., drug use, presence of depression, history of suicide in family or peer network) and proximal activating events (e.g., interpersonal, family, academic events or interactions) that lead to any escalated SI. Such an analysis also helps identify the youth's thoughts, feelings, and behaviors in reaction to these activating events. The therapist and youth complete chains collaboratively, including in the analysis both internal (e.g., thoughts, feelings, memories) and external (e.g., people, places, events) cues and triggers. Any conclusions drawn from the analysis are considered hypotheses to be tested (Rizvi & Ritschel, 2014).

To conduct a chain analysis of an SA, NSSI, or specific set of SIs, the therapist asks the youth to describe the events that lead to and follow typical escalations of SI or NSSI for them. Some have likened this process to freezing frames of a film (Stanley et al., 2009) at a specific point in time so that the therapist and youth can learn more about the youth's experience at critical junctures. Often, the chain analysis begins with a specific stressful life event. In Luz's case, the therapist noticed that SI and NSSI frequently escalated after peers harassed her about her sexuality. In session, the therapist suggested that they use a chain analysis to follow the sequence of events that followed a specific situation, when a girl posted a nasty comment about Luz on social media (see Figure 7.6; a blank version is available as Worksheet 22 in Appendix A).

WORKSHEET 22. Chain Analysis of Suicidal Ideation and Self-Harm

The goal of chain analysis is to become more aware of the thoughts, emotions, and actions that spiral out of control when you fall into an emotional spiral. Work with your therapist to spell out your emotional spiral and the events that trigger them.

Name: Luz	Date: xx/xx/xx

Vulnerability Factors: Spent all night looking through Instagram photos (some with nasty comments)

Prompting Event: Two girls looked at me in the hall and laughed.

	Action/ Emotion/ Thought	What did you do?	Potential solution or skills to use?
Link 1	Thought	"They wrote those nasty comments on Instagram."	Check thinking traps. Come up with realistic coping thought: "It wasn't about me."
Link 2	Emotion	Anger, shame	Relaxation, reach out to friend for help.
Link 3	Action	Turn around and go another way.	Stay around people I trust/enjoy.
Link 4	Thought	"I can't stand it here. They'll never let me live it down."	Challenge thoughts with coping thoughts: "Things will get better."
What problems does this lead to (e.g., self-harm, SI, risk-taking)?		Thoughts about cutting myself. Running home and crashing in my bed.	
What happened after? Short-term outcome:		Locking myself in my room helped me escape; didn't have to face anyone.	
Long-term outcome:		Feel more isolated. Can't turn to anyone.	

FIGURE 7.6. Chain analysis of suicidal ideation in Luz's case: Can you identify the links in the chain?

In their analysis, the therapist and Luz identify a relatively proximal vulnerability factor—Luz spent all night scrolling online photos, some of which contained nasty comments about her. Vulnerability factors are elements of the person, environment, or life circumstances that leave a person more open to the deleterious effects of specific stressors (Rizvi & Ritschel, 2014). Thus, Luz's exposure to repeated comments primed her for a negative reaction when she later saw two girls walking down the hall who laughed in her direction (prompting event). Despite Luz's initially strong belief that the girls were laughing at her, whether they actually were is unknowable (unless Luz were to ask them). Research suggests that intensive rumination on negative affect can increase the magnitude of that negative affect to the point that the individual engages in dysregulated behavior to distract from the affective rumination (Selby, Anestis, & Joiner, 2008). Thus, Luz's reactions spiral in a negative direction in a cascade of emotions that leads to problematic risk behaviors and undesirable long-term outcomes. Luz's first reaction is to fall into a mind-reading trap (see Chapter 2), where she assumes the laughter was about the content she viewed the prior night. Her natural emotional response is anger and shame, which she leaves unchecked. Luz next avoids the scene by turning around and going the long way to class, leaving her with escalating personalized and hopeless thoughts like "I can't stand it here. They'll never let me live it down." This chain of events leads to increased thoughts about cutting herself and isolating at home. This represents the problematic behavior that the therapist is trying to help Luz address. The isolation may protect Luz for the moment (short-term outcome) but only contributes to increased isolation in the long term.

Generating the individual links in the chain helps both the therapist and youth slow down the "frames" and identify where potential solutions exist. For example, catastrophic and personalized thinking traps call for identifying more realistic coping thoughts. Intense feelings like anger and shame might call for relaxation exercises and soliciting trusted family and friends for support. Impulses to avoid and flee an intense scene could be addressed by finding a competing action that helps the youth tolerate the distress more confidently. For example, starting a conversation with a friend in the hallway could help Luz distract herself from the "gossiping" girls or be a supportive reminder (and data point!) that not "everyone is laughing at me."

Chain analysis serves the same function as functional assessment, as described in Chapter 2. A therapist could have chosen to use Worksheet 1 (see Figure 1.4 for a completed individual functional assessment) to meet the same goals of identifying short- and long-term outcomes of problematic behavior. The benefit of a chain analysis is that it helps the youth isolate the multiple places where they could have helped themself slow down the process and break the chain of risk behaviors. A chain analysis can also be used to identify problematic interpersonal interactions, as we will describe in Chapter 11.

Together, chain analysis and functional assessment help support other treatment goals that aim to teach cognitive-behavioral skills related to specific skills-deficits or emotion dysregulation needs. Both tools are used to determine the causes and functions of SI, NSSI, and SAs and direct the therapist to specific skills that would be most useful for the client.

SUMMARY AND KEY POINTS

SI and NSSI can appear in youth with or without other formal mental health issues. Be open-minded, aware, and flexible when assessing for the presence of SI and NSSI and in incorporating them into treatment plans. A therapist working with a teen experiencing SI and NSSI needs to be prepared to address crises at times when they are unexpected. The interventions described here are compatible with the CBT approaches described for other problem areas and so can be integrated seamlessly. Luz's case illustrated the following key points:

- NSSI and SI affect all kinds of youth, but teens from some vulnerable groups require special attention, including sexual minorities and those with a history of other mental health concerns. Young girls are more at risk for NSSI than boys, and boys account for the majority of completed suicides.
- Asking about SI and NSSI does not create new thoughts about SI and NSSI. Some depressed youth will even feel less distressed and suicidal after assessments that include items or questions on suicide.
- Functional assessment of NSSI is paramount as individuals may self-harm for multiple intrapersonal and interpersonal reasons.
- Build a strong working alliance with your client through active listening and by creating an open space for the youth to speak about difficult topics like SI and NSSI.
- Assessing broader environmental stressors will give you helpful information about the context (e.g., bullying/harassment) of recent, acute self-harm.
- Assessment of risk should include data about severity, history, intent, and plans (SHIP), and designation of acute and/or chronic risk status should account for past and recent history.
- Safety planning includes a personalized suicide intensity thermometer and a formal safety plan that identifies warning signs and coping strategies to keep the youth safe.
- Chain analysis is a key intervention to identify the specific antecedents and functions of SI and NSSI behaviors. These data are essential for selecting proper interventions.

CHAPTER 8

Separation Anxiety Disorder

Anxiety upon separation from a primary caregiver is a developmentally appropriate response expected of toddler and preschool-aged children. However, separation anxiety disorder (SEP) is characterized by extreme, developmentally inappropriate distress that interferes with youth (and family) functioning. While anxiety disorders are the most common class of psychiatric illness diagnosed in youth (Merikangas et al., 2010), SEP is the most often diagnosed of the anxiety disorders, particularly in younger children, with prevalence rates at approximately 4% (Cartwright-Hatton, McNicol, & Doubleday, 2006; Costello, Mustillo, Erkanli, Keeler, & Angold, 2003).

Younger children are more likely to receive a SEP diagnosis, with prevalence rates declining dramatically as children reach preadolescence and adolescence (Cohen et al., 1993; Costello et al., 2003; Merikangas et al., 2010). Relative to most other anxiety disorders, SEP is likely to have a younger age of onset (de Lijster et al., 2016). Whereas some studies have found that girls are more likely to experience separation anxiety and receive such a diagnosis (Fan, Su, & Su, 2008; Shear, Jin, Ruscio, Walters, & Kessler, 2006), other studies suggest that rates of SEP and its symptoms are experienced equally between boys and girls (Cohen et al., 1993; Kendall et al., 2010). Information on youth anxiety and racial, ethnic, and cultural differences is sparse.

Allen and colleagues (2010) found that in a clinically referred sample of youth diagnosed with SEP, caregivers and children were most likely to endorse symptoms regarding difficulties, or refusal, going to sleep without the significant attachment figure or caregiver nearby, and difficulties, or reluctance, being alone without the significant attachment figure or caregiver nearby. Caregivers in this sample also more frequently endorsed the persistent and excessive distress symptom when experiencing separation from the significant attachment figure or caregiver. Further examining the differential contributions of specific symptoms to the diagnosis of SEP, Comer and colleagues (2004) found that experiencing significant distress upon separation and fears of being alone without the significant attachment figure or caregiver were the two symptoms most discriminative of youth with lower- versus higher-severity SEP. Therefore, inquiring about these two symptoms may be critical for screening SEP in youth. Also, there is some indication that children experiencing nightmares with separation themes may be a symptom criterion with a higher threshold for endorsement or lesser chance of being endorsed (Allen et al., 2010; Comer et al., 2004).

Given that the symptomatic feature of SEP includes apprehension and difficulty separating from primary caregivers, it is not difficult to recognize the potential for impairments across domains of functioning. Often, for example, SEP emerges when children are expected to separate from caregivers to go to school, and as a result, youth with SEP can demonstrate extreme distress when tasked with going to school and staying in school, and they may have a tantrum upon separation or even refuse to attend school. Research has shown that up to 80% of children with school refusal behavior may have a SEP diagnosis (Masi, Mucci, & Millepiedi, 2001).

Overall, there is significant overlap in and comorbidity among anxiety disorders in youth (Verduin & Kendall, 2003). Avoidance and distress in anticipation of or upon separating may manifest in disruptive and oppositional behaviors, with children refusing to part from their caregivers, go to school, stay in school, stay with babysitters or other adults, sleep independently, or comply with developmentally appropriate requests.

As with other youth onset anxiety disorders, conceptualizing separation anxiety through a developmental psychopathology framework is warranted. SEP in childhood is related to later psychiatric illness in adulthood, though whether via homotypic versus heterotypic continuity or as a specific versus general risk factor remains inconclusive. The SEP hypothesis of panic disorder suggested early on (e.g., Klein, 1964) proposed that adult-onset panic disorder was preceded by separation anxiety in childhood. Whereas some studies have found support that separation anxiety in childhood is associated with greater risk for developing panic disorder in adulthood (Klein, 1964; Kossowsky et al., 2013), other studies have found childhood separation anxiety diagnoses to confer more general risk for developing many psychiatric conditions, including *any* anxiety disorder and nonanxiety disorders such as depression (Aschenbrand, Kendall, Webb, Safford, & Flannery-Schroeder, 2003; Brückl et al., 2007; Lewinsohn, Holm-Denoma, Small, Seeley, & Joiner 2008). The DSM-5 removed the age-of-onset criterion allowing for SEP to be diagnosed across the lifespan and included under anxiety disorders. While adult SEP can onset in adulthood, there is also evidence for homotypic continuity from childhood SEP and persistence of symptoms into adulthood (Manicavasagar, Silove, Curtis, & Wagner, 2000).

INDIVIDUAL AND FAMILY FACTORS

Cognitive Variables

Threat-related selective attention has been found to be a relevant feature of youth anxiety and even predictive of cognitive-behavioral therapy (CBT) response, such that children who experience difficulties disengaging their attention from severely threatening stimuli do not respond as well to CBT intervention (Legerstee, Garnefski, Jellesma, Verhulst, & Utens, 2010; Legerstee et al., 2010). That is, youth who have a hard time pulling themselves away from threatening images and thoughts present a unique challenge for therapists who aim to teach cognitive and behavioral strategies aimed at approaching such fears. Therefore, when considering cognitive factors, it may be useful for the therapist to target having children actively disengage their attention from threatening stimuli. This is not the same as promoting avoidance. For example, when conducting an exposure, a therapist will want the youth to behaviorally approach a fearful situation (e.g., sit in a separate room from the caregiver), but the therapist will also work to ensure the youth does not overly focus on threat cues and interpretations.

When examining differences between the cognitive styles in anxious and nonanxious youth, research indicates that anxious youth are less likely to use positive reappraisal or planning and more likely to catastrophize and ruminate than their nonanxious counterparts (Legerstee, Garnefski, et al., 2010). When considering and adjusting for the possibility that anxious youth may experience more negative events in their lives, it appears that anxious youth are less likely to utilize more adaptive cognitive coping strategies during these negative events.

Caregiver Factors

As with youth anxiety disorders in general, evidence suggests a familial basis to separation anxiety. The etiology of SEP includes genetic, shared environmental, and nonshared or unique environmental influences (Scaini, Ogliari, Eley, Zavos, & Battaglia, 2012). Given this familial basis, separation anxiety likely aggregates in families (Manicavasagar et al., 2001; Silove et al., 1995). In one study examining parent–child concordance for the existence of separation anxiety, 63% of youth with SEP had at least one caregiver with adult separation anxiety, with caregivers reporting significant separation anxiety in their own childhoods (Manacavasagar et al., 2000). Stated somewhat differently, in this study, youth with SEP were 11 times more likely to have one caregiver with adult SEP. Higher levels of separation anxiety symptoms in younger children have been associated with maternal depression, prenatal smoking, and unemployment (Battaglia et al., 2016). There is increased family dysfunction associated with youth anxiety (Côté et al., 2009; Ginsburg et al., 2015).

Anxiety disorders in youth may be transitory (Ginsburg et al., 2015). Most children exhibit relatively mild to moderate and developmentally appropriate levels of separation anxiety that resolve as they progress through infancy and early childhood. For example, while anxiety about strangers that normatively emerges in 8- to 10-month-old infants resolved for most children, there is some evidence that an exaggerated stranger anxiety response may be an early predictor of separation anxiety (Lavallee et al., 2011). Furthermore, one study examined the specific trajectories of children's separation anxiety from 1.5 to 6 years, and found that most children who experience separation anxiety will be unaffected by the time they enter school; however, a subset of children are on a potentially clinically distinguishable trajectory if they demonstrate high and increasing levels of symptomatology starting at 1.5 years through 6 years (Battaglia et al., 2016).

THE CBT MODEL OF SEP

Utilizing the CBT model to formulate and treat SEP requires identifying and helping the client and their caregivers to understand the interplay between the youth's thoughts, feelings, and behaviors. See Figure 8.1 (a reproducible version is available as Handout 16 in Appendix A) for a sample of the model for youth with SEP. Youth with SEP may experience catastrophic thoughts about separating from their caregivers, such as "My parents will get into an accident" or "A robber will break in and steal me," and helpless beliefs about their ability to handle aspects of a separation like "I can't sleep on my own" or "If I get lost, I won't know what to do." The physical feelings that they describe may include acute or intense panic-like sensations, including heart-racing and crying or sensations of dread or stomach upset in anticipation of separation. As such, they may cling to a caregiver, refuse to leave a caregiver's side, refuse to attend school or any activity, or avoid sleepovers and playdates altogether. It is important to identify and help the youth and caregivers identify not just behaviors associated with SEP but behavioral avoidance, escape, and/or rescue that have become associated with SEP. Asking a caregiver, "What does your child do when she becomes separation anxious?" as well as "What does your child refuse to do or avoid doing when

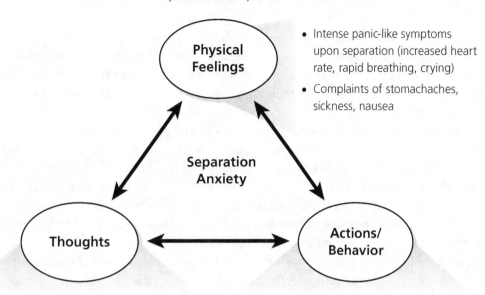

Physical Feelings

- Intense panic-like symptoms upon separation (increased heart rate, rapid breathing, crying)
- Complaints of stomachaches, sickness, nausea

Separation Anxiety

Thoughts

Actions/Behavior

- "My parents will get into an accident."
- "A robber will break in and steal me."
- "I *can't* sleep on my own."
- Worry about harm to self or parent upon separation, or being able to handle self or problems when separated.

- Clinging behavior, reassurance, and attention seeking
- Protests, arguments, complaints, oppositionality
- Refusal to separate at home, school, or elsewhere

FIGURE 8.1. Cognitive-behavioral model of separation anxiety.

he becomes separation anxious?" may be helpful. By extension, ask caregivers, "What do you do in response to your child when they become separation anxious?" and "What have you stopped doing or what do you avoid doing to prevent your child from becoming separation anxious?"

The case formulation allows you to develop a working hypothesis about factors that may be triggering and maintaining the youth's presenting problems (see Chapter 1). For youth-based conditions, it is especially important to include parental, familial, neighborhood, and school contexts in the formulation—of course, in addition to race, ethnicity, culture, and religion-based considerations. For example, some caregivers have described cultural, religious, or socioeconomic reasons for not allowing their children to engage in certain activities perhaps more common in the dominant culture (e.g., sleepovers, overnight camps), which may need to be differentiated from fear-based avoidance. Assessment forms the basis of diagnostic and case formulation and guides the selection of treatment strategies. For children with SEP, assessment should target child-specific physiologic experiences and level of distress (e.g. stomachaches, crying), particular worry thoughts in anticipation of separation (e.g., "What if my parents never come back?"), and situational areas of interference and avoidance, rescue, or escape (e.g., academic, social, family). As with all youth conditions, impairment and interference should be determined in terms of developmentally appropriate expectations. For example, many children may be anxious when attending a classmate's birthday party or playdates; however, a 9-year-old who cries, clings to his mother, or refuses to enter the party or playdate setting may experience significant impairment and interference in functioning. Similarly, most children during the course of their childhoods may experience anxiety at bedtime for several developmentally appropriate reasons (e.g., fear of monsters, fear of the dark, transient school worries); however, youth who have nightly difficulty falling asleep, putting themselves to sleep, and staying asleep without their caregivers being physically present, or "need" to sleep in their caregivers' bed, may be evidencing significant impairment and interference.

Data gathering is key to case conceptualization, and since a cognitive-behavioral case conceptualization targets essential thoughts, feelings, and behaviors, it is crucial for therapists to gather specific data on the child's thoughts, feelings, and behaviors. For SEP, gathering these data on the primary caregivers' thoughts, feelings, and behaviors in anticipation of, and during, separation is essential. Since SEP de facto includes fears and distress related to the presence and safety of another person or persons, gathering data via functional assessment should take care to include parental reactions and responses to separation situations.

Functional assessment begins with the initial intake and is carried through treatment with youth and their caregivers. Caregivers of SEP youth will likely present with several target problem situations that may include child-elevated distress associated with, or outright avoidance of, various situations. A goal of functional assessments is to lay out these problem behaviors in terms of contexts, trigger, antecedents, maintaining mechanisms, and consequences. What happens when a separation situation is impending? How do caregivers respond to a youth's distress?

Context in the functional assessment of SEP may be especially important, as a youth's anxiety may be compartmentalized. That is, some youth might tolerate separation when going to school, but they do not attend camp or sleepovers or sleep in their caregivers' bed. Or, some youth may evidence significantly more distress and protest with one caregiver but not the other. Antecedents or triggers for SEP youth may occur in response to actual in-the-moment situations that call for separation or anticipated situations that may be scheduled in the near or more distant future. Caregivers may describe not disclosing information about impending separation situations until the last minute to prevent (and avoid) protracted anxiety reactions, anticipatory worries, or reassurance seeking and pleas.

Youth with SEP may identify automatic thoughts relating to harm befalling themselves or their caregivers, such as getting lost or kidnapped, or "bad things" happening. Or, since SEP often onsets in younger children, they may have difficulty articulating or expressing specific thoughts in conjunction with their distress, physiologic arousal, and clingy behaviors. Youth's ability and awareness of cognitive aspects of their emotions will guide subsequent use of cognitive strategies. Similarly, as separation anxiety and arousal in youth may trigger a caregiver's own experience of separation anxiety (Hock, McBride, & Gnezda, 1989) or other experiences, ascertaining the caregiver's own beliefs about separation, safety, and their child's ability to cope with or handle a situation is critical.

When considering a behavioral formulation of SEP, gather information regarding behavioral responses to particular triggers and antecedents. Once a child's problem behavior is triggered in anticipation of a separation situation or during an actual separation situation, what happens? How does the child behave? Is the child throwing a tantrum, clinging to caregivers, refusing to physically separate, refusing to get out of the car for an activity, or repeatedly entering the caregivers' bedroom? Is the child asking repeated reassurance-seeking questions or texting multiple times with increasing frequency? Is the child trying to escape potential separation scenarios or avoiding them altogether? Does the child try to be rescued by the primary caregiver if they are already experiencing a separation by calling or having the caregiver "come early" to pick them up? How do other relevant adults, such as babysitters, sibling, teachers, or school nurses, respond to the child in distress?

How does the caregiver behave? Does the caregiver report "giving in" if the child protests to a separation? Does the caregiver rescue the child from school or sleepovers? Have other family members been asked to accommodate the child's behavior, for example, having a sibling attend activities with the child? Do caregivers encourage anxious avoidance or coping responding in their child? How do caregivers respond to reassurance-seeking questions? Do they answer every phone call or text immediately? Have caregivers changed their plans or declined their own activities in advance to avoid potential upset for the child?

Answering these questions—in terms of the potentially dysfunctional response patterns by the child, the caregiver, and the system—is paramount for developing the ongoing formulation and mapping the treatment intervention plan. Understanding the role of avoidance, escape, and rescue in maintaining the child's anxieties and problem behaviors is essential. Relatedly, and perhaps as important, the therapist must explain and communicate to the youth and caregivers the function of these negatively reinforcing patterns as central to the rationale for proposed cognitive and behavioral treatment strategies.

CASE VIGNETTE: CHARLIE

Charlie is a 12-year-old Caucasian cisgender boy who lives with his parents in a three-bedroom home in a suburban middle-class neighborhood. He was brought to treatment at an outpatient center after his parents voiced concerns about his extreme difficulty separating from his parents at school and when being dropped off at friends' houses. Every morning before school, Charlie reports having a stomachache, and he often begs his parents to allow him to stay home from school. More than most kids, Charlie reports dreading September. His dread starts on August 1 every summer, because as he describes, "It is the beginning of the end of summer." During the school year, he also dreads most Mondays, returning to school after a long holiday, Tuesdays after a long weekend, and Thursdays because he has after-care at school and tutoring (i.e., he does not get home until after 5 P.M.).

Charlie is a good student and enjoys reading and math. While Charlie's parents can often get him to school (after significant struggle and distress for all), he will make frequent trips to the school nurse. During the previous school year, his parents left work early 22 times to pick him up and bring him home, leading both parents to receive warnings from their employers because of their extensive absences. Charlie used to take the school bus; however, his morning upset became so significant and constant that he would miss bus pickup. As a result, his mother started driving him, and she gives him a daily pep talk while in the school parking lot. Charlie's mother also picks him up after school. Most days, Charlie reports worrying whether or not she will be late. He insists that she stand in a specific spot at the edge of the parking lot at dismissal because it is visible to him from the school door window where his class lines up to exit the building. Charlie has also arranged with his teacher to be the first in line each afternoon.

Charlie is socially engaged and enjoys hanging out with friends, as long as they come to his house. He will reluctantly schedule a time to hang out with a neighbor, but his contact with peers and friends has decreased substantially over time, as have reciprocal invitations from his peers. Charlie used to play Little League baseball but reportedly thought the coach was "mean," leading him to quit. His parents admit to being relieved because Charlie required significant accommodations to participate (e.g., one of his parents had to be present in the bleachers for all practices and team events). Bleacher duty also included sitting in a specific seat in a specific row more visible to the playing field.

Charlie's parents rarely go out together or hire a babysitter. They indicate that when they did so in the past, Charlie's anticipatory worry and questions would escalate so dramatically, it was "not worth the stress." When they did go out to dinner or some other event, they had to provide Charlie with a detailed timeline and the exact address and location of their whereabouts. When he was younger, he would cry, and he would make several calls to their cell phones. As he got older, he began texting repeatedly while they were out. They also knew that despite clear instructions, Charlie would remain wide awake until they got home.

On an average night, Charlie's sleep routine included the following: his father would read him a story, then his mother would come into his room for "talk time" and sit on the edge of his bed until he fell asleep. Typically, this lasted 60 minutes. While his parents had attempted to allow Charlie to fall asleep on his own, he would come out of his room with various questions and excuses that further delayed his bedtime: "I'm thirsty." "I have to go to the bathroom." "I forgot to tell you something," and so on. Once he was asleep, his mother would attempt to tiptoe very quietly out of the room, being sure not to turn off the night light, not to close the door, and to keep the hall light on. Most nights, Charlie would wake up at some point and slip into their bed. This often resulted in their waking up. Occasionally, they would play what they described as "musical beds," and one parent would go into Charlie's bed. Eventually, they just put a bedroll and blanket on the floor at the foot of their bed, which satisfied Charlie as he could make his way there without waking his parents. They learned to look before bounding out of bed in the morning because he was often curled up on the floor.

ASSESSMENT OF SEP

At the diagnostic intake evaluation, the therapist completed the Anxiety Disorders Interview Schedule with Charlie's parents (ADIS-P, Parent Version) and with Charlie (ADIS-C, Child Version). Notably, the therapist observed that Charlie became distressed when she indicated that they would separate for a portion of the evaluation. He immediately became tearful and climbed into his father's lap. When it came time to separate, Charlie's parents indicated that they would be sitting "right outside the office," and the therapist and parents moved their chairs outside the office rather than having the parents sit in the waiting room. At the conclusion of the assessment, Charlie met the criteria for SEP and specific phobia, situational type, the dark.

Charlie met more than three of the eight required DSM criteria for clinically significant SEP. He described significant worry about "something bad happening" to his parents, including being in a car accident, illness, and even death. He worried that if they went somewhere, they would not come back or they would forget to pick him up. He expressed worry about several bad events happening if apart from his parents, including "freaking out if they don't pick me up," or being kidnapped. He demonstrated persistent resistance to attend developmentally appropriate activities (e.g., school, hang-outs) and his willingness to participate in various activities was decreasing. He evidenced difficulty most mornings, often complaining of stomachaches, emotional upset during the morning routine, which had changed from previously riding the school bus to being driven to school by his mother. Charlie further evidenced disruption in his ability to concentrate while in school because of his anticipatory worry about being picked up and associated stomachaches, resulting in multiple visits to the school nurse, calls to his parents, and many early departures from school.

His parents also noted that their own participation in activities had decreased because of Charlie's SEP. Another significant disruption for the family was the bedtime routine. As noted, sleep disturbance in the form of inability to sleep alone or be away from the primary caregiver is a prevalent marker of youth with SEP. When asked about bedtime, Charlie reported that he used to think there were monsters in his room. Then he worried that since his bedroom is closest to the top of the stairs, burglars would take him first. He also said that "if mom and dad aren't there, I just can't fall asleep." Charlie's parents described that allowing Charlie to sleep in their room and on a bedroll "seemed like a good compromise so all of us could get some sleep." According to his parents, Charlie "always" had difficulty separating starting in kindergarten, and his symptoms had begun to worsen over the past 2 years. When asked about potential differences in Charlie's anxiety over the summer, his parents noted that he appeared to be much less anxious; however, since his mother is a teacher, he stayed home with her most days. He "opted out" of going to day camp.

In reviewing Charlie's lifetime history, it appeared that he experienced several subclinical fears and phobias that caused prolonged periods of disruption for him and his family and then appeared to fade over time. Most notably, these included fears of bees, thunderstorms and loud noises and throughout his childhood caused him to become anxious, tearful, and especially clingy in these situations. These circumstances did not cause ongoing disruption; however, his parents noted that for short periods he would refuse to leave their sides if, for example, he believed there might be bees at the park, thunderstorms in the forecast, or fireworks at a summer celebration. Charlie and his parents denied any current fears of animals, thunderstorms or loud noises. However, both Charlie and his parents endorsed ongoing fear of the dark that began when he started school. According to his parents, Charlie can only sleep if there is a nightlight, which includes when he is sleeping in his parent's room. He refuses to enter a dark room or the basement. He often expresses fears of a blackout, and checks to be sure he knows where the flashlights are and if the batteries are operational. As his parents described it: "He leaves on every light in the house." When asked about his fear of the dark, he described having a "creepy feeling that something will jump out" of the dark. See Figure 8.2 for more SEP diagnostic clarification considerations.

In addition to the semi-structured ADIS-C/P interviews, several other sources of diagnostic data helped to support the SEP diagnosis. First, attending to both Charlie's response to the separation challenge and to his parents' response to his anxiety informs functional assessment. Second, Charlie and his parents completed several objective measures, including the Revised Children's Anxiety and Depression Scale (RCADS; Table 8.1). According to his mother's report, Charlie's *T* score for SEP was in the clinical range, whereas Charlie's self-reported separation anxiety on the RCADS was slightly below threshold. Notably, also approaching clinical threshold according to Charlie's self-report was panic disorder. Although Charlie did not meet the criteria for panic disorder according to the diagnostic interviews in that he did not report experiencing panic attacks "out of the blue" or anticipatory worries about having panic attacks per se, Charlie did report having significant physiological distress, stomach upset, and "freak outs." Elevation on the panic disorder subscale may indicate that the therapist will want to monitor further to rule out formal diagnosis, or it can indicate that elevated somatic symptoms are characteristic of Charlie's SEP and deserve attention as a target problem.

☐ Is there an underlying medical condition triggering somatic symptoms (e.g., gastrointestinal) or behavioral responses (e.g., clinging behaviors)? If "yes," consider anxiety disorder due to a general medical condition. Consult with pediatrician.

☐ Is the separation anxiety developmentally appropriate? Consider the youth's age, full developmental range, and family context.

☐ Is the separation anxiety time-limited and a result of transient life changes (e.g., caregiver separation, divorce, deployment, etc.)? If "yes," consider normative response or adjustment disorder with anxiety.

☐ Is the separation anxiety better explained by grief (e.g., from a primary caregiver's death) or trauma reaction? If "yes," consider normative response, posttraumatic stress disorder (PTSD), or complicated bereavement.

☐ Are safety concerns better explained by general worries in generalized anxiety disorder (GAD)? If "yes," consider GAD.

☐ Is separation anxiety behavior better explained by acute phobic responses (e.g., extra clinging with needle phobia)? If "yes," consider specific phobia and five types.

FIGURE 8.2. Diagnostic clarification checklist: SEP.

Goal Setting and Defining Target Problems

In reviewing the diagnostic assessment with Charlie and his parents, the therapist provided a summary and overview of the large amount of data collected via the interviews, observations, and paper-and-pencil measures. The goal of the feedback session is to convert diagnostic information into a preliminary treatment plan with concrete goals and objectives. To that end, the therapist worked collaboratively with the family to identify specific goals, and when necessary, convert goals into objective and operationalized targets. Be mindful that during this conversation, the child may evidence increased anxiety, especially if the parents and therapist are naming goals that are at the core of the child's fears or very high on the fear and avoidance hierarchy. Similarly, parents may

TABLE 8.1. Charlie's Symptom Profile at Intake Using the RCADS

	Mother		Father		Youth	
	Raw scores	T scores	Raw scores	T scores	Raw scores	T scores
Separation anxiety	19	> 80**	19	> 80**	18	> 80**
Generalized anxiety	11	73**	12	76**	10	59
Panic disorder	10	> 80**	8	> 80**	10	61
Social anxiety	2	33	7	46	7	44
Obsessions/compulsions	0	42	1	46	2	37
Depression	5	54	12	78**	7	47
Total anxiety	42	70**	47	75**	47	60
Total anxiety and depression	47	68*	59	78**	54	58

*T scores higher than 65 indicate borderline clinical threshold. **Scores of 70 or higher indicate scores above clinical threshold. T scores are normalized based on the youth's age and gender.

exhibit their own nervousness related to being able to handle their child's elevated distress given a history of "having tried everything." As such, it is important for the therapist to validate what Charlie and his parents may be feeling and state that goal setting and defining target problems provide the roadmap for a treatment that will match the family's readiness. In Charlie's case, parent, child, and therapist goals were devised as follows:

Parents' Goals

- Go to school on time and ride the bus there.
- Stay in school for a complete day.
- Make plans to hang out with friends outside of the home.
- Join baseball or another sports team or club, and learn to have fun.
- Sleep in his own bedroom and be able to stay there all night.
- Go to day camp during the summer.
- Decrease number of phone calls and texts to us.
- Be able to go out for an evening and hire a babysitter.

Child's Goals

- Decrease feelings of nausea about going to school.
- Make sure Mom and Dad are on time.
- Spend more time with friends after school.

Therapist's Goals

- Decrease school day morning distress, increase on-time and full-day attendance.
- Decrease reassurance-seeking behaviors (e.g., phone calls, texts, conversations at bedtime).
- Increase use of coping behaviors to manage anxious distress.
- Teach parents skills to decrease rescue and accommodation behavior.
- Increase social activities with peers outside of the home.
- Increase ability to tolerate being in dark room.

Child, caregiver, and therapist goals transect multiple developmental academic, social, and emotional targets (see Figure 8.3 for child and caregiver goals; a blank version is available as Worksheet 11 in Appendix A): attending and transitioning to and from school and age-appropriate activities; reciprocally participating in extracurricular activities and social activities with peers; practicing self-efficacy and the ability to use skills to manage states of emotional distress; and increasing autonomy in sleep and other daily behaviors. Although neither Charlie nor his parents identified a goal regarding his phobia of the dark, the therapist added it to her goals for Charlie as this fear appeared to interfere with an expected developmental task above and beyond his SEP interference. Since Charlie's SEP impaired so many areas of his and his family's daily functioning, the issue of his significant fear of the dark could otherwise be easily overshadowed.

SEP goals can be established and quantified in terms of time (e.g., staying in school for the full day, amount of time separated from caregivers); frequency (e.g., increase on-time arrival, full-day attendance, decrease number of texts when separated from caregivers); skill building (e.g., learn and practice somatic management, deep breathing skills). Also, goals can be child-focused as well

WORKSHEET 11. Goals Tracker

Work with your therapist to brainstorm possible specific, meaningful, and achievable goals. Think through what outcomes you expect to see. And then, keep track of how your child does each week.

Parent Goals:	Desired Outcomes	Week 1	Week 2	Week 3	Week 4	Week 5
Go to school on time.	Walk in the building by 8:20 A.M.	1/5 days	3/5 days	3/5 days	5/5 days	4/5 days
Ride the bus to school.	Be at bus pickup by 7:50 A.M. and ride bus 5/5 days.	0	2/5 days	3/5 days	5/5 days	3/5 days
Make playdates with friends outside of the home.	1 weekday & 1 weekend playdate	0 weekday; 0 weekend	0 weekday; 1 weekend	1 weekday; 0 weekend	1 weekday; 1 weekend	1 weekday; 0 weekend
Sleep in his own bedroom and be able to stay in his room (7/7 days).	# nights of sleep in room (including leaving & prompt return)	0/7	0/7	0/7	0/7	2/7
Decrease number of phone calls and texts.	# of phone calls & texts per day	approx. 30	22	15	16	12

Youth Goals:	Desired Outcomes	Week 1	Week 2	Week 3	Week 4	Week 5
Decrease feelings of nausea about going to school.	Anxiety nausea rating (0–10)	10	9	9	6	6
Make sure Mom and Dad are on time.	Reduce worry rating about whether Mom & Dad are on time (0–10)	10	10	8	7	5
Spend more time with friends after school.	Frequency of hang-outs with friends outside of school.	0 weekday; 0 weekend	0 weekday; 1 weekend	1 weekday; 0 weekend	1 weekday; 1 weekend	1 weekday; 0 weekend

FIGURE 8.3. Initially devised Goals Tracker worksheet for Charlie.

as caregiver- and family-focused. As stated above, it will be important to work with the family to prioritize goals, recognize and acknowledge any discordance of goals, validate anxiety around particular goals, and emphasize that the family and therapist will work as a team gradually tackling goals. For example, Charlie stated one of his goals was to "make sure Mom and Dad be on time." The therapist will be sure to discuss this goal with the family on multiple levels in that: (1) Of course, it is not realistic that one can *always* be on time; (2) it is a goal for other peoples' behavior, not one's own; (3) it will require an honest understanding regarding the reality of Charlie's parents' general timeliness (i.e., are they frequently late?); and (4) the exposure phase of treatment will likely require having Charlie practice the scenarios of coping if or when his parents are late. For tracking purposes, it may be useful to assess his worry ratings about the possibility of their lateness, gather data regarding the occurrence of their on-time or late behaviors, follow the use of self-talk when he has this thought, and analyze degrees of "tolerating" this worry, and the like. Goals can be assessed weekly and adapted as necessary.

CASE CONCEPTUALIZATION

CBT Model

Emerging from comprehensive assessment with an enormity of data from multiple stakeholders who have individual goals can be overwhelming. Helping the child and family understand the nature and scope of the problems in a CBT lens may assist in clarifying both the problem and the plan for treatment. Standardized questionnaires suggest SEP as a key problem area, and both caregiver and youth goals indicate this as a primary focus of concern. Self-report from standard diagnostic interviews (ADIS-5-C/P) provided detailed history and behavioral patterns useful for conceptualization. The therapist understood Charlie's long-standing SEP to be triggered by fears of negative events befalling him or his parents, which is then followed by significant surges of internal and external emotional distress. His anxiety is met by certain responses that maintain his avoidance and fear, including reassurance giving and accommodations from the parents and school. Helping the parents and youth to understand this conceptualization will enhance engagement for therapy. As part of initial psychoeducation, the therapist diagrammed the CBT triangle using individual examples that highlighted Charlie's cognitive, behavioral, and affective responses to separation challenges, as shown in Figure 8.4.

For example, Charlie described that as soon as he wakes up and his mother tells him to get ready for school, he worries that she will forget to pick him up after school and he begins to feel nauseous. He is slow to get dressed for school, which triggers his mother to repeatedly enter his room and he begs her to stay home. When she explains that she and his father have to go to work, he makes her promise that she will be on time for pickup. This Q&A repeats approximately 8–10 times every morning, taking increasing amounts of time. Charlie reports that he continues to worry about his mother's punctuality and safety (e.g., she might get into a car accident). Charlie also reports that his heart races and he becomes tearful when he pictures himself getting upset at school, which then prompts him to worry about the reaction from his peers. Often, Charlie's mother winds up helping to dress and feed him "to move things along."

Drawing the CBT model, the therapist helps Charlie identify his thoughts ("My Mom will forget me"), their impact on his feelings (nauseous, heart racing), and his behavioral response (asking for reassurance). The therapist notes that this process cycles in a loop because the youth is increas-

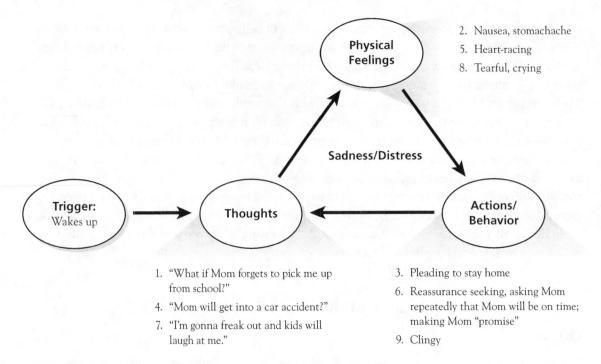

2. Nausea, stomachache
5. Heart-racing
8. Tearful, crying

1. "What if Mom forgets to pick me up from school?"
4. "Mom will get into a car accident?"
7. "I'm gonna freak out and kids will laugh at me."

3. Pleading to stay home
6. Reassurance seeking, asking Mom repeatedly that Mom will be on time; making Mom "promise"
9. Clingy

FIGURE 8.4. Individualized CBT conceptualization for Charlie. His thoughts, feelings, and behavior cycle continuously in a downward spiral (follow the numbers in order: 1, 2, 3, etc. to see how the thought–feeling–action cycle flows into another).

ingly catastrophizing outcomes. For example, when his mother's reassurance does not alleviate anxiety, his subsequent thoughts ("She's only telling me that, but she can't guarantee she'll be there") only escalate his nausea and heart rate, which trigger further reassurance and oppositionality. The goal, at this point, is not to intervene but to highlight how the youth's current reactions lead to a downward spiral and to have him become aware of the places where change could occur. The therapist might also have the parents complete their own CBT triangle to increase awareness of their thought–feeling–action cycles.

Having caregivers and child review Handout 16 can assist in breaking what are likely chaotic and challenging daily episodes into more digestible components. The CBT conceptualization can be used for assessment as well as a means to validate how difficult and overwhelming daily anxious distress can be for all members of the family. Given the expressed worries and time demands associated with having to get to school and work, certain resulting behaviors "make sense." Often, caregivers feel shame in their perceived inability to effectively soothe and coach their child; helping them to clarify episodes via the CBT model is a starting point for understanding the interplay among thought, emotions, and behaviors (and avoidance), as well as for laying the groundwork for areas of skill building and intervention.

Functional Assessment

An integral aspect of case conceptualization is the functional assessment. As discussed above, the functional assessment (see Figure 8.5; a blank version is available as Worksheet 1 in Appendix A) allows the therapist and family to identify the behavioral and emotional responses of concern, and

WORKSHEET 1. Trigger and Response

Tell us about your triggers and how you reacted. Describe your feelings, what you did (action), what happened right away (immediate outcome), and then what happened later (long-term outcome).

```
┌──────────────┐      ┌─────────────────────┐      ┌──────────────┐
│  Antecedent  │ ───▶ │ Behavioral and      │ ───▶ │ Consequences │
│              │      │ Emotional Response  │      │              │
└──────────────┘      └─────────────────────┘      └──────────────┘
```

Trigger	Feeling (emotional response)	Action (behavioral response)	Immediate Results (What keeps it going?)	Long-Term Results (What gets you in trouble?)
I got invited to a sleepover party.	Nervous	Told my friend an excuse about other plans, texted my mom a few times.	Relief at first; Also felt sad when kids started talking about sleepover plans.	Saw TikTok videos from that night and felt left out.
First day of karate class.	Anxious, worried, felt like I wanted to throw up	Stayed in the car, crying, asked to go home.	Felt better when we went home.	Missed out on karate class, didn't see my friends in the class.
Parents went to dinner party and told me at last minute.	Dread, upset stomach	Followed Mom from room to room, asking questions, crying, begging her to stay, made her promise to text me and come home before bedtime.	Felt OK when I googled and saw the restaurant was 2 miles away and Mom answered my texts.	Got nervous and mad again when they came 15 minutes late.

FIGURE 8.5. Individualized functional assessment of Charlie's avoidance related to separation anxiety.

189

the antecedents of those responses and consequences that may be reinforcing and maintaining them. Completion of these functional assessment worksheets in-session or for home practice can provide significant information clarifying the pattern among specific triggers of a child's distress and avoidance and escape behaviors, as well as rescue and accommodation by people in the child's environment (e.g., caregivers, siblings, school personnel).

For Charlie, multiple automatic thoughts about going to school included harm befalling his parents, his mother being late for pickup from school, and worry about "freaking out" in front of peers and becoming embarrassed. These thoughts triggered significant emotional and gastrointestinal distress, prompting behavioral responses of pleading with his parents to not go to school and delay in dressing and eating breakfast. These delays result in missing the school bus, which brings an immediate consequence of relief (for Charlie), as his mother now has to drive him there instead. Functional assessment can be applied to multiple separation examples to assist the therapist in clarifying patterns of antecedent–response–consequences, and to help illustrate for the family the likely role of avoidance, escape, and rescue in providing short-term relief (negative reinforcement). This will offer the rationale for the proposed exposure interventions to come.

When faced with other separation challenges unrelated to school, similar patterns emerge (Figure 8.5). When Charlie is invited to a sleepover, he feels nauseous and immediately makes up an excuse to decline the invitation and texts his mother who reassures him that he does not have to attend the sleepover. These actions provide immediate relief from the distress of his emotional response (nervousness) and his worry thoughts about not being able to fall asleep at his friend's house, starting to cry in front of peers, and having to call his parents to pick him up in the middle of the night. These automatic thoughts occurred, well, *automatically!* As soon as he received the invitation, Charlie's nervousness and somatic responses (e.g., butterflies, nausea) were triggered and he experienced a swirl of thoughts (e.g., "What if I can't fall asleep and all the other kids are asleep?" "What if I start to freak out and they all make fun of me?" "What if it gets too late for Mom and Dad to come pick me up and I'm awake all night alone?"). These thoughts further escalate his distress. In order to cope and feel better, Charlie responds behaviorally by (1) telling his friend he is unavailable (avoidance), and (2) texting his mother repeatedly for reassurance to "be sure" he did not have to go to the sleepover and to have her tell him he would "be OK." In addition to feeling relief following his text exchange with his mother, Charlie also begins to feel sad because other boys start talking about the sleepover plans and what video games they will play. On the evening of the sleepover itself, Charlie reported that he felt guilty for not attending and "left out" after checking social media and seeing pictures of his friends appearing to have fun. An examination of the other examples on this worksheet reveals the triggers of being away from his parents or home, followed by elevated emotional distress, followed by requests to avoid, eventual avoidance or escape, and texting and reassurance seeking. Again, these functional assessment worksheets can be extremely helpful in elucidating patterns that may by entrenched in the family system and that may seem to "make sense" at the surface (e.g., avoiding social embarrassment, providing reassurance and making promises about being punctual, responding to multiple distressing texts).

In the moment of heightened anxiousness and emotional dysregulation, it is difficult to keep longer-term consequences in mind. When triggered, and especially when experiencing the heightened somatic responses that come with SEP, seeking relief from the discomfort becomes a learned proximal response to the situation at hand. The emotions indeed *feel* intolerable—and kids learn to respond in ways that seek relief and make the feelings tolerable. To this end, avoidance works. Similarly, even when the youth may try to face their fears, for example, in signing up for karate, the drive to the class naturally increases their anxiety. At its peak, when Charlie is crying and uncomfortable, he seeks relief via escaping from the situation. To this end, escape works. Furthermore, when faced with a situation that cannot be avoided or escaped, for example, Charlie's parents having to attend a dinner party, Charlie experiences dread ahead of time, and on the night of the event, complains of significant stomach upset and cries. He begs his mother to stay home (e.g., perhaps this behavioral response has worked before, with his parents canceling their plans). When this is ineffective in avoiding the dreaded separation, Charlie seeks promises, reassurances, and constant text contact to help manage his feelings during the separation. By having his parents promise to return home before bedtime, Charlie was also successful in avoiding having to deal with his nighttime worries of sleeping without a parent present. During the evening, if Charlie experiences an anxious thought about his parents falling ill or failing to return, he would text his mother repeatedly until his mother responded and provided immediate (but temporary) relief. To this end, reassurance seeking works. In this example, note that despite their promises to return on time, they arrived late and Charlie was crying and angry with them. On assessment, the therapist determined that Charlie's parents usually were punctual.

Another way to view this phenomenon is reviewing the habituation curve (see Handout 17 in Appendix A) to illustrate the short- and long-term ineffectiveness of avoidance and escape. In this example, when a separation anxious youth learns that his parents are going out, his anxious distress, reassurance seeking, and clinging behaviors escalate, and after his parents cancel their plans, the youth experiences immediate relief. The escape was effective in reducing distress and therefore escape behaviors (e.g., increased crying, reassurance seeking, tantrum, clinging) are negatively reinforced. The youth also misses out on an opportunity to learn that if his parents went out, the anxiety would have diminished over time (habituation) or, if he had remained highly anxious, that he was able to get through it.

Charlie's parents did not cancel their plans; however, this situation illustrates how Charlie's chronic reassurance seeking via questions and texting throughout the evening also get negatively reinforced. When Charlie learns that his parents are going out, he becomes distressed and immediately seeks reassurance by asking them questions. As his distress escalates, his clinging and reassurance-seeking behaviors escalate as these have become coping strategies, in that they elicit temporary reassurance and relief in the form of his parents providing answers and promises. These answers provide momentary rescue from distress. In repeated responding to his questions and texts, Charlie's parents inadvertently reinforce his maladaptive coping. Therefore, these will be essential treatment targets.

TREATMENT PLANNING

Treatment planning flows directly from the initial diagnostic evaluation and case formulation that includes a working hypothesis. While a general diagnosis can provide general proposed interventions, the treatment plan aims to match the specific interventions to the particular antecedent triggers, emotional and behavioral responses, and consequences. As such, the functional assessment is critical in providing a rationale for each of the interventions for a given youth and family. Tables 8.2 and 8.3 offer a general overview and session-by-session treatment plans.

The proposed treatment plan for Charlie and his family is based on his and his parents' primary areas of concern: impairment and functioning that are prompted by separation fears across

TABLE 8.2. Charlie's Broad Treatment Plan for Separation Anxiety

Treatment goals	Interventions
On time and full-day school attendance	Regulate routines, goal setting, psychoeducation about distress, parent training, cognitive restructuring, exposures to school stimuli.
Decrease distress surrounding parent–child separation across situations.	Psychoeducation about distress, parent training and parent anxiety management, cognitive restructuring, problem solving, tolerating uncertainty, exposures to multiple separation triggers
Reduce family conflict around morning and bedtime routine.	Parent training; contingency management; sleep hygiene; somatic management; exposure
Make more friends, increase social activities.	Graded *in vivo* exposure to social situations, social skills training
Reduce safety fears.	Cognitive restructuring; problem solving; exposure
Reduce fearfulness in the dark (increase ability to tolerate being in a dark room).	Graded imaginal and *in vivo* exposure to darkness

multiple domains. For example, school drop-off and pickup represented the most immediate areas of concern. As such, in the earlier phase of treatment, skills and exposures will target these areas. Although Charlie expresses significant worry about his ability to sleep alone and stay in his room, there is little reported distress at the start of treatment because the family has provided multiple accommodations to soothe Charlie's anxiety, including having Charlie sleep on the floor next to his parents' bed. Therefore, the therapist and family have opted to wait to address this treatment goal during a later phase of exposures. The CBT strategies allow therapists flexible sequencing of intervention components that can be tailored to meet the priorities the family has. Other treatment plans for youth and families presenting with SEP and/or other conditions may opt to introduce skills and exposure targets in a different order. For example, if Charlie's nightly bedtime separation distress and behavioral responses presented with significant disruption, the therapist and family may have decided to use psychoeducation, skills, and graded exposure targets around bedtime sleep separation earlier in treatment.

INTERVENTION COMPONENTS AND PROCESS

Psychoeducation

As discussed, psychoeducation in CBT occurs early and often. Consistent with other conditions, psychoeducation for youth and families with SEP includes providing information on the nature of the disorder itself, the CBT model for understanding SEP (see Handouts 16 and 17 in Appendix A), and a rationale for the upcoming course of treatment. In the early phase of treatment, it is helpful to socialize the youth and family to how treatment is likely to proceed. Handout 18 (Appendix A) provides a useful fact sheet on SEP for caregiver and youth.

TABLE 8.3. Charlie's Detailed Treatment Plan for Separation Anxiety

Sessions 1–2

Assessment
- Assess presenting problems.
- Conduct diagnostic assessment with a focus on impairment (real-life functioning).
- Administer symptom profile measures (e.g., RCADS).
- Assess target problems and treatment goals, focusing on improving daily functioning.
- Assess past attempts (including past treatment) to address the problem.
- Assess parent–child interactions.
- Conduct collateral assessments as needed with the youth's school (e.g., counselor, teacher, school nurse); request parents' complete release of information to speak to school contact(s).
- Evaluate co-occurring medical conditions; consult with pediatrician or specialist (e.g., gastroenterologist) as indicated.
- Assess the need for medication and psychiatric referral (see Chapter 4).

Psychoeducation
- Review assessment and generate target problems with youth and parents.
- Create idiographic target problems tracker.
- Collaborate on case conceptualization: CBT model and functional assessment.
- Provide parents and youth with information handouts on separation anxiety and CBT in general.
- Educate parents on the importance of collaborating with their child's school.

Home practice
- Monitor separation triggers over the week: CBT model and functional assessment.
- Have the youth track their reactions to distress and short- and long-term outcomes (functional assessment) in relation to school routines.
- Track parent–youth interactions around separation episodes.

Sessions 3–4

Assessment
- Evaluate and discuss home practice.
- Complete the target problems tracker.
- Complete the symptom tracker every fourth session (e.g., RCADS).

Interventions
- Implement in-session reward chart for home practice completion.
- Implement in-session reward chart for separation and/or participation.
- Review and refine individual functional assessments.
- Educate youth/parents about function of negative affect/distress in avoidance. Use habituation curve to discuss the role of avoidance/escape in maintaining fears.
- Review and refine parent–youth trackers. Educate parents about caregivers as partners and agents of change. Educate parents on parent–child interaction patterns.
- Reinforce messages about fear/escape in maintaining avoidance behaviors.
- Introduce and teach youth deep breathing or somatic management strategies.
- Teach parents "empathize and encourage" and then "coach and approach" to deescalate conflict and encourage the youth's approach.
- Establish contact with the youth's school as needed; help coordinate school response to youth's in-school anxiety.

(continued)

TABLE 8.3. *(continued)*

Home practice
- Monitor separation triggers over the week: CBT model and functional assessment.
- Have the youth continue to conduct functional assessments. Hone awareness of long-term consequences.
- Have parents continue to monitor parent–youth interactions. Hone awareness of interaction patterns.
- Have youth practice deep breathing or somatic management strategy.
- Have parents practice empathize and encourage and then coach and approach.

Sessions 5–6

Assessment
- As in Sessions 3–4

Interventions
- Continue to monitor parents' understanding of parent–youth interaction patterns and practice of empathize and encourage and then coach and approach.
- Continue to monitor youth's understanding of the role of negative affect in triggering avoidance.
- Create reward chart, negotiating week-to-week goals and corresponding rewards. Focus goals on incremental school attendance. Create rewards that are "daily and renewable."
- Give parents practice at rewarding positive behaviors and responding to noncompliance.

Home practice
- Have parents track their youth's accomplishments and levy rewards.
- Have youth practice deep breathing or somatic management strategy.
- Ask youth to note the accomplishments and rewards they earn each day.
- Create a feedback loop with the school regarding on-time and full-day attendance.

Sessions 7–8

Assessment
- As in Sessions 3–4

Interventions
- Monitor self-talk and cognitive restructuring: teach youth the link between their thoughts and anxiety/distress.
- Teach problem solving.
- Build challenge hierarchy or hierarchies through exposures.
- Practice first steps of hierarchy in session.

Home practice
- Have parents and youth monitor reward chart: parents continue practicing consistent delivery of praise and rewards, and youth monitors accomplishments.
- Direct youth to refine steps of challenge hierarchy, focusing on the core challenges related to separation in different situations: before, during, after school; social and extracurricular activities, sleep/nighttime routine.
- Ask youth to attempt first steps of the hierarchy.

(continued)

TABLE 8.3. *(continued)*

Sessions 9–10

Assessment
- As in Sessions 3–4

Interventions
- Monitor self-talk and cognitive restructuring: teach youth the link between their thoughts and anxiety/distress.
- Review problem solving.
- Continue practicing mild steps of challenge hierarchy through exposures, focusing on the core challenges related to separation in different situations: before, during, after school; social and extracurricular activities, sleep/nighttime routine.

Home practice
- Have parents and youth continue to monitor reward chart.
- Ask youth to complete and monitor a thought–action–feeling chart.
- Have youth complete and monitor their at-home practice of problem solving.

Sessions 11–12

Assessment
- As in Sessions 3–4

Psychoeducation
- Discuss developmental expectations regarding sleep.
- Talk about sleep hygiene (see Handout 4).

Interventions
- Discuss monitoring.
- Monitor sleep hygiene.
- Expand and continue somatic management/relaxation training.
- Practice moderately challenging situations through exposures, focusing on the core challenges related to separation in different situations: before, during, after school; social and extracurricular activities, sleep/nighttime routine.

Home practice
- Have parents and youth continue to monitor reward chart.
- Have youth complete and monitor their at-home practice of problem solving.
- Ask youth to monitor their sleep hygiene.

Sessions 13–20

Assessment
- As in Sessions 3–4

Intervention
- Continue practicing increasingly challenging steps on hierarchy through exposures, focusing on the core challenges related to social anxiety, panic attacks, and depression.
- Practice any individual or parent skills to facilitate exposure success.

(continued)

TABLE 8.3. *(continued)*

Home practice
- Have parents and youth continue to monitor reward chart.
- Ask youth and parent to complete any related skill forms.

Sessions 21–25 (biweekly for maintenance)

Assessment
- As in Sessions 3–4

Psychoeducation
- Introduce the relapse prevention phase.
- Discuss possible termination.

Interventions
- Continue practicing increasingly challenging steps on hierarchy through exposures, focusing on the core challenges related to separation in different situations: before, during, after school; social and extracurricular activities, sleep/nighttime routine.
- Practice any individual or parent skills to facilitate exposure success.

Home practice
- Have parents and youth continue to monitor reward chart.
- Ask youth and parent to complete any related skill forms.

For all anxieties, especially SEP, the therapist can work with the family to normalize anxiety and its evolutionary adaptiveness. Separation anxiety is a *normal* part of child development; it makes sense for growing children, with task demands requiring increasing independence (and parental separations) across situations (e.g., more time at school, falling asleep independently) that may cause the child to experience some nervousness and to seek some reassurance. It is often helpful for youth and families to understand the universality of this phase of development. However, it is also important to assist families in understanding how SEP differs, as it may hinder a child's ability to meet short- and long-term developmental task demands. Charlie's SEP is interfering with his ability to go and stay in school, participate in activities and social activities with peers, self-soothe when distressed, and fall asleep and stay asleep.

To provide psychoeducation on the CBT model for SEP, the therapist is sure to find multiple examples from the caregiver–child intake and functional assessments. A basic understanding of the CBT model and the interplay between a youth's—and caregivers'—thoughts, feelings, and behaviors in separation anxiety–provoking situations provides the fundamentals to comprehending the course of treatment and rationale for interventions. It also helps the therapist to validate the level of distress and impairment. For example, in Figure 8.4, Charlie described his worry this way: "Mom will get into a car accident"; this feeling then triggers hyperarousal, gastrointestinal distress, and clingy and reassurance-seeking behaviors. As such, the therapist can provide validation that given his belief in these thoughts and their certitude, his *perceived threat* makes sense and he is responding accordingly. Psychoeducation also provides the therapist with the opportunity to instill hope by relying on the evidence base supporting CBT for anxiety in youth. Many children experience separation anxiety as part of their development, and for some youth, it may even start to interfere with their ability to get though the day, as in SEP. Youth and families who participate in CBT are likely to benefit by learning to: (1) understand their anxiety and the factors that maintain it; (2) develop and practice skills and problem solving; and (3) change behaviors so they are approaching rather than avoiding what scares them.

To summarize, the therapist can provide information sheets about SEP and the CBT model of SEP (see the reproducible Handouts 16, 17, and 18 in Appendix A; refer also to Appendix B for a list of additional reliable sources).

Affective Education and Somatic Management Skills

Given Charlie's experience with physical symptoms (e.g., butterflies, stomachaches, nausea), affective education can help Charlie to: (1) understand the biology behind his somatic arousal and (2) provide rationale for learning somatic management skills (see the "Affective Education" and "Physical Interventions" sections in Chapter 2). The therapist can also include Charlie's parents in this instruction so they, too, will understand the nature of his hyperarousal as they learn to respond differently, to empathize with and encourage him to practice these skills.

SELF-TALK AND COGNITIVE RESTRUCTURING

The cognitive aspects of anxiety in youth (and adults) include various automatic negative thoughts that may have them stuck in thinking traps (as discussed in Chapter 2; see Handout 2 in Appendix A for a comprehensive list). There may be overlap among the types of cognitive distortions or thinking traps. For youth with SEP, worry thoughts regarding separating from caregivers may anticipate future negative events (fortune-telling), that something bad will certainly happen and it will be very terrible (catastrophizing) and the youth will be unable to handle it. The youth overestimates the bad outcome and its consequences and underestimates their ability to handle it.

When Charlie did not immediately see his mother at the school exit, his anxious self-talk went from believing she forgot to pick him up to fear that she had gotten into a car accident, an example of *catastrophizing* (see Figure 8.6; a blank version is available as Worksheet 5 in Appendix A). Connected to his crying and panic-like experience that he rated a 9/10, he also indicated having a thought about not knowing where to go. In helping Charlie better understand his SEP, the therapist can explain to him that his feeling of being "freaked out" is connected to his catastrophic and *helpless* thinking. Once Charlie is able to identify these specific thoughts, the therapist can work with the child to practice the cognitive restructuring of them. Since Charlie's anxious response occurs rapidly and is accompanied by intense physiological sensations, it will be important to assist him (and perhaps school personnel in this situation; see below) in developing the skills to slow down his breathing and his thinking. In helping him to challenge such anxious self-talk, here are some sample "detective questions" to ask:

"How many times has Mom forgotten to pick you up from school?"
"What are the chances that Mom has forgotten to pick you up from school?"
"What else is possible? What else may be contributing to Mom being late?"

WORKSHEET 5. Thinking Traps Tracker

What thinking traps do you fall into when feeling sad, anxious, or distressed? For each situation, describe and rate how you feel. Describe your automatic thought (the first thought that comes into your head). What thinking trap might you be falling into? How does that make you feel (result)?

Trigger	Feeling (Rate 0–10: "not at all" to "excruciating")	Thought	Thinking Trap	Result?
I got invited to a sleepover party.	Nervous, sad (6)	"I won't be able to sleep and will be the only one awake." "I'll have to call Mom to come get me again." "I'll miss out on another party."	Fortune-telling	Felt worse (9)
I didn't see Mom at the school exit.	Panic, crying (9)	"She forgot to pick me up." "She got into an accident." "I don't know where to go."	Catastrophizing, helpless thinking	Freaked out (10)
My parents told me they are going out of town for a night.	Dread, worry, sick to my stomach (7)	"What if their airplane crashes?" "I need my mom here to be able to fall asleep." "They'll never come back."	Catastrophizing, helpless thinking	Begged them not to go, cried, couldn't stop asking questions (10)

FIGURE 8.6. Completed Thinking Traps Tracker worksheet for Charlie.

198

The therapist can also work with Charlie to develop, practice, and engage in specific coping self-talk. For example:

"If I don't immediately see Mom at the exit, stay calm."
"If Mom is late, wait a few minutes and use the plan we worked out." (See the "Problem Solving" section below.)

The sequence of helping Charlie to work on the cognitive aspects of his SEP includes practicing identifying his specific automatic thoughts, feelings, and behaviors and understanding that his somatic arousal and avoidance are connected to various cognitive distortions, such as catastrophizing that overestimate the actual threat and helplessness that underestimates his ability to handle a situation or distress. Next the therapist works with Charlie to challenge and question some of these anxious thoughts. Importantly, the goal is not positive thinking; rather, it is about helping to set more realistic thinking and expectations: "There are all sorts of reasons caregivers can be late. We cannot expect anyone to be on time 100% of the time." See Figure 8.7 (a blank version is available as Worksheet 16 in Appendix A) for more examples.

Thinking traps can also interfere with attempts to implement later behavior change. For example, two of Charlie's go-to methods for managing his anxiety at after-school pickup are to be sure he is the first person in the school exit line (safety behavior) and to seek reassurance from his parents by texting (safety behavior and parent rescue). As the therapist works with parents and school personnel on exposures, Charlie will need assistance in challenging particular automatic thoughts associated with safety behaviors. That is, in asking Charlie about having to be first in line, it may be useful to gently challenge this belief:

THERAPIST: What would happen if you were the second or third person in line? Or, even fifth or sixth? Last person in line?

CHARLIE: I wouldn't be able to see Mom right away.

THERAPIST: That's true. You'd be a little further back. What do you estimate is the difference in the amount of time to see Mom if you are at the front versus the end of the line?

CHARLIE: I don't know.

THERAPIST: Maybe we can be a detective and investigate this question?

In this example, the therapist is working with Charlie to challenge a safety behavior (having to be first in line). They need to help him recognize that the behavior is tied to a belief that being first in line makes a critical difference in his tolerance of the situation (waiting for his mother and/or father). In working to eliminate safety behaviors during exposures, the therapist works with a youth to tolerate distress without reliance on a particular safety behavior. Helping Charlie "handle" his anxious arousal whether he is at the front, middle, or back of the line improves his self-efficacy and sense that he can manage his own distress in challenging situations. The therapist can help him challenge assumptions that the extra wait will lead to significant outcomes.

When waiting for his mom and beginning to feel anxious (see Figure 8.7), Charlie exclaimed, "I don't know where to go." The therapist can work with Charlie to develop a response plan via problem solving; however, she could also work with him to explore, and learn from, what actually happened in this (and perhaps other) situations.

WORKSHEET 16. Coping Thoughts Tracker

Brainstorm coping thoughts that could answer your thinking trap! Try and come up with coping statements that are more realistic and ask, "How am I not seeing the whole picture?"

Trigger	Thought	Thinking Trap	Coping Thought	Result?
I got invited to a sleepover party.	"I won't be able to sleep and will be the only one awake." "I'll have to call Mom to come get me again." "I'll miss out on another party."	Fortune-telling	"I've never actually been awake all night & will fall asleep eventually." "I don't want to miss out again so I want to try it." "Even if I get upset, my friends will understand."	Felt a little better, then decided to go. Felt happy that my friend was excited when I said "yes." Felt nervous again but then it went down.
I didn't see Mom at the school exit.	"She forgot to pick me up." "She got into an accident." "I don't know where to go."	Catastrophizing, helpless thinking	"I trust Mom will get here when she can." "I know the plan and can go to the main office to wait." "I can wait 15 minutes before calling her."	Felt better and more calm. Mom showed up 2 minutes later.
My parents told me they are going out of town for a night.	"What if their airplane crashes?" "I need my mom here to be able to fall asleep." "They'll never come back."	Catastrophizing, helpless thinking	"They're not even taking an airplane." "Even if I have a hard time sleeping, I can do this." "Duh, they'll come back." "It will be nice to see grandma."	Felt a little better. Still did not want them to go. They went and I was upset, but played with grandma. They came back and it was OK.

FIGURE 8.7. Completed Coping Thoughts Tracker worksheet for Charlie.

200

THERAPIST: So what happened after it felt like you were freaking out and believed you did not know where to go?

CHARLIE: The teacher saw I was crying and pulled me aside.

THERAPIST: So the teacher was there, and he stood with you at the door?

CHARLIE: Yes. A few feet from the door.

THERAPIST: And then what happened? Where did you go next?

CHARLIE: Nowhere. We waited there and then Mom came a few minutes later.

The therapist can work with the youth to recognize that despite significant distress and catastrophic thinking about his mother's whereabouts and helpless thinking about himself, the situation resolved. It also creates an opportunity to plan and problem-solve for a realistic situation: what he can do and where he can go if a parent is late picking him up. Reviewing the situation in this way also allows the therapist and Charlie to identify a potential *coping thought* to reference and utilize in future similar anxiety-producing situations where he is awaiting his parent's arrival.

Problem Solving

Another way to increase a youth's self-efficacy is to teach formal problem-solving skills that will enable the youth to influence change over challenging situations. Charlie expressed helpless thinking in claiming, "I don't know where to go," when his mother was late picking him up. In response to this, Charlie's therapist used problem solving to engage Charlie's own creativity and self-reliance (see Chapter 2 for a review of problem solving using STEPS). In this case, the therapist uses Worksheet 15 (a blank version is available in Appendix A) to brainstorm possible solutions to a common problem for Charlie (see Figure 8.8 for the completed form).

THERAPIST: One of the thoughts you wrote on your Thinking Traps Tracker is that you would not know where to go if your mom is not standing in the specific spot you assigned to her when you walk out of the school building. How about if we work out a plan so you will know where else to go if she's not there? [specifying the problem]

CHARLIE: OK.

THERAPIST: Let's imagine you walk out the school door and do not see Mom right away. What's the first thing we thought it would be good to do? [brainstorming solutions]

CHARLIE: I should tell myself, "Stay calm." And take a few deep breaths.

THERAPIST: Right, good. What are some other options at this point? [encouraging continued brainstorming]

CHARLIE: I can stand there and wait.

THERAPIST: Yes. Where is "there"?

CHARLIE: Right by the door.

THERAPIST: OK. So one option is to stay by the door. Sometimes anxiety wants us to react right away. What's a good amount of time to stay by the door and wait, do you think?

CHARLIE: 5 minutes or 15 minutes?

WORKSHEET 15. Problem–Solving STEPS

To solve problems, take these steps: say what the problem is, think of solutions, examine each solution, pick one solution and try it, and see if it worked!

Say What the Problem Is: *Don't know where to go if Mom is not standing in her spot after school.*

Think of Solutions	Examine Each Solution		Rank
	Pros	**Cons**	
1. Stay calm, take deep breaths.	It'll help calm me in the moment.	Hard to do; and I still don't know where my mom is.	1
2. I can just wait by the door for up to 15 minutes.	Stay in one place.	15 minutes is a long time.	3
3. Tell a teacher.	They can be helpful.	They might tell me to go back outside.	2
4. Go back to the main office.	It's safe; they might be helpful.	They might tell me to go back outside; they might've already left.	4

Pick One Solution and Try It: *Take a breath and then tell teacher.*

FIGURE 8.8. Brainstorming problem solving for Charlie.

THERAPIST: Oh, so that's a range. So up to 15 minutes? [reflecting, not yet deciding on an amount of time] What else may be an option when you're waiting there? [Notice that an evaluation of options is delayed until brainstorming is complete.]

CHARLIE: I can tell the teacher.

THERAPIST: OK, so another option would be to tell the teacher and go with them somewhere else. What's another option? Do other kids sometimes have to wait for their parents?

CHARLIE: Yeah, I guess so.

THERAPIST: Where did they go?

CHARLIE: I dunno. I guess some stay outside, and some kids go back into the main office.

THERAPIST: OK, good, so going back into the building to the main office can be an option. Now let's take a closer look at this list of options we've come up with and pick a solution you can plan to use if you don't see Mom when you exit. [Pick a potential solution and plan to use it.]

In this example, the therapist and Charlie have worked together to brainstorm possible options for the feared (and actual) situation, that his mother is late picking him up from school. Brainstorming is conducted without evaluating individual solutions because premature judgments often derail the brainstorming stage. Self-monitoring and home practice exercises have helped

Charlie to better identify the SEP thoughts, feelings, and behaviors. This will then help yield specific beliefs about, as well as identify potential deficits in, problem solving as a skill. For more generalized deficits, the treatment plan can target improving problem solving more broadly; deficits may be related to higher arousal, distress, and difficulty in recognizing alternatives. As such, the therapist and youth can work to develop a targeted coping plan.

Exposures

As evidenced by the comprehensive functional assessment, Charlie's significant separation anxiety affects several areas of his personal, family, academic, and social functioning. The therapist will work with Charlie and his parents to identify these various areas and develop fear and avoidance hierarchies that guide the exposure phase of treatment. There may be general areas for intervention (e.g., school, peers, social activities, bedtime) and specific safety behaviors cutting across all or most situations (e.g., calling or texting, reassurance seeking) that will need to be targeted during exposures. For Charlie and his family, the school-related aspects of his SEP are connected to his getting to school, going to the nurse's office, staying in school, and his elevated distress at dismissal time. While Charlie has maintained social friendships, his SEP keeps him from hanging out with his peers at their homes and away from his own. He has also begun to decline invitations to birthday parties and other peer gatherings that have a sleepover component. Relatedly, an especially difficult area of anxiety for Charlie is separation at bedtime and anxiety related to his belief that he will be unable to fall asleep on his own. Consistent with anxious youth, Charlie attempts to manage his anxious distress by avoiding or escaping from situations that cause him anxiety (e.g., sleeping on his own at home, taking the school bus, sleepovers) or having his parents rescue him (e.g., being picked up early from school). Charlie and his parents tend to engage in a pattern of behaviors that serve to reinforce his anxiety; safety behaviors serve to further reinforce Charlie's anxiety and anxious responding. These include the pervasive Q&A of reassurance seeking and the phone calls and texts to and from his parents.

In developing a plan for the exposure phase of treatment, the therapist works with the family to identify a hierarchy of meaningful exposures across the varied domains of Charlie's anxieties. These can be arranged in a graduated fashion with increasingly challenging and anxiety-provoking situations; the order can also be varied especially as naturally occurring situations may present themselves (e.g., an invitation to hang out). Given the particular nature of SEP and Charlie's age, parents are essential for orchestrating the exposure plans *and* practicing their own new empathize and encourage and coach and approach responding (see Chapter 5, "Working with Caregivers and Parents"). Below are sample exposure hierarchies. Additional examples of exposures for morning and school routines may be found in Chapter 11, "School Refusal and Problematic Attendance."

Challenge Hierarchy A: Morning Routine Regulation

1. Regulate morning routine with waking time (connected to sleep routine exposures of getting up in his own room).
2. Pick out his own clothes and get dressed.
3. Sit at the kitchen table and eat breakfast (catching urges to follow a parent from room to room).
4. Limit reassurance questions in the morning to three (then two, then one, then none).
5. Walk out the door by an agreed-upon time each morning.

Challenge Hierarchy B: Fear of Separation, the Bus-Ride Routine

1. Have Charlie stand at the bus stop for an increasing amount of time (5, 10, 15 minutes) before his mother drives him to school.
2. Arrange to have Charlie picked up at one of the later pickup spots on the bus route so that Charlie has a short ride to school. Mother can meet Charlie at school at the bus drop-off, before fading away. As Charlie's anxiety gets better, the family can lengthen the school bus ride.

Challenge Hierarchy C: Fear of Separation at School

1. Stand second or third in line at dismissal.
2. Have mother progressively move out of Charlie's sight from classroom.
3. Stand in the last position in line at dismissal.
4. Have Mom intentionally arrive 5 minutes late for pickup.
5. Take the school bus to school.
6. Talk to peers at the bus stop.
7. Talk to teacher at the bus stop.

Challenge Hierarchy D: Fear of Separation at Social Activities

1. Hang out at peer's house for 30 minutes (parent present).
2. Hang out at peer's house for 1 hour (parent present).
3. Hang out at peer's house for 30 minutes (parent drop-off and pickup).
4. Hang out at peer's house for 1 hour (parent drop-off and pickup).
5. Hang out at peer's house for 2–3 hours (parent drop-off and pickup).
6. Sleep over at cousin's house.
7. Sleep over at peer's house.

For any of these actions, the therapist can start by incorporating safety signals (e.g., a limited number of texts to mother) before fading them out. The goal is to make each challenge possible so that the youth has a successful experience as the challenges grow harder.

Challenge Hierarchy E: Fear of Separation at Nighttime and Sleep

1. Sleep in his own bedroom with a parent sitting on the bed until he falls asleep.
2. Sleep in his own bedroom with a parent sitting on a chair near the bed until he falls asleep.
3. Sleep in his own bedroom with a parent sitting on a chair near the bed for 30 minutes.
4. Repeat the same action as above while progressively decreasing the amount of time a parent sits on a chair near the bed (e.g., 20 minutes, 10 minutes, 5 minutes).

Challenge Hierarchy F: Fear of Separation from Mom and Dad

1. Stay with Grandma and Grandpa for 1 hour at home (both parents leave for 1 hour).
2. Stay with Grandma and Grandpa for 2 hours at home (both parents leave for 2 hours).
3. Stay with Grandma and Grandpa at their house for 2 hours (drop-off and pickup).

4. Stay with Grandma and Grandpa at their house between 3 and 4 hours (drop-off, variable pickup).

5. Stay with Grandma and Grandpa at home, including at bedtime (parents go out until after bedtime).

The therapist would similarly work with Charlie and his parents to develop and integrate graduated exposures regarding his fear of the dark. They may opt to target the sleep and nighttime separation-based fears in the middle phase of treatment and then target the phobia of the dark. They can also consider some of the fear-of-the-dark targets (e.g., using a nightlight) for variability while working on the sleep and separation targets.

Having initiated morning and school-related exposures, the therapist and family can move toward the goal of helping Charlie (and his parents) cope with nighttime separation anxieties and challenge the expectation that he requires their presence to fall asleep. The goal is to teach Charlie developmentally appropriate skills regarding falling and staying asleep while increasing independent coping and self-soothing.

As noted in the challenge hierarchy for nighttime and sleep, initial exposures can target Charlie's return to his own room, gradually reducing the amount of time his parents spend in his room and increasing the physical distance between them and Charlie as he falls asleep. The eventual goal is to have the parents leave the room *before* Charlie falls asleep so that he can cope with falling asleep without being "rescued" by his parents. The therapist works collaboratively with Charlie and his parents to plan bedtime exposures. The therapist can introduce somatic management to aid Charlie generally with the physical aspects and emotion dysregulation of his SEP, and they can also work on somatic and relaxation strategies, and/or mindfulness strategies for bedtime calming routines (see Chapter 2). See Figure 8.9 (a blank version is available as Worksheet 6 in Appendix A), paying particular attention to helping Charlie prepare early coping self-talk (e.g., "Mom and Dad are just down the hall" "I'm OK and will fall asleep eventually") and strategies for transitioning to sleep (e.g., reading, relaxation, music).

When planning bedtime exposures, the therapist should also help parents identify anticipated challenges (e.g., "What do we do if . . ."). Advanced planning might include contingency management plans and reward charts to systematically reinforce Charlie's efforts to sleep in his room independently for progressively longer periods of time. Therapists will need to prepare the family for a likely extinction burst. As the family begins implementing the plan, the youth may experience initial increased distress that can disrupt the family's sleep. As discussed, helping parents to identify their own expectations and predictions can aid in exposure planning. Parents may require assistance in challenging their own beliefs about Charlie's ability to fall asleep on his own, and their own abilities to assist him:

MOTHER: What if he is up all night? He has to go to school tomorrow and can't function if he doesn't sleep. He'll keep us up all night, too, and we have to work.

THERAPIST: Yes, this may happen at first. How often did this happen before?

MOTHER: Never all night but until 2 A.M. a couple of times.

THERAPIST: And what happened?

FATHER: (*sheepishly*) We let him come into our bed.

THERAPIST: At 2 A.M. when everyone is exhausted, that can be really difficult. It *is* easier to

WORKSHEET 6. *In Vivo* Exposure/Behavioral Experiment

> Complete this worksheet with the youth as you are preparing for a behavioral experiment.

1. Situation (What's the situation?):

Sleeping and staying in my own room with Mom and Dad in their bedroom

2. Feelings: **Distress Rating:** 10/10

Anxious

3. Anxious/Negative Thoughts:	**Thinking Traps (See list below.)**
"If Mom and Dad aren't there, I just can't fall asleep."	What ifs
"What if I get freaked out, and can't sleep all night?"	Fortune-telling
"I'm gonna be the only one awake."	Catastrophizing
"What if something really bad happens tonight?"	

Thinking Traps: mind reading, fortune-telling, catastrophizing, jumping to conclusions, what if's, discounting the positives, looking for the negatives, overgeneralizing, all-or-nothing thinking, should statements, taking things too personally, blaming.

4. Coping Thoughts (How do you respond to your anxious thoughts?):

"Mom and Dad are just down the hall, and I know they are rooting for me."
"I'm OK and will fall asleep eventually. I don't have any evidence that I will be up all night because it's never happened."
"I probably won't be the last one awake, but even if I am, I can do it."
"The anxiety is sending me the danger signal."
"If I stay in my room, I'll earn my points."

Challenge Questions: Do I know for certain that _____? Am I 100% sure that _____? What evidence do I have that _____? What is the worst that could happen? How bad is that? Do I have a crystal ball?

5. Achievable Behavioral Goals (What do you want to accomplish?):

Goal	Accomplished?
a. Stay in my room and call out one time to Mom.	Yes
b. Listen to my mindfulness app.	Yes
c. Stay in my room until morning wake time at 6:30 A.M.	No, but I went right back in when Dad brought me.

6. Rewards:

Reward	Earned?
a. Two points for Fortnite time	Yes
b. Earn in-app sticker	Yes
c. Two points for Fortnite time	One point for trying and going back right away

FIGURE 8.9. Exposure worksheet for separation anxiety.

let him in the bed! The tricky part is that you then missed the opportunity to learn that he may have fallen asleep eventually on his own.

The therapist will want to validate the caregivers' experiences, frustration, and likely exhaustion if there is chronic sleep disturbance. Caregivers generally know that redirecting a child back to their bed might be best, but when everyone is tired and worried that the child may not get enough sleep for school, they may just give in. This makes sense given their experiences. Therapists can model how to empathize and encourage with the parents themselves and then provide the psychoeducation and planning for the family system to get to longer-term adaptive coping.

Role playing imagined scenarios with caregivers and developing potential scripted responses and guidelines may assist their preparedness for follow-through with the exposure.

FATHER: What do we do if he comes into our room?

THERAPIST: We can probably predict that he will at first come into your room so let's plan for it! When he comes into your room, you can use empathize and encourage statements like we have discussed: "I know you're nervous, and I know you can work to settle yourself down." Then guide him back to his room, using coach and approach, reminding him to use his coping skills and that he will earn points for staying in his room. Let's practice that, OK?

FATHER: OK.

THERAPIST (*pretending to be Charlie*): Dad, I can't sleep. Can you please come lie down with me?

FATHER: I know you're having a hard time, but remember we are practicing. So, let me walk you back to your room, and you can practice reminding yourself that you don't really need me to lie next to you. You can do this. I'm proud of you for trying. You'll get a point on your chart for practicing again tonight.

THERAPIST (*as self*): Good use of empathize and encourage! Way to keep it brief, and validate and highlight problem solving and the reward plan.

FATHER: OK, I can try that. I'm not sure it will work. What if he's up all night long? Sometimes I worry that he is, and we just don't know.

THERAPIST: Let's check that out. But even if he does stay up, what ultimately happens?

FATHER: He's usually exhausted in the morning and refuses to get up.

THERAPIST: OK, that's when we'll have to rely on our reward plan and routine regulation efforts. [See Chapter 11 for more examples of how to use contingency management to address morning routines.] For the first few days, we're going to have to embolden you to get Charlie up any way you can, give him immediate rewards, and then trudge him off to school.

FATHER/MOTHER: But then he'll be exhausted all day at school.

THERAPIST: The first few days or week, yes. He'll be tired at the end of the day, and over time falling asleep likely will be easier at a normal time. I'm sorry there's no magic bullet here, but he will not get on a regular schedule unless we have a few disrupted nights. How can *we* make sure your family's prepared for that? [Therapist can problem-solve how to help the family cope and prepare for some sleepless nights and help Charlie persist through the change process.]

While Charlie has his own room and lives with both parents, other families and contexts may appear to complicate a family's ability to execute nighttime SEP exposures. For example, how should therapists help families to implement these types of exposures when, say, the family lives in a one-bedroom apartment or the youth shares a bedroom with a sibling or other family member? In these situations, therapists have to rely on the case conceptualization and the functional assessment of antecedents and consequences that may be triggering and maintaining the anxiety. If, for example, Charlie lived in a small apartment with his parents, the therapist could work with them to shape Charlie's ability to independently initiate and continue his bedtime routine. Most importantly, the therapist should focus on the area of greatest impairment and attend to the needs represented here. If it's necessary to have the youth sleep in the same room as the parents or another family member, target areas where the separation anxiety is interfering with daily life (e.g., the youth continues to follow the parents around during the day; the youth frequently asks for reassurance during sleep time). Separation per se is not the required outcome so much as independent functioning.

IDENTIFYING PARENT–CHILD INTERACTION PATTERNS

Given the very nature of SEP in youth and its core fears related to separating from and harm befalling a primary caregiver, assessing and intervening at the level of caregiver–child interaction are likely essential. As noted above, the functional assessment worksheets will provide a roadmap for understanding how caregiver–child interactions in anxiety-provoking situations may be maintaining youth anxiety via escape, rescue, or avoidance (see Figure 8.5). In identifying these, the therapist can work to provide corrective psychoeducation, coping self-talk for the child and caregiver, scripts for empathize and encourage approach behavior for the youth, limiting rescue behaviors on the part of caregivers, and exposures that account for safety behaviors in the caregiver–child interaction (e.g., reassurance seeking via multiple questions or texts).

Empathize and Encourage

To aid caregivers in coaching their child with SEP, therapists should first teach them to empathize with the youth's experience before encouraging them to approach a scary situation (see Chapter 5, as well as Handout 11 in Appendix A). Empathizing first serves to validate and label the child's experience before moving too quickly toward problem solving or pushing a youth. It also reinforces the coaching role for caregivers. Some caregivers identify strongly with their youth's anxiety and overshare their own past experiences or distress in the moment. Such disclosures tend to escalate the youth's own anxiety and communicates that avoidance is a legitimate solution to anxiety. Having the caregiver focus on the youth's anxiety serves the purpose of communicating understanding and validation of emotions while avoiding escalating the situation. See Chapter 5 for more examples of empathize and encourage.

Validating the youth's feelings is necessary but not sufficient. Once Charlie's parents were able to learn to expressly empathize (e.g., "I know how upset your stomach must feel in this situation"), they could next learn to encourage active coping, problem solving, and approach behaviors. Over the course of treatment, the therapist can first coach the family, then transfer coaching and problem solving to caregivers, and then the caregivers can transfer the same techniques to the child while providing *scaffolding*. Ultimately, the child can use the skills independently. As in the example above, Charlie's father provided an initial empathic and validating remark, then encouraged Charlie to use his coping strategies while reminding him of the reward plan and physically guiding him back to his room.

Reward Charts and Contingency Management

The therapist, Charlie, and his parents developed weekly out-of-session contingency management plans that paralleled the targets of each week's session. As discussed, reward charts should be kept simple and easy for parents and child to track and consistently maintain (see daily renewable reward plans in Chapter 5). During the exposure phase, the therapist was able to work with Charlie and his parents to develop a reward chart that targeted the specific exposure from the challenge hierarchy. For example, when Charlie stood in the third place in the school exit line, he was able to earn 2 points daily and exchange those points at the end of each week for a desired prize. Initially, these prizes were small items Charlie could earn quickly (ideally, daily). Prizes later transitioned into experiences (e.g., getting to pick the movie on family movie night) and saving points for larger prizes (e.g., video games, going out to a movie). See Figure 8.10 for a sample (a blank version is available as Worksheet 10 in Appendix A).

In-session reward charts developed by the therapist and Charlie targeted between-session home practice completion. Charlie was able to earn points for completion of each week's home practice, focusing first on skills worksheet and then on exposure practice logs. The in-session contingency management plan also allowed the therapist to reinforce Charlie's in-session participation, separation exposures from his parents early in treatment and practice exposures conducted in the office.

Collaborating with the School

Youth with SEP like Charlie often experience aspects of their anxious distress in connection with going to and staying in school (see Chapter 11 for examples). Case conceptualization will include understanding the intersection of a youth's anxiety and the school setting to determine recommended collateral work with the school. In the context of the conceptualization and caregiver consent, the therapist and caregiver can work together to include relevant school personnel. In Charlie's case, given his frequent trips to the school nurse and requests for early pickups, the therapist, parent, and nurse can work together to develop guidelines for Charlie's visits to the school nurse. For example, they will want to agree on the circumstances under which he can go to the nurse's office, for how long, and how the nurse can empathize and encourage and prompt his return to class. Similarly, the group will agree on clear limits around parent phone calls. To aid these efforts, the therapist can tailor relevant worksheets to help the nurse translate coping skills to the nurse's office, ensuring everyone involved is speaking the same language regarding Charlie's anxiety. Since one of Charlie's fear and avoidance hierarchies centered around Charlie's worry that he had to be first in line to exit the classroom and school, the therapist, parent(s), and teacher ought to be in contact to prepare for and execute the exposures. They should identify

WORKSHEET 10. Daily Renewable Rewards Chart

Brainstorm step-by-step goals and rewards to go with each level. Then track success!

Theme: _Riding the Bus_

Goals (incremental levels)	Reward (incremental levels)	Sun	Mon	Tue	Wed	Thu	Fri	Sat	# of Days Achieved
Get on bus by 7:30 A.M.	Get phone leaving out the door. Keep all day	–	N	N	N	✓	✓	–	2
Mom/Dad drive to school by 10:00 A.M.	Pick up your phone at counselor's at lunchtime	–	N	N	✓	–	–	–	1
Get to school by lunchtime (noon)	Get your phone when you get home after last school period.	–	N	✓	–	–	–	–	1
Don't get to school at all	No phone	–	✓	–	–	–	–	–	1

Theme: _School Dismissal_

Goals (incremental levels)	Reward (incremental levels)	Sun	Mon	Tue	Wed	Thu	Fri	Sat	# of Days Achieved
Stand in last spot in school dismissal line.	5 points toward Fortnite time	–	N	N	N	N	–	–	1
Stand in fifth spot in dismissal line.	3 points toward Fortnite time	–	N	N	N	N	–	–	0
Stand in third spot in dismissal line.	2 points toward Fortnite time	–	N	✓	✓	✓	–	–	3
Stand in first spot in dismissal line.	0 points toward Fortnite time	–	N	✓	–	–	–	–	1

FIGURE 8.10. Daily renewable rewards example to encourage Charlie's school attendance.

the roles each might play to facilitate implementation, coach Charlie through the exposure, and reward him afterward.

Progress Monitoring

With the many domains across which Charlie's SEP impacted him and his family, the exposure phase of treatment required several months of intervention within and across these domains. The therapist collaborated with the family to gradually and systematically approach some targets (habituation-based) while variably introducing and combining other exposure targets (inhibitory learning-based) (see Figure 8.11; a blank version is available as Worksheet 11 in Appendix A). Primary goals included school-based exposure, starting with the morning routine of getting Charlie to school on time, decreasing the number of times he goes to the nurse and leaves school early, and decreasing safety behaviors (e.g., where he stands in the dismissal line). Progress monitoring included periodic collateral phone calls with the school nurse and Charlie's teacher to assist them in coaching Charlie to use certain skills and redirecting his requests to leave school and make phone calls to his parents.

Social activity exposures included scheduling hangouts and extracurricular activities that required drop-offs and pickups. As more of these were scheduled and completed, despite initial anticipatory worries, Charlie learned that he could ride out his anxiety and the expectancy that he would "freak out" without Mom diminished; these hang-outs became intrinsically motivating for him. Family-based exposures included targeting the bedtime routine and having Charlie return to sleeping in his own room. While initially this was very difficult, requiring multiple evenings of disrupted sleep, Charlie was successfully able to sleep in his own room, first with his parents present and then without them. Charlie's parents increased their effectiveness in praising him and setting firm limits, persisted in redirecting him back to his room, and implemented a behavior plan whereby he could earn desired rewards. Another family-based goal included Charlie's parents helping him (and themselves!) to practice their leaving and returning home in the evenings, and they scheduled various events of increasing duration for themselves outside the home (e.g., dinner, the theater, concerts), each time arranging for Charlie to stay with a babysitter. A few months into treatment, Charlie's parents spent a weekend away from home—progress indeed!—and though challenging at times, they all completed the exposure skillfully.

Charlie's self-report and his mother's parent report at Week 12 of treatment indicated significant improvements, especially with regard to the separation anxiety subscale of the RCADS (see Table 8.4). Notably, while subclinical across the subscales, the SEP domain remains elevated. The therapist can examine specific items to better understand response pattern (i.e., multiple items rated 1–2, or fewer items rated at a higher frequency of 2–3). In any case, both reports are very encouraging (the father's report was unavailable for this assessment).

TERMINATION AND RELAPSE PREVENTION

The varied domains of Charlie's SEP required significant planning and coordination of exposures outside of the therapy office. That's not to say the therapist and Charlie could not work on exposures in the office (such as separating from parents to come to the office, drop-off rather than staying, returning late). Even over telehealth, "office"-based exposures could include parents

WORKSHEET 11. Goals Tracker

Work with your therapist to brainstorm possible specific, meaningful, and achievable goals. Think through what outcomes you expect to see. And then, keep track of how your child does each week.

Parent Goals:	Desired Outcomes	Weeks 6–17	Week 18	Week 19	Week 20
Go to school on time.	Walk in the building by 8:20 A.M.	...	5/5 days	4/5 days	5/5 days
Ride the bus to school.	Be at bus pickup by 7:30 A.M. and ride bus 5/5 days.	...	5/5 days	5/5 days	5/5 days
Make playdates with friends outside of the home.	1 weekday & 1 weekend playdate	...	2 weekdays; 1 weekend	1 weekday; 2 weekends	1 weekday; 2 weekends
Sleep in his own bedroom and is able to stay in his room (7/7 days).	# of nights sleep in room (including leaving & prompt return)	...	6/7	5/7	6/7
Decrease number of phone calls and texts.	# of phone calls & texts per day	...	7	3	4

Youth Goals:	Desired Outcomes	Week x	Week 18	Week 19	Week 20
Decrease feeling nauseous about going to school	Anxiety nausea rating (0–10)	...	4	2	3
Make sure mom and dad are on time	Reduce worry rating about whether mom & dad are on time (0–10)	...	4	5	3
Spend more time with friends after school	Frequency of hangouts with friends outside of school	...	0 weekday; 1 weekend	1 weekday; 1 weekend	2 weekday; 1 weekend

FIGURE 8.11. Completed Goals Tracker worksheet for Charlie at the end of treatment.

TABLE 8.4. Charlie's Symptom Profile at Week 12 Using the RCADS

	Mother		Father		Youth	
	Raw score	*T* scores	Raw scores	*T* scores	Raw scores	*T* scores
Separation anxiety	10	69	—	—	10	63
Generalized anxiety	7	60	—	—	6	47
Panic disorder	4	61	—	—	8	57
Social anxiety	5	41	—	—	7	44
Obsessions/compulsions	1	46	—	—	1	34
Depression	7	61	—	—	7	47
Total anxiety	27	56	—	—	32	49
Total anxiety and depression	34	58	—	—	39	49

T scores higher than 65 indicate borderline clinical threshold. Scores of 70 or higher indicate scores above clinical threshold. *T* scores are normalized based on youth's age and gender.

leaving the room or home as appropriate and for increasing durations. Charlie's parents were key in orchestrating and executing the at-home and school-based exposures and needed additional coaching and support in the later phase of treatment. As they were able to implement and follow through on the behavior plan for bedtime, no early pickups from school, date nights, and the ability to coach him to use his skills (especially cognitive challenging), they could begin to discuss tapering sessions and eventual termination.

Relapse prevention for Charlie and his parents focused on continuing to practice separation challenges and identifying possible future challenges (e.g., an upcoming sleepover, going to day camp), and preparing for possible extinction bursts.

Prognosis and Follow-Up

Charlie and his parents made significant improvements, but he continued to experience elevated anxiety. Charlie's anxiety includes a quick, emotional sensitivity and somatic (especially gastrointestinal) response. Though this has improved, he and his parents will want to continue to monitor and assist him when he feels nauseous. The therapist and family agreed to follow-up booster sessions starting mid-Spring to prepare Charlie for his first attempt at summer camp and a friend's sleepover party, an event he had missed last year.

Challenges in This Case

As with many cases, Charlie's anxiety, overall distress, and multidomain impairment can feel overwhelming. Where does a therapist begin when SEP impairs a youth across so many domains, and the youth's distress impacts the family's functioning throughout the day: in the morning before school, getting to school, staying in school, exiting school, hanging out at friends' houses, sleeping independently and comfortably? We selected Charlie's case precisely because of its complexity. It makes sense for the therapist to start with the areas of greatest impairment and match the family's treatment goals. The therapist's case conceptualization then helps the therapist connect the multiple areas of impairment by understanding the common thought, action, and feeling processes that underlie them all. In this way, the youth can experience gains in multiple domains even as therapy activities are concretely focusing on one or two areas. It was important to work with Charlie's parents to set realistic expectations and to understand that treatment gains would progress gradually. It is critical to remind caregivers that it took years for the problems to build; it would be unrealistic to expect resolution in days. Starting with one or two main goals, achieving some progress, and then moving on to another one or two goals provide a steadier approach. Often, Charlie's parents would present to treatment with a weekly "crisis" related to his anxiety, for example, a meltdown or tantrum associated with an anxiety-provoking situation or a sense of urgency based on an external task demand (e.g., invitation to a sleepover, deadline for reserving a spot in camp). Any of the skills we've discussed here can be applied to these kinds of weekly events, and it is a very powerful experience to demonstrate that the skills you have been teaching can apply to such seemingly novel challenges. At the same time, one should not hesitate to "table" or "put on hold" certain events and challenges for later discussion in order to maintain continuity of treatment plan or to remain focused on a particular goal. Relatedly, it was important to simultaneously assure Charlie that he would not have to complete all of the tasks at the top of his hierarchies at once and that he could handle (and would learn to handle) the anticipated distress.

SUMMARY AND KEY POINTS

Given the de facto role of caregivers in SEP, carefully assess for caregiver accommodation behaviors that rescue SEP youth (e.g., nighttime and bedtime routines, early school pickups, reducing or eliminating separation events by not going out, staying at friends' houses).

- Additional collateral sessions may be required for caregiver involvement and coordination of at-home exposures.
- Note and teach the youth about negative self-talk, in particular about thinking traps that include negative fortune-telling and catastrophizing.
- Separating at bedtime and concomitant sleep onset troubles are also a common presenting concern for youth with SEP. Identify and challenge the youth's potential beliefs regarding sleep skills: "I can't sleep if my mom's not there" or "I need my dad sitting there to be able to fall asleep."
- Target and teach somatic management strategies for somatic symptoms (e.g., deep breathing, mindfulness), hyperarousal, and emotion dysregulation symptoms (e.g., stomachaches, crying).
- Assess oppositional behaviors in conjunction with separation scenarios and teach caregivers limit setting, empathize and encourage, and contingency management strategies.
- Collaborate with school regarding SEP interference with youth drop-off and visits to school nurse and provide guidelines that will keep the child in school.
- Design exposures to challenge excessive checking in and reassurance-seeking behaviors (e.g., excessive contact); provide scripts to and role-play them with caregivers.

CHAPTER 9

Social Anxiety Disorder

Normative development includes increasing emphasis on peers and social evaluation, with transient social anxiety common at various points of childhood. Social anxiety disorder (SAD) typically onsets in early adolescence between the ages of 10 and 13 years (Kessler, Berglund, et al., 2005; Rapee & Spence, 2004), and often is diagnosed in younger, pre-pubertal children in clinically referred youth anxiety samples (Kendall et al., 2010). SAD may be related to the multiple changes associated with this transition period, which includes pubertal and cognitive development and changes in the youth's environment (Rapee & Spence, 2004). Prevalence appears to increase over the course of youth development (Beesdo et al., 2007; Costello et al., 2011), and there is evidence that younger onset may be related to the disorders continuing into adulthood (Beesdo et al., 2007). SAD is among the most common psychiatric disorders, affecting approximately 13% of the general population (Kessler, Chiu, Demler, Merikangas, & Walters, 2005; Ruscio et al., 2007), and among the most prevalent disorders in youth, with approximately 7.4% prevalence (Kessler, Petukhova, Sampson, Zaslavsky, & Wittcehn, 2012).

Clinical presentations in younger versus older children with social anxiety appear to share many core symptom features and levels of reported distress. However, when compared to younger children, adolescents with SAD appear to experience broader and greater social functional impairments consistent with the increasing social demands and domains of adolescence (Rao et al., 2007). As previously noted, youth anxiety disorders can be highly comorbid with other anxiety disorders as well as mood and externalizing conditions. Research suggests notably higher comorbidity of youth social anxiety and generalized anxiety disorders (Leyfer, Gallo, Cooper-Vince, & Pincus, 2013) as well as selective mutism (Dummit et al., 1997). Social anxiety and alcohol and substance use and abuse in adolescence also have been linked (Merikangas et al., 1998; Wolitzky-Taylor, Bobova, Zinbarg, Mineka, & Craske, 2012). As with other disorders, etiological and maintenance models of youth SAD postulate an interplay among relevant genetic, temperamental, environmental, cognitive, and behavioral factors (Halldorsson & Creswell, 2017; Ollendick & Hirshfeld-Becker, 2002; Rapee & Spence, 2004; Spence & Rapee, 2016).

BEHAVIORAL INHIBITION AND TEMPERAMENT

Behavioral inhibition (BI) to new and unfamiliar situations or people has been proposed and studied as a temperamental precursor to anxiety and social anxiety (Kagan, Resnick, & Snidman,

1988; Kagan, 1994). Youth observed to be higher in BI are more likely to evidence fearfulness, restraint, and avoidance in novel situations. Prospectively and retrospectively, higher BI scores have been associated with greater likelihood of anxiety conditions (e.g., Biederman et al., 2001; Hayward, Killen, Kraemer, & Taylor, 1998). While there has been some consideration regarding whether BI is a unique precursor to SAD (see Degnan, Almas, & Fox, 2010), longitudinal work seems to indicate that BI may confer a significant and particularly unique risk factor for SAD (Muris, 2011; Rapee, 2014).

Physiologic correlates of BI have also been established (Hirshfeld et al., 1992), and studies demonstrate the heritability of inhibited behaviors as a factor that may be transmitted (e.g., Robinson, Kagan, Reznick, & Corley, 1992). Unsurprisingly, temperamentally BI youth will interact with their early environments and may elicit certain responses; as such, caregiving, caregiver styles (e.g., overcontrol, overprotectiveness), and caregiver psychopathologies may interact with a child's inhibited presentation to reinforce and maintain inhibition or avoidance of social interactions (Lewis-Morratty et al., 2012; Rubin, Burgess, & Hastings, 2002; see also Hirshfeld-Becker et al., 2008; Spence & Rapee, 2016).

Genetic research links youth BI and environmental factors such as parenting styles and later social anxiety (Spence & Rapee, 2016). In their interactions, caregivers may model cognitive biases associated with anxious behaviors (e.g., expecting negative outcomes, selective attention, emphasizing perceived threatening social cues). As opposed to intrusiveness and overcontrol, caregivers can model adaptive and possibly protective behaviors by encouraging problem solving, social approach behaviors, and use of coping skills (Ollendick, Benoit, Grills-Taquechel, & Weeks, 2014).

Cognitive Variables

There is significant interplay among factors in the development and maintenance of SAD in youth (see Halldorsson & Creswell, 2017; Spence & Rapee, 2016). Maladaptive thinking affects how youth engage with their environments and, in turn, how the environment responds. Cognitive aspects in youth with SAD can include interpreting social situations as dangerous, with negative and judgmental self-focused attention, and negatively valenced anticipatory processing of upcoming social events as well as negatively valenced postevent processing. Furthermore, these cognitive biases regarding social tasks may be associated with missed information and misinformation; elevated physiological anxiety states may further reinforce some of the thinking errors.

As children advance through development into adolescence, they normatively shift to emphasizing socioevaluation from their peers (Sumter et al., 2010). Socially anxious youth are more likely than nonanxious youth to interpret ambiguous social information in a negative fashion (Miers, Blöte, & Westenberg, 2011). Also, socially anxious youth are more likely to be self-focused in ways that are self-critical (Inderbitzen-Nolan, Anderson, & Johnson, 2007; Miers, Blöte, Bokhorst, & Westenberg, 2009).

Behavioral Variables

There may be some validity in youth perceptions and evaluations of their own social proficiency. That is, some youth with SAD may indeed have poorer social skills and exhibit social deficits when they interact with others (Inderbitzen-Nolan et al., 2007; Miers et al., 2009). These potential social skills deficits therefore require assessment and targeted intervention. Various behaviors may be associated with SAD, including speech-related behaviors (e.g., shaky voice, mumbling, stuttering), disrupted social skills (e.g., poor eye contact), and nail biting (Albano, 1995; Beidel & Turner, 1998). In efforts not to draw attention to themselves, these youth may behave reticently, avoiding eye contact and social interactions (Kley, Tuschen-Caffier, & Heinrichs, 2012). Safety behaviors can include: hiding behind books or their smartphones, wearing oversized or certain clothing to hide themselves, and sitting or standing in peripheral areas.

Socioacademic task demands may also be difficult for socially anxious youth, and some youth may fear and attempt to avoid certain performance elements (e.g., reading aloud, presenting in front of a class, being called on by the teacher, participation, classmate interactions). This may impact skill development, perceptions of competence, and, of course, *actual* performance (Blöte, Miers, Heyne, & Westenberg, 2015). Overall, given the increasing importance of socioevaluative feedback, a lack of social skills can interact with avoidance and safety behaviors to adversely impact the course and trajectory of youth social anxiety (Miers, Blöte, de Rooij, Bokhorst, & Westenberg, 2012).

Interpersonal Processes

Interpersonal models emphasize that behavioral patterns in socially anxious individuals elicit negative responses from others (Alden & Taylor, 2004; see also Spence & Rapee, 2016). For example, some research indicates that several behavioral correlates of social anxiety (e.g., poorer eye contact, lack of conversational reciprocity in social interactions) may be associated with others being more likely to disengage with socially anxious versus nonanxious individuals (Alden & Taylor, 2004). Shy individuals are frequently rated as less intelligent (Paulhaus & Morgan, 1997).

Evidence suggests that SAD youth are more likely to be rejected by their peers and may experience peer victimization (see Spence & Rapee, 2016). These factors might come together to disrupt and further impair socially anxious youth in the formation of relationships. Youth with SAD experience lower perceived peer acceptance as well as lower friendship quality (Festa & Ginsburg, 2011). These adverse interpersonal experiences likely contribute to the etiology and maintenance of SAD and ongoing transactional feedback, cognitive biases, selective attention, and avoidance (Blöte et al., 2015; see also Spence & Rapee, 2016).

In treating youth for SAD, the clinician can assess for these etiologic and maintenance variables, especially specific safety behaviors, social skills deficits, and information-processing biases. Treatment can be augmented to incorporate social skills training (e.g., social effectiveness therapy for children [SCET-C]; Beidel, Turner, & Morris, 2000) and targeted attentional strategies (e.g., reducing self-focused attention, mindfulness; Bögels & Mansell, 2004). Given the very nature of SAD, group-based cognitive-behavioral therapy (CBT), if available, can also be considered (e.g., Stand Up, Speak Out; Albano & DiBartolo, 2007).

CASE VIGNETTE: SHELBY

Shelby is a 14-year-old Black cisgender female whose family identifies as African American. She is completing the eighth grade and resides with her parents and two older brothers in a suburban town. Her parents described that she has "always been shy," especially compared to her outgoing brothers. Over the past couple of years—in middle school—she became increasingly self-conscious and anxious. She used to have a small group of friends, both boys and girls, with whom she hung out at the playground and after school. Then, according to Shelby, "They just stopped being my friends in seventh grade." She worries that kids do not like her, about not knowing what to say, and that she will say something "stupid or immature." She hates when teachers call on her, and she often stares at her desk to avoid eye contact with the teacher. She NEVER raises her hand even if she knows the answer to a question. If she is called on, she is generally prompted to "speak up" and raise her voice from its usual soft volume. While she generally gets good grades, teacher comments on her report card often note her lack of participation.

Shelby can "be herself" with her immediate family, but even large family gatherings make her nervous as aunts, uncles, and cousins "ask so many questions." According to her parents, as a young child, Shelby would hide behind their pant legs when approached by new or unfamiliar adults, and even today, she will sometimes avoid reciprocating a "hello" if a familiar adult greets her.

Until the fifth grade, she used to play clarinet, but stopped. The performances became "too terrifying," and she remembers when she "freaked out" at a spring concert. She begged her parents to let her skip it, but they made her go, and she "froze" during the clarinet section's performance. She has not quit dance, yet, but really wants to. When she does attend dance practice, her heart races, and when she's there, she tries to stand in the back of the studio. What she really enjoys these days is playing video games with her brothers if they are home and watching movies on her computer. She can spend hours on social media. She never posts content or makes comments but occasionally she will "like" a photo posted by a peer. She reports feeling "mortified" when her mother posts family pictures and Shelby refuses to be "tagged." In addition to feeling "mortified," she also describes herself as "awkward" and "weird."

This coming fall, Shelby will be graduating from middle school and attending the local high school. She's already predicting "it will be a disaster." She and her parents were encouraged to seek treatment by Shelby's aunt who is a social worker and to whom Shelby confided her feelings of isolation and significant worries about high school. Shelby's aunt convinced her sister, Shelby's mother, that Shelby was not "just shy" and that this was not "just middle school stuff."

ASSESSMENT OF SAD

Shelby attended the diagnostic intake evaluation with her parents. She appeared anxious upon meeting the therapist, speaking in a low volume and avoiding eye contact initially. Like Shelby, her mother spoke in a low volume but engaged in the assessment interview, and her father did most of the talking throughout it. The therapist completed the Anxiety Disorders Interview Schedule—Parent Version (ADIS-P) with Shelby's parents and the ADIS-C (Child Version) with Shelby. During the first half of the interview, Shelby made variable eye contact with the therapist and although she answered questions when asked, she did so with one-word responses and did not elaborate on her responses. Over the course of the interview, she appeared to become slightly more comfortable, smiling at the therapist and providing more detailed answers to questions. When asked why she came to the clinic, she expressed a desire to improve her situation, stating, "I wish I had more friends."

Following the comprehensive assessment, Shelby met the criteria for SAD. She experienced anxiety across multiple social and performance situations as she chronically feared negative evaluation, rejection, and embarrassment. She evidenced increased avoidance of situations, from fairly minor daily interactions (e.g., greetings and conversations with familiar and unfamiliar people) to situations that called attention to her specifically (e.g., answering a question in class, having her picture taken), to performance-related activities (e.g., playing the clarinet, participating in dance class). For unavoidable situations, Shelby reported a feeling of "barely surviving" or enduring with significant distress and physiological arousal. It was clear, from the assessment with both Shelby and her parents, that her level of social anxiety had interfered with her daily functioning in multiple ways. For example, it was starting to impact her grades, her ability to make and keep friends, and to have fun or even feel comfortable day-to-day. Furthermore, her symptoms appeared to be worsening. Although Shelby did not meet the criteria for depression, she did express increasing sadness connected to feelings of rejection and isolation, which is a common experience in youth with SAD. See Figure 9.1 for additional factors to consider for diagnostic clarification.

The ADIS provided significant information on Shelby's SAD. Also, in support of the diagnostic criteria, the clinician observed her behaviors during the initial introduction, open-ended questioning and conversation, and semi-structured question-and-answer (Q&A) segments. As noted, Shelby had difficulty maintaining eye contact, speaking audibly at first, and engaging in spontaneous and ongoing dialogue outside of the clinical Q&A segment. In general, the clinician wants to observe the youth's social engagement behaviors and assess social skills (see Figure 9.2; a blank version is available as Worksheet 23 in Appendix A). As observed and confirmed during the parent portion of the assessment, Shelby's mother disclosed her experiences with social anxiety in her own childhood and into the present day. As a result, her parents often disagree on how much to "push" Shelby to be social, answer questions from adults, be "like her brothers," and not quit activities. According to Shelby's father, her mother "lets her out of things"; according to Shelby's mother, her husband does not understand the intensity of his daughter's anxiety and says he "pushes too hard." Understanding these parental behaviors and family context (as well as biological vulnerability given her mother's family history of SAD) provides further information for functional assessment and case formulation.

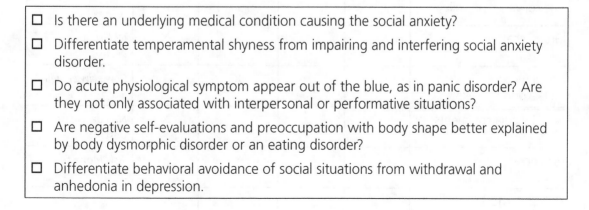

□ Is there an underlying medical condition causing the social anxiety?

□ Differentiate temperamental shyness from impairing and interfering social anxiety disorder.

□ Do acute physiological symptom appear out of the blue, as in panic disorder? Are they not only associated with interpersonal or performative situations?

□ Are negative self-evaluations and preoccupation with body shape better explained by body dysmorphic disorder or an eating disorder?

□ Differentiate behavioral avoidance of social situations from withdrawal and anhedonia in depression.

FIGURE 9.1. Diagnostic clarification checklist: SAD.

WORKSHEET 23. Social Skills Checklist

Use behavioral observation and report from the youth, family, and other reporters to assess social skills strengths and concerns.

	Notable Strength	Never a Problem	Sometimes a Problem	Always a Problem	Comment
Nonverbals, Cues, and Posture					
Eye contact				X	*In class; gets better over time*
Expressing interest Smiling, nodding			X		
Shrinking and hiding				X	
Hiding behind clothes Hiding behind smartphones, headphones, books, electronics				X	
Standing in the periphery				X	
Handshakes					*Not sure*
Spoken Conversations: Starting, Joining, Maintaining					
The conversation volley: responding, reciprocity				X	*Sometimes doesn't even say hello back*
Volume and tone				X	
Expressing interest			X		
Written "Conversation:" Texting and Social Media Communication					
The conversation volley			.	X	
Group chatting				X	*Not in any groups*
Social media To like or not to like			X		*Sometimes will like*
Social media comments				X	*No comments or posts*
Writing an email			X		*Ask Mom to do it*
Other Target?					

FIGURE 9.2. Social skills checklist and targets for Shelby.

Additionally, Shelby and her parents completed the Revised Children's Anxiety and Depression Scale (RCADS). Their reports were discordant. As can be seen in Table 9.1, according to her father's report, Shelby demonstrated clinically elevated scores for social anxiety and borderline symptoms for depression. An examination of Shelby's RCADS profiles does not indicate any such elevations, and a closer look at her item responses indicates she did not endorse any item higher than a "1." The therapist may want to consider such responses given the very nature of Shelby's social anxiety and the potential for underreporting given self-presentational demands and concerns.

Goal Setting and Defining Target Problems

At the conclusion of the assessment, the therapist has accumulated a large amount of data to be converted into a case conceptualization, treatment goals, and targets. The feedback session affords the opportunity for the therapist to collaboratively set goals and operationalize and prioritize these targets. Caregivers and children may have expressed discordant goals; furthermore, the youth may experience anxiety in a discussion of treatment goals when anxiety-inducing situations are identified as targets for practice and exposure. For the individual with SAD in particular, the intake with the therapist is in itself an evaluative situation with an unfamiliar adult. It may help the clinician to validate this anxiety and perhaps even utilize the situation of the intake as illustrative for the feedback session and in providing an overview on the proposed course of treatment. That is, as in Shelby's case, the therapist can inquire about her anticipatory anxious self-talk, possible physiological arousal, and possible desire to avoid the intake assessment interview. The therapist can further share behavioral observations regarding initial speaking volume, eye contact, and as appropriate, improvements over the course of assessment with the therapist and encourage Shelby to "hang in there" despite her urges to "escape" their initial meeting. Upon reviewing all the feedback, work with the caregivers and youth to set specific, concrete, and realistic expectations. Also, acknowledge that there are likely differences in what "realistic" expectations mean to each person. For example, Shelby may not become "more like her brothers" in their reported ease and facility in socializing. Rather, the therapist can find possible points of overlap and work with the

TABLE 9.1. Shelby's Symptom Profile at Intake Using the RCADS

	Mother		Father		Youth	
	Raw score	*T* scores	Raw scores	*T* scores	Raw scores	*T* scores
Separation anxiety	3	53	4	58	0	40
Generalized anxiety	7	49	4	52	1	32
Panic disorder	9	66*	3	55	1	40
Social anxiety	15	55	20	74**	4	33
Obsessions/compulsions	1	39	0	43	0	35
Depression	10	56	9	65	0	29
Total anxiety	35	54	31	61	6	31
Total anxiety and depression	45	55	40	63	6	29

*T scores higher than 65 indicate borderline clinical threshold. **Scores of 70 or higher indicate scores above clinical threshold. *T* scores are normalized based on youth's age and gender.

caregivers and youth to operationalize their expressed goals (e.g., "We want her to be more social" or "We want her to be more like her brothers"). In Shelby's case, parent, child, and therapist goals were devised as follows:

Parents' Goals

- Participate in class when the teacher asks a question.
- Raise her hand in class.
- Ask teachers for help if she does not understand or know something.
- Respond to and have conversations with adults.
- Join activities and participate.
- Make plans to hang out with friends.
- Spend less time in her room on her computer.

Teen's Goals

- Make more friends.
- Get Mom and Dad (mostly Dad) "off my back."

Therapist's Goals

- Increase social activity, engagement, and practice with peers in person and on social media.
- Increase social activity, engagement, and participation with familiar and unfamiliar adults.
- Monitor, practice, and improve social skills.
- Monitor, practice, and improve conversation skills.
- Increase the use of coping behaviors to manage anxious distress.
- Teach parents skills to decrease rescue and accommodation behavior.
- Prepare for transition to high school.

Shelby did not express many goals, but her primary goal has intrinsic value and can be addressed by making progress on other caregiver and therapist goals. Practicing conversations with family and unfamiliar adults can assist—though not replace—practice in having conversations with same-age peers. Also given the social anxiety inherent in the initial evaluation and sessions of treatment, Shelby's reluctance to list concrete goals was not surprising. The therapist can list goals for socioacademic activities (e.g., raising her hand in class, asking the teacher a question or for help), knowing that Shelby acknowledged these as problematic areas during the intake, and align them with the parents' goals.

As can be seen in Figure 9.3 (a blank version is available as Worksheet 11 in Appendix A), identifying and tracking youth and caregiver goals can provide targets across multiple domains. Goals targeting social anxiety can be framed in various forms. That is, goals can address other-focused social skills acquisition and practice (e.g., eye contact, speech volume), self-focused anxiety and distress-management skills, peer-focused in-person social activities (e.g., initiating contact, texting for live interactions), social media interactions, and more general socialization goals (e.g., saying hello to different people). Caregiver-focused goals help parents to better understand, validate, and coach Shelby in realistic ways (e.g., reframing Shelby's goal of getting her father to "back off") and catch possible rescue behaviors that may have functioned to maintain some of her SAD.

WORKSHEET 11. Goals Tracker

Work with your therapist to brainstorm possible specific, meaningful, and achievable goals. Think through what outcomes you expect to see. And then, keep track of how your child does each week.

Parent Goals	Desired Outcomes	Week 1	Week 2	Week 3	Week 4	Week 5
Increase class participation.	Raise her hand 1/day. Ask teacher 1 question/day.					
Decrease avoidance/isolation (hanging out in room all day).	Frequency of hang-outs with friends (inside and outside house)					
Join or rejoin one activity.	Join or rejoin one activity and attend weekly meetings.					
Mom & Dad goals: increase empathize & encourage skills	Dad: increase "empathize" talk; Mom: increase "encourage" talk					
Improve social skills & increase conversations.	Respond to adults ("Hello" and "How are you?") & initiate ("Hello" and "How are you?").					

Youth Goals	Desired Outcomes	Week 1	Week 2	Week 3	Week 4	Week 5
Make more friends	Join or rejoin one activity and attend weekly meetings					
Make more friends	Respond to peer texts and social media posts					
Make more friends	Initiate texts and social media posts to friends					
Get Mom and Dad "off my back"	Notice and comment on Dad's increased efforts with validation					

FIGURE 9.3. Completed Goals Tracker worksheet for Shelby.

223

CASE CONCEPTUALIZATION

CBT Model

Following assessment, summarize the varied data sources and provide a preliminary framework for the youth and their caregivers to understand social anxiety. In this case, the therapist described Shelby's SAD from a CBT perspective. Recall that although Shelby and her parents may have acknowledged her difficulties across situations, it was her aunt who suggested they seek professional help because she thought Shelby's SAD was increasingly interfering with her development. Shelby had a longstanding childhood experience of shyness; biological and temperamental vulnerability (behavioral inhibition); increasing rescue, escape, and avoidance behaviors; and eventually a clinical level of SAD. Helping Shelby and her parents understand CBT conceptualization will assist in validating her experience, understanding the nature and scope of the problem, and, of course, laying the groundwork for cognitive-behavioral interventions. Shelby experiences significant fears of negative evaluation by others that is connected to surges of physical distress and "freezing up" or "shutting down." In addition to these fears and her increased focus on the perspectives of others, especially peers, Shelby's self-consciousness is maintained and exacerbated by internal dialogue filled with self-criticism and doubt. As such, she avoids social situations (e.g., from eye contact to conversations) as much as possible. Her anxiety-related behaviors have been met by some accommodations from her parents and certain teachers, her brothers who sometimes respond for her, neighbors who no longer greet her directly "because she is so shy." A portion of the interference from Shelby's SAD is conflict between her parents on how to respond to Shelby to encourage, not overwhelm, her. Shelby's father described multiple examples where he attempted to push Shelby to enter a social situation, but Shelby's mother would intervene after seeing her distress and allow her to escape. The therapist's initial feedback aims to incorporate a broad view of SAD and provide a framework for the interplay among Shelby's (and the family's) cognitive, behavioral, and emotional responses to social tasks, demands, and interactions (see Figure 9.4).

In one example of the CBT model applied to one of Shelby's social anxiety episodes, Shelby notes that as soon as her math teacher asks the classroom, "Who knows the answer to Question 1?," she feels a surge of anxiety that includes her heart racing and a lump in her throat. She describes thoughts such as "Oh no! I hope she doesn't call on me," "I'll be mortified if she calls on me," and "I don't know the answer. I don't even remember the question." Shelby has a pattern of avoiding eye contact with her teachers, and she will slouch her shoulders and try to hide her body behind the classmate sitting in front of her. At times, she tries to go to the bathroom during class before the teacher reviews the homework and asks for student participation. Another time, when she was paired with a peer for a small-group project, she felt intense physical sensations and worry thoughts, such as "She doesn't want to be paired with me," "She must think I'm such an idiot," "I don't know what to say," and "I don't really care, she can be in charge." In these situations, Shelby's teachers have reported observing that she remains quiet with her peers and does not assert herself in group projects.

The therapist uses the CBT model in Figure 9.4 to help Shelby identify and recognize the interplay among her thoughts, preevent processing, and negative self-talk (e.g., "She must think I'm such an idiot" or "I'll be mortified if she calls on me"), physical symptoms (heart racing, lump in throat), and her behavioral responses (avoiding eye contact, not speaking up, trying to escape to the bathroom). With multiple examples and using Handout 19 (a reproducible version is available in Appendix A), the therapist teaches the CBT model and begins to note how Shelby anticipates her distress in situations that have real social demands and how her own thinking and behaviors may escalate her distress and maladaptive behaviors. In these initial feedback sessions, the goal

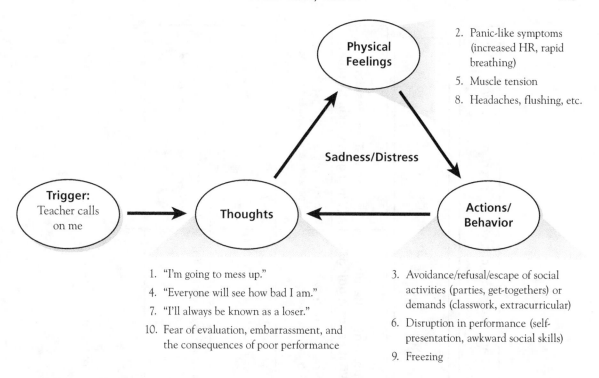

FIGURE 9.4. Individualized CBT conceptualization for Shelby. Her thoughts, feelings, and behavior cycle continuously in a downward spiral (follow the numbers in order: 1, 2, 3, etc. to see how the thought–feeling–action cycle flows into another).

is to provide an understanding of the CBT conceptualization without necessarily intervening directly. Given the differing roles played by Shelby's parents, it may be useful to ask them to review the CBT model for situations triggered by Shelby's SAD so they can begin to identify their own specific cognitive, behavioral, and affective experiences. Their responses may reveal their own physiological responses, beliefs about Shelby's anxious experiences, and expectations regarding her behavior and what she can handle. Given their noted pattern of differential responding and conflict, having them each review the CBT model may help the therapist to highlight the family aspects of the conceptualization.

Functional Assessment

Functional assessment is a central component of case conceptualization (see Figure 9.5; a blank version is available as Worksheet 1 in Appendix A). Given the multitude of daily social demands and interactions, Shelby is contending with ongoing potential anxiety triggers. Consider the sheer number of direct and indirect social demands encountered over the course of a day. Introducing and utilizing functional assessment allow the therapist, Shelby, and her parents to begin to identify her particular triggers; associated cognitive, emotional, and behavioral responses; and consequences. Completion of this worksheet provides important data regarding patterns of avoidance, escape, and rescue that may be reinforcing social anxiety.

Shelby described being recently made to go to school by her father on the day of her speech for English class. Her anxiety intensified in the morning, and despite attempts Shelby aimed at her mother, begging her to stay home, the teen went to school. Shelby said she could not eat or

WORKSHEET 1. Trigger and Response

Tell us about your triggers and how you reacted. Describe your feelings, what you did (action), what happened right away (immediate outcome), and then what happened later (long-term outcome).

```
┌──────────────┐          ┌──────────────────┐          ┌──────────────┐
│  Antecedent  │ ───────▶ │  Behavioral and   │ ───────▶ │ Consequences │
│              │          │ Emotional Response│          │              │
└──────────────┘          └──────────────────┘          └──────────────┘
```

Trigger	Feeling (emotional response)	Action (behavioral response)	Immediate Results (What keeps it going?)	Long-Term Results (What gets you in trouble?)
The girl before me starts her speech.	Fear, heart pounding, nauseous, panic	Hide behind my friend. Ask if I can go to the bathroom.	Nothing; still miserable; teacher said to wait.	The feeling just kept getting worse as the girl's speech went on.
The girl's speech ends.	Full-out panic	I asked the teacher if I can do my speech another day.	Temporary relief, felt hopeful she'd say "yes."	???
Teacher asked if I was OK?	Felt hopeful	I said I was sick to my stomach—asked to go to the nurse.	Teacher agreed! Total relief!	Now I have to do the speech another time. Teacher seemed annoyed at me.

FIGURE 9.5. Individualized functional assessment of social anxiety for speech fears.

concentrate all day, and her anticipatory automatic thoughts centered on messing up, stuttering or mumbling, and freezing when it came time to present, thereby becoming "mortified" in front of her classmates. She noted her heart racing. As such, her immediate behavioral responses included trying to avoid being seen by the teacher (hiding behind her friend) and then trying to escape the room while the presenter preceding her was speaking. When the teacher denied her bathroom request, she described increasing anxiety and panic-like sensations. After the teacher relented, agreeing to allow Shelby to postpone her speech, Shelby described "total relief" as the immediate consequence and then recognized that she would have to present the speech in the future. She also described additional worry that the teacher was now annoyed and mad at her.

The functional assessment applied to this single situation helps the therapist begin to apply the CBT model to Shelby's thoughts, feelings, and behaviors and to observe how her avoidance and escape (actual and attempted) and others' rescue behaviors indeed provide relief. At the same time, it's important to emphasize the short-term nature of this relief. The functional assessments demonstrate how these actions negatively reinforce and maintain her anxiety in the long term. Furthermore, an assessment lays the groundwork and rationale for eventual *in vivo* exposures. The therapist can use the habituation curve (see reproducible Handout 20 in Appendix A) to illustrate that youth with SAD learn escape from a fearful event is an effective way to cope—in the short run—even at the cost of long-term impairment. It also highlights the roles that others play. For example, Shelby attempted to avoid school altogether, but her attempts were blocked by both her father and mother (e.g., she reported it was mostly her father who objected). Immediately prior to the speech, she attempted to hide from the teacher and then escape by going to the bathroom, and this attempt was blocked when the teacher instructed her to wait. Her final effort to escape was successful when the teacher allowed her to postpone her speech to another day. However, as Shelby discovered when she completed the "secondary (long-term) consequence" box, an additional automatic thought triggered a new worry: that her teacher was annoyed with her. Over time, Shelby would come to see similar patterns emerge over repeated functional assessments.

TREATMENT PLANNING

With the diagnostic evaluation and feedback completed and the preliminary case conceptualization formulated, treatment planning introduces the cognitive-behavioral interventions. As described above for Shelby and other youth with SAD, functional assessment (as intervention) provides the rationale for the selected interventions, as illustrated in Tables 9.2 and 9.3.

The therapist starts with the domains that represent the greatest areas of impairment, matched with youth and caregiver goals to maximize treatment motivation. In Shelby's case, social anxiety inhibits her functioning most in academic settings (e.g., answering questions in class, pursuing needed help), maintaining friendships (e.g., responding to invites and peer communication), and sustaining extracurricular activities (e.g., quitting clarinet due to social embarrassment). Thus, initial sessions will focus on the assessment of these impairments and formulating a conceptualization that identifies specific cognitive, emotional, and behavioral processes and social skills. Interventions are then chosen that help address these specific deficits. For example, the therapist will emphasize cognitive restructuring as Shelby evidences significant thinking traps (e.g., catastrophizing, mind reading); social skills training will be incorporated as Shelby's anxiety leads to and is exacerbated by noticeable social deficits.

TABLE 9.2. Shelby's Broad Treatment Plan for Social Anxiety

Treatment goals	Interventions
Increase participation in classes.	Psychoeducation; cognitive restructuring; exposures to in-school social demands; daily report card
Increase socializing with adults and peers, make more friends, increase social activities.	Psychoeducation; parent training; cognitive restructuring; problem solving; exposures to varied social situations; social skills training
Reduce family conflict.	Psychoeducation; parent training; contingency management; empathize and encourage; communication skills training; exposure
Make more friends, increase social activities.	Exposure to social situations; social skills training
Reduce distress and panic sensations.	Psychoeducation about distress; somatic management; cognitive restructuring; problem solving; exposure
Prepare for transition to high school.	Goal setting; problem solving

Functional assessment helps identify potential barriers and facilitators. For example, early assessment identified Shelby's use of escape to the nurse's office as a means of reducing distress (negative reinforcement). Safety behaviors and people (e.g., school nurse, mother) can then be identified and incorporated into treatment planning. For instance, suspecting that Shelby's mother identified with her anxiety and often allowed Shelby to escape social situations, the therapist decided to incorporate caregiver education and training early in therapy. Functional assessment also identified the incentives and facilitators of approach behavior. Her parents reported that Shelby enjoys video games and idolizes her brothers. They also reported that Shelby seems at peace when dancing at home and only becomes nervous in groups. Given these findings, the therapist can incorporate the brothers into behavioral exposures to provide support and to incentivize Shelby's participation. The therapist also considered using dance as a starting point where Shelby could gradually increase her social presence.

Likewise, behavioral observations identified several social deficits that could reinforce avoidance functions. Poor eye contact could serve to avoid social engagement or unwanted attention, and Shelby may be perceived as stand-offish or aloof when others try to engage her in conversation. Behavioral practice, of course, is integrated throughout treatment (not just after skill-building lessons) so that the youth can practice social skills and challenge cognitive assumptions. Caregivers are involved throughout to manage incentive programs and to reinforce skill building outside of session.

Throughout treatment planning, the therapist is trying to prioritize the domains of greatest impairment and to target key cognitive-behavioral processes. Sequencing of treatment interventions tends to emphasize the strategies the therapist believes will be most effective in targeting the most critical processes, while also considering the barriers and facilitators that impact effectiveness. SAD presents a multitude of potential daily demands and challenges, especially for a teen. As treatment progresses, the therapist can vary the planned sequence of interventions based on emerging situations or observed deficits. For example, the therapist might create a series of behav-

TABLE 9.3. Shelby's Detailed Treatment Plan for Social Anxiety

Sessions 1–2

Assessment
- Assess presenting problems.
- Conduct diagnostic assessment with a focus on impairment (real-life functioning).
- Administer symptom profile measures (e.g., RCADS).
- Assess target problems and treatment goals, focusing on improving daily functioning.
- Assess past attempts (including past treatment) to address the problem.
- Assess parent–child interactions.
- Conduct collateral assessments as needed with the youth's school (e.g., counselor, teacher, school nurse); request parents' complete release of information to speak to school contact(s).
- Evaluate co-occurring medical conditions; consult with pediatrician or specialist (e.g., gastroenterologist) as indicated.
- Assess need for medication and psychiatric referral.

Psychoeducation
- Review assessment and generate target problems with youth and parents.
- Create idiographic target problems tracker.
- Collaborate on case conceptualization: CBT model and functional assessment.
- Provide parents and youth with information handouts on social anxiety and CBT in general.
- Educate parents on the importance of collaborating with their child's school.
- Educate parents about the potential benefits of medication.

Home practice
- Monitor social triggers over the week: CBT model and functional assessment.
- Have the youth track their reactions to distress and short- and long-term outcomes (functional assessment) in relation to social anxiety.

Sessions 3–4

Assessment
- Evaluate and discuss home practice.
- Complete the target problems tracker.
- Complete symptom tracker every fourth session (e.g., RCADS).

Interventions
- Implement in-session reward chart for home practice completion.
- Implement in-session reward chart for social goals (e.g., eye contact/volume, participation).
- Review and refine individual functional assessments. Conduct motivational interviewing to highlight the trade-off between short-term gains and long-term consequences.
- Educate youth/parents about function of negative affect/distress in avoidance. Use habituation curve to discuss the role of avoidance/escape in maintaining fears.
- Educate parents about three common parent–youth interaction cycles (accommodation, passivity–discouragement, coercive). Reinforce messages about fear/escape in maintaining avoidance behaviors.
- Teach parents "empathize and encourage" to deescalate conflict and encourage the youth's approach. Given differential parent responses, focus on "empathize" for father and "encourage" for mother.
- Determine need to establish contact with youth's current school as well as high school to which Shelby will transition. Help coordinate school response (e.g., may include specific teachers, counselor, etc.) to identify possible frontline anxiety coaches and possible exposure targets and assistants.

(continued)

TABLE 9.3. *(continued)*

Home practice
- Monitor social triggers over the week: CBT model and functional assessment.
- Have the youth continue to conduct functional assessments. Hone awareness of long-term consequences.
- Have parents practice empathize and encourage.

Sessions 5–6

Assessment
- As in Sessions 3–4

Interventions
- Continue to monitor youth's understanding of the role of negative affect and physiological arousal in triggering avoidance and escape behaviors.
- Teach, practice, and reinforce in-session social skills.

Home practice
- Use tracking forms for social skills practice.

Sessions 7–8

Assessment
- As in Sessions 3–4

Interventions
- Monitor self-talk and cognitive restructuring: teach youth the link between their thoughts and anxiety/distress, especially fear of negative evaluation.
- Teach problem solving and social problem solving.
- Practice and reinforce in-session social skills.
- Build challenge hierarchy or hierarchies through exposures, practice first steps of hierarchy in session.
- Review goals tracker.

Home practice
- Direct youth to refine steps of challenge hierarchy, focusing on the core challenges related to social demands and anxiety in different situations and/or people: responding to new or unfamiliar adults or peers; social performances; socializing via text, online, and in person; attending extracurriculars.
- Ask youth to attempt first steps of the hierarchy.

Sessions 9–10

Assessment
- As in Sessions 3–4

Interventions
- Monitor self-talk and cognitive restructuring: teach youth the link between their thoughts and anxiety/distress.
- Review cognitive distortions with particular attention to "mind reading."

(continued)

TABLE 9.3. *(continued)*

- Review problem solving; practice and reinforce in-session social skills.
- Continue practicing mild steps of challenge hierarchy through exposures, focusing on the core challenges related to social demands and anxiety in different situations and/or people: responding to new or unfamiliar adults or peers; social performances; socializing via text, online, and in person; attending extracurriculars.

Home practice
- Have youth continue to attempt first steps of hierarchy.
- Ask youth to complete and monitor a thought–action–feeling chart and exposure worksheet.

Sessions 11–12
Assessment
- As in Sessions 3–4

Psychoeducation
- Discuss family conflict.

Interventions
- Teach communication skills, empathize and encourage, coach and approach, and interpersonal effectiveness skills.
- Conduct chain analyses of conflict situations.
- Practice moderately challenging situations through exposures, focusing on the core challenges related to social demands and anxiety in different situations and/or people: responding to new or unfamiliar adults or peers; social performances; socializing via text, online, and in person; attending extracurriculars.

Home practice
- Have youth complete an exposure worksheet.
- Ask parents to continue practicing consistent delivery of empathize and encourage, praise and rewards, and youth-monitored accomplishments.

Sessions 13–20
Assessment
- As in Sessions 3–4

Intervention
- Continue practicing increasingly challenging steps in the hierarchy through exposures, focusing on the core challenges related to social anxiety.
- Practice and reinforce in-session social skills.
- Practice any individual or parent skills to facilitate exposure success (with, as needed, check-ins or sessions).

Home practice
- Direct the youth to complete moderate to challenging exposures from the hierarchy and exposure worksheets.
- Have parents and youth monitor a reward chart; ask parents to continue practicing consistent delivery of praise and rewards, and youth-monitored accomplishments.
- Have parents and youth complete any related skill forms.

(continued)

TABLE 9.3. *(continued)*

Sessions 21–25 (biweekly for maintenance)

Assessment
- As in Sessions 3–4

Psychoeducation
- Introduce relapse prevention phase.
- Discuss possible termination.

Interventions
- Continue practicing increasingly challenging steps on the hierarchy through exposures, focusing on the core challenges related to social interactions in different situations.
- Practice any individual or parent skills to facilitate exposure success.

Home practice
- Review goal tracker.
- Ask youth and parent to complete any related skill forms.

ioral practices around a social challenge coming up (e.g., a dance recital) and may have to introduce interventions targeting newly revealed barriers or social deficits (e.g., conversational skills, self-awareness of nonverbal cues, posture, and body language).

INTERVENTION COMPONENTS AND PROCESS

Psychoeducation

Psychoeducation begins with providing to youth and their families information on the nature of SAD itself and an overview of the CBT model that will guide the course of treatment. To assist in talking with youth and caregivers, the therapist can provide handouts highlighting key points about SAD and its treatment (see reproducible Handouts 19, 20, and 21 in Appendix A; also refer to Appendix B for a list of additional reliable sources). Psychoeducation serves to normalize anxiety broadly, to explain its adaptiveness, and to set realistic expectations. That is, given biological vulnerabilities and temperament, Shelby may not be as outgoing as her brothers, and it will be important to educate her parents on areas of impairment and developmental functioning and to assist them in goal setting. As described earlier, the therapist may be able to draw on examples that occurred during the intake to highlight how social anxiety impacts the youth (e.g., Shelby's difficulty in making eye contact).

Another target for psychoeducation for youth with SAD is to explain that *some* social anxiety is normal. One can expect to get anxious before a performance whether on a stage or in front of a classroom for a speech. It's normal to feel *some* anxiety when speaking to a new person or an authority figure. It's normal to feel *some* anxiety about the social drama in middle school or about starting a new class or school. It's normal to feel *some* anxiety about having to engage in small talk or feel uncomfortable during awkward silences. The therapist can utilize self-disclosure as appropriate with their own examples of contending with social anxiety experiences. We all have had to face them at one point or another. Relatedly, psychoeducation helps youth and their families recognize how social anxiety may be impairing functioning as well as developmental growth. While socially and academically Shelby may still say she is fine, her increasing avoidance may begin to impact her grades more directly as she likely encounters teachers who require participation or presentations as part of grading, and her increasing withdrawal may deprive her of meaningful friendships and lead to growing isolation.

Figure 9.4 (the CBT model) highlights the multiple automatic thoughts Shelby has: hoping the teacher would not call on her, asserting to herself that she does not know the answer, and predicting that she will be mortified if called on. These thoughts were associated with multiple physical panic-like symptoms, avoidance, and planning-for-escape behaviors. Psychoeducation helps Shelby and her family understand this interplay of thoughts, emotions, and behaviors. It will also (1) create awareness and identify the role of this internal, critical, negative self-talk, (2) validate her experience of anxiety and distress based on this internal filter, and (3) note that avoidance and escape have been learned over time as "coping" strategies to provide immediate relief.

Self–Talk and Cognitive Restructuring

Youth with SAD may have anxious externally focused self-talk that is focused on the perceived negative evaluation of others as well as internally focused negative self-judgments. Helping youth to identify their automatic thoughts will assist them in understanding their negative predictions regarding social situations, their cognitive distortions connected to anticipatory anxiety, and their patterns of wanting to avoid. Socially anxious youth often worry about what others may think of them or what they "know" others are thinking (mind reading). They predict negative outcomes from social interactions (fortune-telling) and anticipate they will be completely awful (catastrophizing). Treatment includes helping youth to identify these thoughts, predictions, and thinking traps (see Figure 9.6; a blank version is available as Worksheet 5 in Appendix A).

Shelby's first example is useful for outlining a familiar pattern when confronted with an in-school class presentation. Whenever a teacher announces a report or presentation assignment, Shelby has multiple automatic negative thoughts predicting negative outcomes with regard to the presentation (e.g., messing up, freezing, stuttering), response of others (e.g., kids will make fun of her and think she is an "idiot"), and her go-to coping plan (e.g., avoid or escape!). The therapist can work with Shelby to recognize this pattern of self-talk and thinking traps and begin to slow down and *realistically* challenge some of these thoughts.

The therapist can work with Shelby to ask herself some questions, such as:

"Have you messed up before?"
"What would happen if you mess up during the presentation?"
"What is the worst that can happen?"
"Do other kids mess up during their presentations? What happens when they mess up?"
"What have other kids said to you before? How do you know they would notice?"

Importantly, the therapist is not aiming to have Shelby believe that she will not mess up or stutter. She may. The goal is not merely positive thinking—a common myth regarding CBT. Rather, a goal is to help Shelby in decatastrophizing her predictions and in testing assumptions about what others think. Another goal is to aid Shelby in problem solving how she might handle these situations differently:

THERAPIST: The last time you had a presentation, how did you mess up?

SHELBY: The teacher told me to speak up.

WORKSHEET 5. Thinking Traps Tracker

What thinking traps do you fall into when feeling sad, anxious, or distressed? For each situation, describe and rate how you feel. Describe your automatic thought (the first thought that comes into your head). What thinking trap might you be falling into? How does that make you feel (the result)?

Trigger	Feeling (Rate 0–10: "not at all" to "excruciating")	Thought	Thinking Trap	Result?
Teacher said we would have to present report next week.	Fear, panic (9)	"I'm gonna mess up." "I'll stutter and freeze up." "They'll all make fun of me and think I'm an idiot." "I have to get out of it."	Fortune-telling, mind reading, catastrophizing, looking for the escape hatch	Felt worse (9).
Saw Ella's party on Snapchat.	Anxious (7), sad (7)	"I wish I was invited." "We used to be friends." "They don't like me." "I have no friends." "High school is going 2 suck." "Ugh, now they know I viewed it."	Mind reading, catastrophizing, all-or-nothing thinking	Cried, played video games (6).
Got into another fight with Dad about not saying "hi" to his coworker.	Mad (9), nervous (7)	"He doesn't get me." "I'm an embarrassment to them." "I'm always awkward."	Mind reading; all-or-nothing thinking	Slammed my door and stayed in my room; felt bad all night (8 or 9).

FIGURE 9.6. Completed Thinking Traps Tracker worksheet for Shelby.

234

THERAPIST: OK, and then what happened?

SHELBY: I started freaking out. My voice was shaking, and my heart was racing.

THERAPIST: And what did you do?

SHELBY: I tried to raise my voice. And then we finished and it was so hot. Everyone was looking at me.

THERAPIST: So in this situation, messing up meant the volume of your voice was not loud enough?

SHELBY: Yeah.

THERAPIST: And then when you got feedback from the teacher, it sounds like you got anxious, which makes sense. And then your voice got shaky, and you addressed the feedback and successfully made it through the presentation?

SHELBY: I guess.

THERAPIST: Did the teacher tell anyone else to speak up?

SHELBY: Yeah.

THERAPIST: Did you think that kid was an idiot because he or she didn't speak up?

SHELBY: Um, no.

THERAPIST: OK, so it's possible to have the teacher ask some other students to speak up and NOT think those kids are idiots. Good information! Is there anything you can do to prepare for this kind of situation in the next presentation?

SHELBY: I don't know.

THERAPIST: How is it that we get better at doing something?

SHELBY: Practice?

THERAPIST: Right, practice. Maybe one thing we can have you do when you prepare for a presentation is to practice raising your volume? [Problem solving and skill building].

SHELBY: I guess.

The therapist can also work with Shelby to generate more active coping self-talk. In her initial evaluation and through self-monitoring homework completion, Shelby has provided salient examples of trying to avoid or escape socioacademic demand situations. One of Shelby's most consistent automatic thoughts is "I have to get out of here" or "Get out of this," or some form of avoidance. She cannot always "get out of it" as her teachers sometimes refuse her requests or her father refuses to let her avoid the situation. However, her automatic self-coaching directs her to the nearest escape routes. As Shelby and her therapist work on cognitive aspects of her social anxiety, it may be useful to help Shelby develop a modified internal script that recognizes and validates her anxiety, recognizes the desire to escape or avoid, and deliberately identifies a coping thought and plan. For example:

THERAPIST: Notice that when you get nervous about something in school, you often think about getting out of it or avoiding it?

SHELBY: Yeah. I don't want to freak out or be mortified in front of people.

THERAPIST: Yeah, one of the ways you've learned to cope with getting nervous is by telling yourself, one, "I have to get out of here," and two, "I can't handle this, so before I fall apart in front of anyone, I better get out of here." So when you have those kinds of thoughts, it makes sense that your behavior is to ask the teacher or your parents to get out of the situation.

SHELBY: Uh-huh.

THERAPIST: Instead of telling yourself to get out, what else might you say to yourself?

SHELBY: Um, stay. Don't leave. Hold it in.

THERAPIST: OK, how about if you start with describing your thoughts and feelings to yourself?

SHELBY: OK. I know I'm super-nervous and want to get out of here.

THERAPIST: Yes, good. And then labeling your thinking traps?

SHELBY: I'm fortune-telling and catastrophizing.

THERAPIST: And then a coping thought?

SHELBY: It's not the end of the world.

THERAPIST: Even though . . .

SHELBY: . . . even though it feels really uncomfortable.

THERAPIST: Yes, that's a good first step at decatastrophizing. That feels fair. Good. And coaching yourself through the next steps?

SHELBY: I have to practice. I'll survive.

THERAPIST: Can you handle it?

SHELBY: I think so.

THERAPIST: How do we test it out?

SHELBY: I know, I know. I have to do it.

THERAPIST: And when that escape thought comes up again, you can recognize it and say to yourself something like "There is that get-out-of-here thought again. That's the anxiety talking. It doesn't mean I have to escape."

Socially anxious youth also tend to engage in self-talk that is concerned with what others may be thinking about them. They may even be *certain* that someone does not like them, is making fun of them, thinks they are dumb, stupid, weird, awkward, and the like. See Table 2.2 in Chapter 2 (or reproducible Handout 2 in Appendix A) for a complete list of thinking traps. *Mind reading* is a common and powerful thinking trap that keeps kids (and adults) stuck in their social anxiety and often worsens situations. The goal of cognitive restructuring around automatic thoughts in the mind-reading domain is not necessarily to dispute what someone is or is not thinking about them—this is unknowable. We cannot know what others are thinking of us unless they verbalize it. Therapists can assist the youth in recognizing this thinking trap and dispute the associated all-or-nothing certainty: "Everyone thinks I'm stupid."

"If we are working on being a detective of your thoughts, how do you *know* that everyone thinks you're stupid?"

"Can you really know what other people are thinking?"
"What else is possible?"
"If they are laughing, does it mean that they are laughing at you?"

It is also important to recognize and validate that people are often judging each other, whether we are attending to it or not. You may have some peers who are indeed reacting to or making fun of others. Helping youth cope includes helping them to acknowledge this as well as to recognize that not *everyone* is judging us negatively and, further, others are reacting to us much less than we think.

One strategy might be to ask the youth how they react in relation to other kids:
"What do you think about other kids when they mess up or stutter?"

Again, the goal is not to sell the youth on the idea that the world is perfect, or that other people approve of everything that we do. Rather, the therapist hopes to ingrain a window of flexibility in the youth's thinking such that their natural instincts are less harsh, negative, and critical than they have been so far. The therapist helps Shelby generate more flexible and open-minded coping thoughts that challenge her thinking traps (see Figure 9.7; a blank version is available as Worksheet 16 in Appendix A).

Problem Solving

Teaching Shelby problem-solving skills may allow her to consider options other than escape or avoidance in coping with her anxiety. Considering Shelby's identified goal of making more friends, it may be useful to connect psychoeducation regarding her beliefs about others (and their beliefs about her), her beliefs regarding her own self-efficacy in social situations with peers, her physiological distress that makes socializing uncomfortable, and her efforts to decrease this discomfort with avoidance and increasing withdrawal. Problem solving aims to have youth develop an ability to generate options, and think about possibilities overlooked, never considered, or simply dismissed (see Chapter 2 for a complete review of problem solving, or STEPS). Consider this conversation:

THERAPIST: One of the goals you set is to make more friends.

SHELBY: I guess.

THERAPIST: OK, so if the problem is making more friends, let's come up with some possible solutions that could help with that. What are some ways that people make friends?

SHELBY: (*shrugs*) Um, not sure.

THERAPIST: OK, how did you meet the friends you used to have or have now?

SHELBY: At school. In class, I guess.

THERAPIST: So there are people in your classes you could talk to. How else?

SHELBY: In dance class, too.

THERAPIST: So doing activities together? Are there other activities where you made friends? Or, things you used to do that you gave up because it made you too nervous?

WORKSHEET 16. Coping Thoughts Tracker

Brainstorm coping thoughts that could respond to your thinking trap! Try and come up with coping statements that are more realistic and ask, "How am I not seeing the whole picture?"

Trigger	Thought	Thinking Trap	Coping Thought	Result?
Teacher said we would have to present report next week; already thinking how to get out of it.	"I'm gonna mess up." "I'll stutter and freeze up." "They'll all make fun of me and think I'm an idiot." "I have to get out of it."	Fortune-telling, mind reading, catastrophizing, looking for the escape hatch	"The anxiety always tells me to look for the escape hatch." "Last time I messed up a little and kept going and got it over with." "They're probably focusing on me less than I think, and I can only control my own stuff anyway."	Felt less panic, even a little proud for catching it; thought about asking Mom to help me practice.
Saw Ella's party on Snapchat.	"I wish I was invited." "We used to be friends." "They don't like me." "I have no friends." "High school is going 2 suck." "Ugh, now they know I viewed it."	Mind reading, catastrophizing, all-or-nothing thinking	"Ella invited me last year, and I bailed because of my anxiety." "I can reach out to her and wish her a happy belated birthday." "I have friends and am working on making more friends." "My anxiety can be SO dramatic sometimes I need to call it out."	Felt better; still sad I missed it; more determined to make friends.
Got into another fight with Dad about not saying "hi" to his coworker.	"He doesn't get me." "I'm an embarrassment to them." "I'm always awkward."	Mind reading; all-or-nothing thinking	"He can be pushy, and I know he's been practicing the empathize skill. He needs more practice, ha ha." "I'm not always awkward. Sometimes I feel like that." "I will practice saying 'hi' to his coworker."	Felt a little less mad; went to talk to Dad; we agreed to keep practicing our skills.

FIGURE 9.7. Completed Coping Thoughts Tracker worksheet for Shelby.

238

SHELBY: I used to play clarinet but hated the shows.

THERAPIST: Did you enjoy playing clarinet?

SHELBY: Kinda.

THERAPIST: Are there kids from dance class or from when you played clarinet who seem like people you'd like to try to talk to or get to know? [Notice the option is not "be friends with" but steps in service of "making" friends.]

SHELBY: There are a couple, I guess.

THERAPIST: Let's list their names so we are sure to be specific. How would you reach out to them? Call them?

SHELBY: (*stares blankly at therapist*) Text? Snap maybe.

THERAPIST: (*remembering that youth rarely call each other these days*) Right, good. You can also consider talking to one of them at the next dance class.

SHELBY: Yeah.

THERAPIST: It's true that doing activities together is a great way to get to know people. Are there are other activities you've considered doing but maybe didn't because of anxiety?

SHELBY: The school play.

THERAPIST: Great. What has gotten in the way of you signing up or auditioning?

SHELBY: Being on the stage.

THERAPIST: If you're not feeling ready to have an acting part, are there ways to be involved with the play?

SHELBY: I guess with the set design or tech stuff.

THERAPIST: That's a really solid option that challenges all-or-nothing thinking about participating in the play. Way to think in a flexible way. Love those ideas.

Clearly, a goal of making friends is multi-tiered. In this example, the therapist works with Shelby to identify the ways in which people make friends (e.g., shared activities), possible peers with whom she might engage in her current social orbit (e.g., dance class), how she might approach or communicate (e.g., a text or on social media), and other potential activities previously avoided (see Figure 9.8; a reproducible version is available as Worksheet 15 in Appendix A). Notice the therapist works to identify broad strategies and steps for socializing, such as spending time together and communicating. She also works with Shelby to be specific, name names, and over time, when she selects an option, they hone in on an even more specific how-to plan. Importantly, and especially with SAD, the therapist may need to target social skills more directly. Figure 9.2 (a reproducible version is available as Worksheet 23 in Appendix A) provides an overview of social skills to assess, target, and practice in session as needed. These may be actual or perceived deficits expressed in automatic thoughts (e.g., "I don't know what to say"). It is also critical to remember that problem solving should be conducted in an iterative process that involves brainstorming ample possible solutions, trying out solutions, and then returning to the list if choices do not fully resolve the problem. No idea is meant to be successful on the first attempt, nor should any solution solve an entire problem. Rather, the steps of problem solving help move the youth toward a goal in a constructive direction to avoid getting stuck.

WORKSHEET 15. Problem–Solving STEPS

> To solve problems, take these steps: say what the problem is, think of solutions, examine each solution, pick one solution and try it, and see if it worked!

Say What the Problem Is: *Trying new places to start conversations/meet people*

| Think of Solutions | Examine Each Solution | | Rank |
	Pros	Cons	
Talk to people in class.	I see them every day. There's lots of options.	No one talks in class. Everyone has their friends already.	3
Meet people at dance class.	We have the same interests. I have fun there.	I don't know if they want new friends. They might live far away.	1
Text/Snap people who I used to play clarinet with.	We had common interests.	They might think it's weird for me to call out of the blue. They might wonder why I dropped out of the group.	4
Be on stage crew for the musical.	Low pressure. You hang out while working on a project.	People are running around.	2

Pick One Solution and Try It: *I'll start with dance class because I'm already doing that and know people there.*

FIGURE 9.8. Brainstorming problem solving for Shelby.

Exposures

Given Shelby's significant social anxiety, level of avoidance, and the lack of social interactions and opportunities in any given day, ample skills practice, rehearsal, behavioral experiments, and exposures to socially anxiety-provoking situations will be key within-session and home practice interventions. Broader domains to target in Shelby's hierarchy can include: peer social activities, general and creative performance, academic performance with graduated approach, and participation rather than escape. As described in Chapter 6, and exemplified in the functional assessments, it will be important to enlist Shelby's parents during the exposure phase of treatment. A noted therapist goal is to teach parents how to coach Shelby more effectively and reduce their accommodation and rescue behaviors in order to best optimize exposure. Parents may need their own coaching on how best to accomplish this steady backing off from managing Shelby's social life (e.g., suggesting that she "do this" or "call this friend") and developmentally scaffolding the transition. Appropriate to her developmental phase and the increasing prominence of peers, Shelby is placing priority on the social goal of making more friends and expressing discomfort in her increasing isolation, while also showing a competing discomfort in staying in social situations that make her extremely uncomfortable. Like many anxious youth, she is stuck. To aid her in getting unstuck, the therapist provides a path via the conceptualization that provides (1) the skills to monitor her anxious self-talk and thinking traps that promote negative self-judgments and avoidance behaviors, (2) the skills to address actual or perceived deficits in problem solving or social interactions, and (3) opportunities to practice approaching and staying in anxiety-provoking situations (either novel or previously avoided). The therapist works with Shelby and her parents to generate relevant challenge hierarchies:

Hierarchy Challenge A: Speaking to Peers and New/Unfamiliar People

1. Say hello to a peer at dance class.
2. Text a peer from dance class to ask a question.
3. Text a classmate asking a question about the homework assignment.
4. Say "yes" when asked to join other dance class students for pizza.
5. Start a conversation with the clinic receptionist.
6. Say hello to, and ask at least one follow-up question of, a neighbor.
7. Ask a person on the street for directions.
8. Email drama teacher about the timeline and options for signing up for the school play.
9. Sign up for the stage or tech crew for the school play.
10. Make eye contact with passers-by on the street while walking.
11. Call restaurant to order family take-out.
12. Start conversation with a student who has neighboring locker.
13. Sign up for the environmental club and attend its next meeting.

Hierarchy Challenge B: Interacting in Socioacademic Context

1. Walk up to teacher after class and ask a question about homework assignment.
2. Raise hand to answer a question in math class.
3. Raise hand to answer a question in science class.
4. Sit up and make eye contact with teacher in English class.
5. Go to librarian and ask for help with a research topic.
6. Read aloud to my therapist for 5 minutes, 10 minutes, 15 minutes.
7. Give an impromptu talk about myself to therapist for 5 minutes.
8. Present a research project to my therapist (while sitting, then while standing).
9. Present a research project to my parents and brothers.

Hierarchy Challenge C: Facing Performance Fears, Fears of Being the Center of Attention, Fears of Embarrassment or Feeling "Mortified"

1. Attend dance class weekly.
2. Stand in second row during dance class instead of back row.
3. Stand in front row at the end nearest the door during dance class.
4. Stand in front row middle of the class during dance class.
5. Play one song on the clarinet for my therapist in the office.
6. Play one song on the clarinet for my therapist and their colleagues.
7. Walk through the clinic wearing a silly hat.
8. Walk down the street wearing a silly hat.
9. Drop books in the middle of the sidewalk as people walk by.
10. Walk down the hall with toilet paper stuck to my shoe.

For better or worse, social anxiety exposures are plentiful as social demands are common for preteens and adolescents. Perhaps trickier is creating enough exposures that involve same-age peers, as it can be challenging to arrange for volunteer confederates or locate groups of teens in naturalistic settings that are feasible for a practice setting and effective for the youth's target goals. Shelby and her therapist can collaboratively decide on the order of exposures based on her goals, the hierarchies targeting certain domains of her worry, and/or naturally occurring and less hierarchy-driven social situations that emerge over the course of treatment (e.g., a school presentation, a party).

In-session exposures can include various tasks that require Shelby to present to her therapist and provide her with the opportunity to trigger various somatic symptoms and automatic negative thoughts associated with social performance situations, as well as to recognize and challenge the urges to avoid or escape such situations. In so doing, Shelby can possibly habituate to initial surges in her anxiety while also learning to inhibit the avoidance response. Additionally, she practices specific presentations skills and social skills, and strategies for getting through presentations even if a feared outcome occurs. Figure 9.9 (a blank version is available as Worksheet 6 in Appendix A) illustrates an example in which Shelby agrees to give a 5-minute impromptu speech to her therapist. Immediately, Shelby becomes anxious and notes physical symptoms and automatic thoughts related to what she will say, how she will say it, how it will be received, and how she could cope by getting out of it. The therapist helps Shelby to slow down and write up her thoughts and sensations. The therapist works to connect the thoughts to Shelby's typical thinking traps, especially her tendency to "look for an escape hatch," and then to help her practice coming up with coping self-statements. In going through this exercise, Shelby starts to build and strengthen her ability to feel her own anxiety, challenge her negative thinking, and engage in the social task at hand. The exposure is less designed to help her be good at 5-minute impromptu speeches; rather, it is designed to give her practice in testing out her thoughts as hypotheses, not facts, and to push through her somatic arousal and avoidance to gather data on her ability to handle social demands. The specific behavioral goals (starting without protests, lasting 5 minutes, making eye contact 10 times) direct Shelby's actions, and when successful, they help counter preexposure assumptions.

As noted, therapists can incorporate creativity into the technical aspects of exposure design. With social anxiety exposures, therapists can vary the difficulty level for patients depending on their particular concerns by varying aspects of the social situation. For example, in-session exposure presentations can be varied by audience size (e.g., therapist, caregivers, colleagues); duration (10 seconds, 10 minutes); level of preparation (e.g., impromptu, planned topic); subject matter (e.g., topic with which the patient is familiar, "tell me about yourself," an unknown or more challenging topic, topic designed to have patient mess up on purpose, humorous topic); assertiveness (e.g., stating an opinion on a given topic, expressing an unfavorable or minority opinion); physical aspects (e.g., sitting while presenting, standing at the front of a room); social skills (e.g., focus on increasing volume, making eye contact); evaluative elements (e.g., with corrective feedback on performance, without feedback); embarrassment targets (e.g., wearing a silly hat while presenting, messing up on purpose), and so on. The goal for the therapist is to create challenges that (1) produce sufficient activation of the fear structure and (2) provide diverse and generalizable counterevidence to feared assumptions.

To address Shelby's primary stated goal that has particular intrinsic value to her, exposures that target friend making can be broken down into multiple related exposures in service of this goal. That is, in-session and home practice–based exposures have Shelby start or join conversa-

WORKSHEET 6. *In Vivo* Exposure/Behavioral Experiment

Complete this worksheet with the youth as you are preparing for a behavioral experiment.

1. Situation (What's the situation?):

Impromptu speech of therapist's choosing

2. Feelings: **Distress Rating:** _85_

Anxious, sweaty palms, butterflies in stomach

3. Anxious/Negative Thoughts:

Anxious/Negative Thoughts	Thinking Traps (See list below.)
a. *"I won't know what to say."*	a. Fortune-telling
b. *"You're going to think I'm stupid."*	b. Mind reading
c. *"Everyone can do this and I can't."*	c. Overgeneralizing, all-or-nothing
d. *"I'm going to stutter and mumble."*	d. Fortune-telling, looking for the negative.
e. *"I can't do this. My therapist said I don't have to do this if I don't want to."*	e. Looking for the escape hatch (The Avoider)

Thinking Traps: mind reading, fortune-telling, catastrophizing, jumping to conclusions, what if's, discounting the positives, looking for the negatives, overgeneralizing, all-or-nothing thinking, should statements, taking things too personally, blaming.

4. Coping Thoughts (How do you respond to your anxious thoughts?):

"If my mind goes blank, I can just pause and take a deep breath."
"You've been supportive so far. You're not here to judge me."
"Most people get anxious during speeches."
"If I stutter or mumble, just keep going."
"I need to hang in there if I want to get better at this. It's only 5 minutes."

Challenge Questions: Do I know for certain that _____? Am I 100% sure that _____? What evidence do I have that _____? What is the worst that could happen? How bad is that? Do I have a crystal ball?

5. Achievable Behavioral Goals (What do you want to accomplish?):

Goal	Accomplished?
a. *Just start talking instead of trying to get out of it.*	
b. *Last 5 minutes.*	
c. *Make eye contact at least 10 times.*	

6. Rewards:

Reward	Earned?
a. *Earn open talk time at the end of session.*	
b. *Get a new bitmoji app for phone.*	
c.	

FIGURE 9.9. Exposure worksheet for social anxiety.

tions (with adults or peers, but with an emphasis on peers), initiate social contact (e.g., say "hello," text, "like" or post online, or make eye contact), join conversations, join activities, ask questions, participate and contribute (in an activity or a group chat). We cannot make people be our friends; however, increasing our socialization might increase the likelihood that we meet people and spend time with them.

Shelby was able to identify peers from her dance class with whom she could start to engage and those who had been nice to her in the past. For a home practice exposure, she agreed to try to say "hello" and start a conversation with a peer and send a follow-up text asking a question. Prior to the exposure, she and her therapist made a plan and prepared for the exposure:

THERAPIST: So you're cool with saying hello to her in class and then sending her a text?

SHELBY: I guess so.

THERAPIST: What is some of the anxious self-talk going on in your head?

SHELBY: She'll think I'm weird. She won't want to talk to me. I'll look like an idiot.

THERAPIST: What thinking traps are those?

SHELBY: Mind-reading?

THERAPIST: Yep. What else?

SHELBY: Fortune-telling.

THERAPIST: Yes, good. So what can you do with those thoughts?

SHELBY: Challenge them. Question them.

THERAPIST: Good. What are some questions to ask and some coping thoughts?

SHELBY: What's the worst that can happen? I don't know what she is thinking but she's been nice before.

THERAPIST: So what is the worst that can happen?

SHELBY: She won't want to talk to me.

THERAPIST: How do we find that out?

SHELBY: Ugh. Test it out.

THERAPIST: And if she doesn't want to talk to you?

SHELBY: That'll suck.

THERAPIST: Yes. And?

SHELBY: And I have to try to find out.

THERAPIST: What are the chances she'll think you're an idiot?

SHELBY: 50 or 60%.

THERAPIST: That high? Are you an idiot?

SHELBY: Sometimes.

THERAPIST: That's harsh, self-judgy, and probably not so helpful to your cause, right? I'm an idiot too sometimes, right? No need to answer that!

SHELBY: (laughs).

THERAPIST: What if you think she's an idiot? Or, not nice? Or, what if she's really nice? Or, what if you make her day because she is sad about something? Or, what if you have a pleasant exchange? Or, what if it's fine? Or, what if she says "hi" to you next class because you said "hi" to her this time? Or, what if she doesn't think you're an idiot but she thought you were unfriendly or too shy because you avoided eye contact or talking to her in the past? There are SO many possibilities the anxiety does not let you see sometimes.

SHELBY: I guess.

THERAPIST: What can you tell yourself to encourage yourself to do the exposure and get through it?

SHELBY: I want friends and I have to try. I won't know unless I keep practicing.

THERAPIST: How good will you feel in trying to talk to her? How can you reward yourself for doing this exposure?

In the above exchange, the therapist can opt to go in various specific directions; however, the general skill in preparing for the exposure is to assist Shelby in identifying her automatic thoughts and thinking traps, recognizing their connection to her anxiety and avoidance and to devise her coping plan. Notice that in helping Shelby to challenge and question anticipatory negative thoughts, the goal is not to reassure her that everyone will be nice and all outcomes will be positive. The therapist uses validation of Shelby's discomfort (and it would "suck" if her feared outcome occurred) and humor and irreverence (we're all "idiots" sometimes and calling ourselves that in our private thoughts is not so helpful). The therapist also helps to generate potential alternative outcomes. Socially anxious youth have many assumptions and attentional biases at play and are focused on the possibility of evaluation and rejection while also making their own negative self-judgments. They often miss the many other possibilities in attempts at social engagement (e.g., "What if YOU don't like THEM!") Importantly, the therapist has previously worked to remind Shelby that these exposures are in service of her goal of making friends so she may use this value as intrinsic motivation to try the exposure. The emphasis is on the effort of attempting to speak to her peer, and less on the outcome itself, and self-rewarding should be contingent on this effort. (One cannot know if one wants to be friends with someone else, unless one gets to know the other person!) Of course, working with younger youth can include a reward chart for exposure completion that includes stickers, points, tokens, small prizes, for example, to enlist extrinsic motivation. It will be important to enlist and incorporate parents as appropriate: for coaching, praising approach over avoidance, developing a reward chart for exposures, and offering positive parent feedback based on *effort,* not outcome.

At the next session during this phase of treatment, Shelby and her therapist review the home practice exposure:

THERAPIST: How did it go?

SHELBY: Fine, I guess.

THERAPIST: So you did it? That's terrific, good for you for doing something that was scary for you. Take me through it.

SHELBY: Um, I said hello at the end of dance class. She was nice.

THERAPIST: More specific, please.

SHELBY: She said "hi" or something to that effect, and she said she liked my tights. And I said I liked her outfit, too.

THERAPIST: Did she call you an idiot? Or, Weirdo? Did she whisper behind your back?

SHELBY: (*smiling*) No.

THERAPIST: OK and then what happened?

SHELBY: She said "Bye, see you next week" or something like that, and then I said "bye" and waved.

THERAPIST: Good. Nice work! Did the ol' Escape Hatch Trap show up?

SHELBY: Oh, yeah.

THERAPIST: And, how did you deal with it?

SHELBY: I don't know. I just told myself to do it and walk up to her. I ignored it.

THERAPIST: It sounds like you heard it, ignored it, AND actually defied it. Way to go! Now you've started something. What could be a next step?

SHELBY: Talk to her next week. Maybe send her that text?

The therapist praises Shelby for completing the home practice and attempting the exposure, *regardless of outcome*. Specific, positive, labeled praise is important as we are trying to shape her approach behaviors (over usual avoidance), focus on effort, and model a potential script for her own self-appraisals. Then it's important to elicit a bit of a play-by-play with as many details as possible, while also comparing anticipated outcomes from those automatic thoughts that were generated to the actual outcomes and any expectancy violations. We cannot mind-read and know if the dance class peer thought she was "weird" or "an idiot," but we can (1) help Shelby to self-praise and reward herself for starting a conversation, and (2) recognize otherwise overlooked information: that the peer responded and even commented on her outfit. The therapist also works to identify the coping strategy Shelby used to push through the self-talk, encouraging avoidance so she can begin to script future coping, approach self-talk (e.g., "I just told myself to do it and walk up to her. I ignored it.").

Let's say the above example had gone differently, or another home practice exposure was less "fine."

THERAPIST: How did it go?

SHELBY: Horrible?

THERAPIST: So you did it?

SHELBY: Yeah. It sucked.

THERAPIST: First, that's terrific that you did it. Good for you for doing something that was scary for you. Take me through it.

SHELBY: Um, I said hello at the end of dance class. And she smiled and walked away.

THERAPIST: More specific please.

SHELBY: She didn't say anything.

THERAPIST: Did she call you an idiot? Or, weirdo? Or, whisper behind your back?

SHELBY: No, but she was probably thinking it.

THERAPIST: Do you know that for sure?

SHELBY: No.

THERAPIST: What's that trap?

SHELBY: Mind reading. But she didn't say anything.

THERAPIST: That must have felt tough. I can understand why you thought it sucked. Though, we don't know what she was thinking.

THERAPIST: What did you observe? What happened next?

SHELBY: I don't know; she left.

THERAPIST: You said she smiled?

SHELBY: I guess.

THERAPIST: OK, that's some information. What was your volume like?

SHELBY: Usual I guess.

THERAPIST: So, it was low? Do we know for certain that she heard you?

SHELBY: I think. I don't know.

THERAPIST: We can see what happens next week then, when you go back to dance class. Did the ol' Escape Hatch Trap show up?

SHELBY: Oh, yeah.

THERAPIST: And, how did you deal with it?

SHELBY: I don't know. I just told myself to do it and walk up to her. I ignored it.

THERAPIST: It sounds like you heard it, ignored it, AND actually defied it. Way to go! Now you've started something. What can you tell yourself?

SHELBY: At least I tried. She smiled. Maybe she didn't hear me. It was right at the end at the exit.

THERAPIST: And even if she did hear you? What else is possible?

SHELBY: Maybe she was nervous. Or, surprised because I don't usually speak up.

THERAPIST: Yeah, those are good alternative thoughts. And what if she did ignore you, which, of course, does suck?

SHELBY: I don't know.

THERAPIST: Either way you have good information, right? One, you tried something scary and survived it. Two, you found out you CAN approach someone. Three, maybe it will be important to try a different time, like before class, or at a higher volume, or a different person. That's good information.

SHELBY: OK.

THERAPIST: Did you praise yourself?

SHELBY: For what, she didn't say anything?

THERAPIST: (*laughing*) That wasn't the home practice. The home practice was for YOU to say something. And you did!

Thus, in this scenario, the therapist and Shelby collaboratively reviewed the exposure and processed a play-by-play of what "sucked." The therapist made sure to identify possible negative postevent processing biases that could affect a youth's recall of exposure home practice while not invalidating experiences, which may have indeed felt like they "sucked." The play-by-play review serves to (1) compare predicted and actual outcomes; (2) note expectancy violations; (3) recognize, label, and challenge cognitive distortions; (4) reinforce the effort, not the outcome, and provide a model for self-reinforcement; and (5) establish the frame of exposures as methods of hypothesis testing and information gathering. It's all data.

We do not know what effect this exchange will ultimately have, regardless of how successful it appeared after one attempt. Maybe Shelby and the other teen never talk again; maybe they become best friends; or maybe anything in between happens. We do not know, but we know that Shelby and this girl could never become friends if Shelby avoided ever talking to her. Given those choices, it was worth the shot. This commitment to the process is what deserves praise.

IDENTIFYING CAREGIVER–CHILD INTERACTION PATTERNS

As emerged over the course of the assessment and importantly was highlighted in the conceptualization, Shelby's parents respond somewhat differently to Shelby's social anxiety, distress, and avoidance behaviors. In the early phase of treatment, the therapist works with them on goal setting and clarifying realistic expectations (e.g., Shelby may not be able to be "more like her brothers" socially). Their identified goals share some overlap with Shelby's goals, though they emphasize socioacademic aspects as well as peer-related goals. Working on functional assessments will aid in understanding how parental responding has been involved in reinforcing some of Shelby's escape/ avoidance behaviors and maintaining her anxiety. The therapist provided Handout 11 (a reproducible version is available in Appendix A) to help educate Shelby's parents about various parenting traps, including examples of where the parents might fall into one of the common traps. As described below, the mother and father tend to fall into independent traps, such that the mother tends to rescue Shelby from anxiety (Accommodation Spiral) and her father tends to become critical (Aggressive–Coercive Spiral). The therapist next acts to help the parents increase awareness of their own patterns in responding to Shelby (see Figure 9.10; a blank version is available as Worksheet 9 in Appendix A).

Importantly, the variability in her parents' responses creates an opening for intermittent reinforcement, which is the most powerful form of reinforcement. Like the power in slot machines, Shelby's parents intermittently allow her anxiety to win the "jackpot" of escaping scary situations from time to time. They may not allow escape all the time (continuous reinforcement), but they reinforce it enough to maintain the anxiety. The therapist has to work with the caregivers to recognize these patterns, understand how they are (inadvertently) maintaining the anxiety, and establish the rationale for the exposure phase. In service of these steps, the therapist works with Shelby's parents to identify their own thoughts, feelings, and behaviors in response to Shelby's anxiety, which are likely serving as antecedents to accommodating the avoidance behaviors.

During the exposure phase, the therapist worked with Shelby's parents to set up exposure opportunities (e.g., requiring Shelby to place orders for take-out), agree on expectations regarding school and activity attendance, praise her efforts on therapy-related home practice, and commend her when she approaches or stays in any social situation that she is tempted to leave. The

WORKSHEET 9. Parent–Child Chain Analysis

	Can you identify any parenting traps? What alternatives could you try?		
	Action/Response	**Parenting Trap**	**Potential Solution or Skills to Use?**
Prompting Event:	Shelby has an upcoming oral report in social studies.		
Child Action:	Shelby asks parents for a note to be excused from giving an oral report.		
Parent Response:	Mom: I say, "Maybe," because I don't want to set her up for failure.	Accommodation	Empathize and encourage; prompt child to use problem solving
Child Reaction:	Shelby pushed her case. "Why shouldn't I be excused?!"		
Parent Response:	Dad: I blurted out something about her taking the easy way out and never getting better.	Aggressive–coercive	Empathize and encourage
Conflict/Problem Behavior:	Shelby slammed her door and didn't come out the rest of the night.		
Outcome 1 (What happened)?	We didn't see her.		
Outcome 2:	She didn't work on her report.		
Outcome 3:	She was even more anxious and upset the next day.		

FIGURE 9.10. Chain analysis of caregiver–child interactions in Shelby's case.

therapist can work to understand the parents' differential responses as illustrative of the cognitive-behavioral model (i.e., the thoughts, expectations, and feelings they have when Shelby becomes anxious, withdraws, and wants to avoid social interactions). With Shelby, for example, the therapist learns that both parents are worried about possible failure and Shelby's reaction to it:

THERAPIST: So what do you think will happen when Shelby goes to school and has to give that report?

FATHER: She'll try to get out of it. She's a smart kid and can get away with that now. At some point though, she's gonna have a professor or boss who doesn't care about her nerves. Then what? I don't want her to be some millennial snowflake.

MOTHER: Don't call her that. She may get so upset that she cries in front of the other kids, and that will be even more horrible for her. She'll never get over that. Maybe the teacher can just let her present to her alone after school.

THERAPIST: It sounds like you're both worried about some negative outcome for Shelby, which helps me to understand how and why you respond to her in different ways sometimes. Dad, it seems like you think she's giving in and taking the easy way out. And looking into the future she won't have the skills she needs to succeed. Mom, it seems like you're more worried that something horrible will happen to her if she tries to go through with the presentation and that will have serious personal and social consequences for her right now.

By shedding light on their pattern of responding in light of their fears for Shelby, the therapist can utilize psychoeducation as well as prescriptive interventions for each parent to recognize, challenge, and problem-solve around their own self-talk. In Shelby's case, each parent has strengths, particularly with empathize and encourage skills. Shelby's mother evidences a good ability to empathize with her daughter's anxiety and, on occasion, encourage approach behaviors. On other occasions, however, she permits avoidance behaviors and sometimes rescues Shelby because of her own distress. The therapist can coach Shelby's mother to challenge her own catastrophic thinking and conceptualize exposures as opportunities to practice skills and avoidance as missed opportunities to practice such skills and possibly get favorable feedback.

Shelby's father, on the other hand, has his own version of feared outcome that drives his encouragement without sufficient empathizing. The therapist can work with him to better understand Shelby's anxiety, and can perhaps use examples of other anxieties he may have experienced if not social anxiety. The therapist can further work with Shelby's father to provide nonjudgmental statements validating her anxious experiences (e.g., "I know that raising your hand in class makes you really nervous and makes you not want to do it"). In this and other cases, the therapist wants to work with the caregiver to actively listen, empathize, and provide validating statements without necessarily problem solving. Note that for Shelby's father, his instinct to prevent avoidance is in line with the therapist's conceptualization and planned exposures. However, in the absence of empathy and sufficient support, his stylistic approach has become a source of contention and produced another "escape hatch" whereby Shelby "goes to mom" to get "dad off my back" (one of Shelby's two stated therapy goals). Coaching Shelby's father with scripts for specific labeled praise and positive reinforcement facilitates both the parents' and youth's goals by making the father an ally for change. Chapter 5 gives more examples of how to move caregivers toward an active and supportive stance while promoting change.

Reward Charts and Contingency Management

Given Shelby's negative self-talk and her age, the therapist will want to pay particular attention to Shelby's self-reward and self-praise. As noted, the therapist can model scripts for self-rewarding for effort rather than outcome (e.g., "I'm proud that I tried that"), approach over avoidance, coping (e.g., "It was hard to stay, but I hung in there for the whole time and I am proud of myself"), catching negative self-judgments (e.g., "I caught myself when I thought I was being awkward"). That's not to say she cannot come up with a plan for external rewards for working on exposures (e.g., "After I complete my three exposures this weekend, I will treat myself to ice cream on Sunday"). For this exercise, the therapist brainstormed options for goals and rewards (see Figure 9.11; a blank version is available as Worksheet 14 in Appendix A).

Of course, working with Shelby's parents can include helping them to provide specific labeled praise for Shelby's approach behaviors, home practice completion, and exposure efforts. Rewards can be built into weekly exposures (e.g., "If you order pizza on the phone, you pick the movie for family night"). Praise can come in the form of earning tokens for other rewards (e.g., a behavior chart where Shelby earns 1 point for every social exposure that can be traded in for iPad app purchases) or earning rewards requiring accumulating points over time (e.g., purchase of a new video game). Parents can be taught to use existing youth requests as leverage for contingency management planning (see Chapter 5 for examples of parent-facilitated reward plans).

Collaborating with the School

When working with socially anxious youth, it can be helpful to identify key liaisons at the youth's school to assist in supporting the teen's therapy goals. Given the sheer number of social interactions that occur at school, the therapist can work with Shelby to identify potential in-school social interactions where she can incorporate her at-home exposure practice. With Shelby's increasing interference and impairment related to her socioacademic and performance anxiety goals, it may be beneficial to connect with teachers or in-school personnel to functionally assess and better understand how Shelby presents in school generally, review her class participation (or lack thereof), and derive examples of actual and attempted avoidance in response to a presentation demand. See Chapter 11 for recommendations on connecting with school personnel and developing a coordinated intervention plan. For example, teachers could fill out their own functional assessment worksheet (see Figure 9.5; a blank version is available as Worksheet 1 in Appendix A) to provide details about Shelby's typical response in academic settings. Teachers may be receptive to psychoeducation and treatment goals, as well as strategies to incorporate in their work with youth. For example, the therapist can teach Shelby's teachers how to incorporate empathize and encourage language into their instruction.

Beyond assessment, teachers or school personnel might be recruited during the exposure design and execution phase. For example, therapist and teacher can coordinate exposures revolving around Shelby initially raising her hand for a question she knows in advance or for setting up a time to meet with the teacher to discuss a certain project. Other coordinated in-school exposures for Shelby can include the following:

- Teacher-facilitated group project pairings
- Knowing in advance what section to "read aloud"
- Practicing a talk or presentation to a teacher in advance for feedback

WORKSHEET 14. Goals and Rewards Chart

Whenever we're trying new skills, we should reward ourselves for making the effort. First, brainstorm achievable, meaningful goals. Then, pick how you would reward yourself for each accomplishment.

Goals I Can Match Myself	Reward	M	T	W	TR	F	Sat	Sun	# of Days Achieved
Texting one friend a day	Get ice cream at Rita's if I do it at least 5 days this week.	Y	N	N	Y	N	Y	N	3
Catching negative self-talk	Give myself a pat on the back for each one.	N	N	Y	Y	Y	N	Y	4

Goals My Parents Can Reward Me For	Reward	M	T	W	TR	F	Sat	Sun	# of Days Achieved
Order take-out.	Pick family TV night show.	–	–	–	–	Y	N	–	1

FIGURE 9.11. Goals and rewards chart for Shelby.

252

- Preparing a question for office hours
- Being approached for an in-school volunteer opportunity

Over time, the preplanned exposures can transition to more naturalistic and realistic ones (e.g., being called on without advanced knowledge of the question, the teacher not knowing that a meeting request is coming in advance). Of course, the level of school collaboration and explicit involvement may vary widely depending on the school system, teacher availability and preference, and caregiver and youth preference. Ideally, incorporating the most youth-relevant people and settings can allow for potent and meaningful *in vivo* exposure work.

Progress Monitoring

Assessment in CBT is ongoing, and when the RCADS was administered at Week 4 (Table 9.4), Shelby's anxiety appeared to have increased on the self-report form, especially in her responses regarding social anxiety. This is noteworthy and could indicate that Shelby (1) likely underreported her anxiety at intake in relation to her social concerns, (2) has increased her self-disclosure of her social concerns, and relatedly, (3) may have better access and understanding of her anxious symptomatology after engaging in treatment. RCADS scores might also reflect an increase in her anxious experience that resulted from actively engaging in treatment. This is understandable given the very nature of CBT in focusing on her, providing psychoeducation on her avoidance/escape, and setting the plan to encourage approach and exposures.

Progress monitoring also includes monitoring improvements in Shelby's social skills (see Figure 9.2), which can include in-session behavioral observation and pre- and postskills rehearsal. Tracking Shelby's home practice exposure completion allows the therapist to see that Shelby is increasing skills practice outside of the office, and increasing social engagement and activities (e.g., attending dance class weekly, approaching peers, raising her hand in class). Collaboration and check-ins with the school are also key in progress monitoring, especially regarding class participation and presentation goals.

TABLE 9.4. Shelby's Symptom Profile Using the RCADS, Weeks 1 to 4

	Youth, Week 1		Youth, Week 4	
	Raw scores	*T* scores	Raw scores	*T* scores
Separation anxiety	0	40	1	44
Generalized anxiety	1	32	2	35
Panic disorder	1	40	3	46
Social anxiety	4	33	18	61
Obsessions/compulsions	0	35	0	35
Depression	0	29	6	46
Total anxiety	6	31	24	45
Total anxiety and depression	6	29	30	45

T scores higher than 65 indicate borderline clinical threshold. Scores of 70 or higher indicate scores above clinical threshold. *T* scores are normalized based on youth's age and gender.

As Shelby's therapy advances into the later phases, her parents have improved their ability to empathize and encourage her social anxiety, without accommodating it and helping her utilize the "escape hatch."

TERMINATION AND RELAPSE PREVENTION

The last phase of treatment includes a steady diet of in-session and out-of-the-office *in vivo* exposures tackling all aspects of Shelby's hierarchy. Of course, over the course of treatment, there are naturally occurring situations that arise (e.g., birthdays, activities, performances) that allow for variability in the collaborative exposure design. After several months of weekly sessions, Shelby is demonstrating improvements in her class participation and no longer trying to get out of oral presentations according to her teacher. She has reengaged in dance class and attends regularly and has made two friends there with whom she socializes. Her parents are reporting less conflict around "getting her to do stuff" or "letting her off the hook." She continues to struggle with some negative self-judgments before, after, and during presentations and she is also able to challenge these more effectively and not get stuck in a spiral for as long. A positive sign emerged when Shelby asked to cancel a session in order to hang out after school.

The therapist, Shelby, and her parents also collaboratively decide on a termination date for treatment, all the while working on a relapse prevention plan. This plan will help Shelby to consolidate her most effective skills (i.e., catching the "escape hatch" trap and challenging it by staying), assist her parents to note theirs (empathize and encourage, coach and approach), and, of course, guide Shelby to keep practicing. Shelby's mother also noted her use of CBT skills to address her own social anxiety, and the desire to model for Shelby by signing up for social activities despite her discomfort. Relapse prevention also focuses on looking ahead to prepare and problem-solve for anticipated challenges that may increase Shelby's anxiety or trigger her desire to avoid (e.g., a switch in teacher the next semester, holiday dance performance) and remind the family of the effective skills they have learned. It also involves focusing on anticipated *opportunities* that may arise to intentionally practice learned skills and challenge her social anxiety (such as a summer job).

Prognosis and Follow-Up

At termination, the therapist conveyed that Shelby's prognosis was positive, assuming Shelby and her parents continue to practice and engage with realistic expectations (e.g., increasing her socializing did not mean that she would become an extrovert, and she would need to continue to be mindful of her negative self-appraisals), and recognize the social challenges of high school. It was also helpful for Shelby and her therapist to schedule booster sessions along the way to aid in these challenges. The therapist additionally began to brainstorm upcoming developmental challenges consistent with emerging adulthood and that would likely be challenging (e.g., making phone calls to schedule your own health appointments, job interviews).

Challenges in This Case

Consistent with the other SAD cases, Shelby presented with significant and worsening anxiety across domains. It would be understandable for the therapist to feel overwhelmed by the many aspects of Shelby's anxiety: her level of distress, negative self-judgments, lack of self-efficacy, escape and avoidance behaviors. The therapist will need to work with Shelby on: social skills; increasing isolation; differential parental responses and parent/family conflict; possible need for ongoing collaboration and collateral work with the teacher and school; and Shelby's transition from middle school to high school. Perhaps the last area will be especially challenging given how difficult and trying this phase can be for even the least anxious teen. Let's take a moment to reflect on our own social experiences in middle school going into high school with a collective nod to the likely near-universal challenges we struggled to manage, bearing in mind the present-day overlay of social contexts to be navigated via social media and its many seemingly constant and ever-present platforms.

As such, the case conceptualization and an ongoing functional understanding of Shelby's anxieties can guide the complexities of these multiple domains and provide a roadmap for interventions at all levels, from improving eye contact to joining a club. Continuing to reformulate the case conceptualization with new and gathered data and skills that progress over the course of treatment can aid in helping all involved participants—therapist, parents, youth—in establishing realistic expectations. Social interaction is a constant in life and can feel overwhelming. As such, it may be especially important to highlight seemingly small increments of progress—remember how anxious Shelby was when she first met her therapist?

SUMMARY AND KEY POINTS

Youth with SAD often present with multiple-domain impairment, including clinical anxiety, deprived peer socialization, social skills' deficits, and academic performance concerns. Treatment should focus on the domains of greatest impairment, matched with youth and caregiver goals, and informed by the therapist's conceptualization.

- Assess specific areas of parental/caregiver/teacher accommodation via escape/avoidance (e.g., answering for socially anxious youth, letting them out of oral reports) that may be negatively reinforcing those very behaviors.
- Assess the youth's potential interpersonal skills and deficits and incorporate social skills training and practice.
- Set realistic outcome expectations in line with the youth's temperament.
- Assess information-processing biases especially with regard to the youth's preevent and postevent negative evaluative processing and self-talk.
- Note any mind reading and other common cognitive distortions in social anxiety.
- Include same-age peers in exposures.
- Assess and incorporate the youth's interests to maximize their intrinsic motivation for social and performance exposures.
- Assess alcohol and substance use in teens in connection with social anxiety (e.g., the urge to "self-medicate," difficulty with assertiveness or peer refusal).

CHAPTER 10

Generalized Anxiety Disorder

Worry is the fundamental aspect of generalized anxiety disorder (GAD) that leads to anxious apprehension, physical tension, and behavioral avoidance and escape. Worry is a cognitive feature of anxiety (Barlow, 1988) that reflects expansive and unconstructive attempts to problem-solve or plan for stressful life hassles and challenges. Worry itself is a natural reaction when the solution to a forthcoming problem is unclear, or the outcome of an upcoming challenge is unpredictable, or when the demands on one's cognitive load exceed one's capacity. When the worry process becomes difficult to interrupt or expands to multiple domains (school, social, work, family, the future), it can significantly limit the youth's natural functioning and performance (Alfano, 2012; Roemer & Borkovec, 1993).

Youth commonly engage in worry, with some evidence suggesting that a majority of children report excessive worrying at various points of childhood and adolescence, with older youth and girls appearing to exhibit higher levels of worry (see Bell-Dolan, Last, & Strauss, 1990; Songco, Hudson, & Fox, 2020). Community data on youth worries indicate that it is developmentally normative for most youth to endorse at least some worries across domains, including health, safety, death, family, school, social issues, and community, and world events (Silverman, La Greca, & Wasserstein, 1995; Muris, Meesters, Merckelbach, Sermon, & Zwakhalen, 1998). The content of such worry is relatively similar between referred and nonreferred youth; what presents differently is the intensity, types, and uncontrollability of the worries (Weems, Silverman, & La Greca, 2000).

Beyond worry, youth who meet formal criteria for GAD will endorse at least one physiological symptom, such as upset stomach, muscle tension, headaches, and difficulty concentrating. Youth and caregivers often differ in their report of somatic symptoms, with caregivers endorsing more of them, suggesting that caregivers may attribute physical symptoms to anxiety more readily than youth do. As expected, older youth experience or endorse somatic symptoms more frequently than younger children (Kendall & Pimentel, 2003).

COGNITIVE VARIABLES

Highly anxious youth evidence consistent cognitive biases, such that they are more likely to interpret threat and anticipate negative outcomes (e.g., Suarez & Bell-Dolan, 2001). Adult models of worry posit that, as a cognitive activity, worry behaviors may serve the function of avoiding emotional experiences (Borkovec, Shadick, & Hopkins, 1991). Similarly, meta-cognitive models of adult GAD propose that both positive and negative thoughts, and beliefs about the worry itself, further reinforces the worry behaviors (Wells, 2006). Many individuals with GAD ascribe positive attributes to worry, such as the belief that their worrying helps them plan for challenges or problem-solve (Gosselin et al., 2007). Adults with clinical anxiety also hold negative beliefs about worry that reinforce its persistence, such as superstitions about its role, or assumptions about its uncontrollability (Cartwright-Hatton et al., 2004). Recent research has also found evidence that youth engage in similar meta-cognitions about worry and the nature of these beliefs predicts the level of worry (Bacow, Pincus, Ehrenreich, & Brody, 2009; Wilson et al., 2009)

BEHAVIORAL VARIABLES

A common behavioral consequence of worry is the reassurance seeking the youth uses at an attempt to address their anxiety. These behaviors may include, for example, asking parents, caregivers, friends, and teachers questions related to their worry topics and seeking their reassurance that feared outcomes will not occur: "Will it rain on the way to school?" "Will the teacher be mad that I'm late?" "Will I catch up if I miss instructions?" These questions presume to innocently seek information, but their more insidious function becomes apparent when no answer seems to quell the youth's anxiety. Reassurance seeking can also take the form of persistent information gathering from external sources, such as news sources, the Internet, friends, and family members. Procrastination and excessive planning are other forms of behavioral avoidance. For example, youth with GAD may study excessively for tests or they may leave exceedingly early for appointments to avoid undesirable outcomes, like lower grades or performance evaluations from others. As with other behavioral avoidance, the youth falls into these traps out of the false belief that such behaviors will protect them from negative outcomes. That brief reduction in anxiety reinforces the persistent worry and behavioral avoidance even if these tactics do not improve the actual meaningful outcomes in the long run (e.g., excessive planning does not necessarily help an individual accomplish more tasks).

PARENT AND FAMILY VARIABLES

Caregiver behaviors may also play a role. Evidence suggests that overprotection and anxious parenting style are commonly associated with youth worry (Muris et al., 2000), and caregivers may model their own anxious behaviors that reinforce those behaviors in their children (Fisak & Gills-Taquechel, 2007). Overprotection may deprive youth of the opportunity to problem-solve on their own or experientially learn that difficult outcomes may indeed occur without catastrophic results. Importantly, there is also evidence that clinically anxious youths' reports of rejection by their parents are associated with higher levels of worry (Brown & Whiteside, 2008). See Chapter 5 for further discussion and a more in-depth description of caregiver interventions.

CBT MODEL OF GAD

As with other anxieties, application of the cognitive-behavioral (CBT) model to GAD requires identifying how the youth's thoughts, feelings and behaviors interact in response to stressors (see Handout 22 in Appendix A). The youth's cognitive processes, characterized by excessive worry, are perhaps most apparent, at first. Youth with GAD experience excessive and uncontrollable worry that reflects, and perpetuates, significant distress. The content of the youth's worries assumes negative catastrophic outcomes and overestimates the likelihood of negative outcomes: "If I get a B, I won't get into college" or "What if I get attacked by a shark when we go to the beach?" The therapist has to be on the alert for presumed negative outcomes that the youth cannot express, such as "I'm gonna be late for the bus." To others this might seem like a plausible but noncatastrophic outcome. To the worried youth, it implies all sorts of catastrophic outcomes. It will be helpful to assist the youth to articulate their concrete fears as much as possible.

Of course, more worry begets further worry as the youth continues to cogitate on the likely bad things to come. As they persist in worrying, somatic agitation builds in the form of tension or inability to relax. Poor concentration may be evident, and they may appear preoccupied or distracted. They may experience disturbance in sleep rituals as the events of the day keep them awake; they may experience restless sleep with worries about upcoming demands. The worried youth tries to accommodate these worries and somatic distress with rigid and perfectionistic planning or performing. The assumption is that catastrophic outcomes can be avoided if they try hard enough or plan for every eventuality. Of course, it is impossible to plan for every possible outcome, so the youth eventually confronts some level of "failure." If the youth cannot tolerate this failure (i.e., any discrepancy between the predicted and experienced outcomes), the youth begins to fear future failures and associated discomfort. Youth with GAD may react to this by "doubling down" on the preparation and/or perfectionism to try and avert "disaster" again. Reassurance from others brings temporary relief relying on the assumption that others can protect the youth from any unpredictable outcome. However, this brings failure, too, as no support person can fully stave off any unwanted events. As such, it is crucial to assess how the youth manages uncertainties and how others accommodate the youth to minimize their worries.

CASE VIGNETTE: JIN

Jin is a 10-year-old Chinese American cisgender boy. He lives with his mother, 8-year-old sister, and maternal grandparents in a modest suburban neighborhood. Jin's father died from illness just after his sister's birth, and Jin has ongoing relations with his paternal grandparents, aunts, uncles, and cousins, most of whom live nearby. The family does not discuss the circumstances around his father's illness or death. Jin was referred to treatment at an outpatient clinic by his pediatrician following his annual checkup and screening for anxiety and mood symptoms. His mother described that he always seems tense and worried about something. He also reported having headaches, which were medically evaluated and thought to be associated with anxiety. Jin's nickname is "Little Man" because he is frequently concerned with adult matters. He worries about family finances, the health of his family, especially that of his mother and both sets of aging grandparents. He frequently asks his mother if she has taken her vitamins and if she is eating healthy foods. He is a good, high-achieving student in the third grade at the local public school. He likes school and loves to read comic books. However, he often worries about school, his grades, tests, and if he will fall behind. Many nights, he has difficulty falling asleep because he is worried about what might happen the next day. Sometimes, he will get out of bed at night and ask his mother several questions about his assignments, or some crime- or weather-related events he overheard while his grandfather was watching the news on TV. For Christmas, he asked for a weather station so he could forecast bad weather. Over the summer, he refused to swim at the beach because he had heard on the news about local shark attacks. Over the past couple of years, he has expressed increasing worries about school shootings.

Jin is quiet and has a couple of friends with whom he rides the bus and sits at lunch. He gets stressed out in the morning because he fears he will miss the bus and be late. Jin is well liked by his teachers and always completes his homework on time. They encourage him to raise his hand more in class, but overall, he participates when called on. They have reported that he sometimes asks questions to which they are sure he knows the answer. Jin generally gets along with his sister, although his mother describes that he can be overprotective. His sister states that he is "always reminding me of the rules and bossing me around."

According to his mother, Jin is always thinking and expecting the worst, and she does not see him having as much fun as other kids his age. She says his second favorite activity to thinking is asking questions. He has been begging her for a mobile phone "because you never know"; however, she is reluctant to purchase one for him, concerned that he will use the phone to read news or text her to ask questions. His mother worries that as he gets older, his worrying and question asking will alienate his peers and he will lose friends. She often feels guilty after snapping at him for asking so many reassurance-seeking questions, especially since she is frequently working and they have such limited time together. Jin has a close relationship with his maternal grandfather who drops him off and picks him up after school. They will also frequently watch TV together and discuss current events, although Jin's mother becomes upset when her father allows Jin to watch the news.

ASSESSMENT OF GAD

Jin was brought to diagnostic intake by his mother and maternal grandparents. The therapist completed the Anxiety Disorders Interview Schedule—Parent Version (ADIS-P) with Jin's mother and, with her consent, his grandparents remained in the room. The therapist then met with Jin to complete the ADIS-C (Child Version). He separated easily from his mother and grandparents and hugged each of them before entering the assessment, saying, as recorded in his report, "because you never know." At the conclusion of the assessment, Jin met all the criteria for GAD. Everyone was in agreement that he is a "worrier" whose worries are indeed out of proportion to most situations. When discussing the onset of his symptoms, his mother noted that Jin has generally been a curious and anxious child "since he could speak." It is worth noting that although they did not consistently participate in the ADIS-P, when the therapist directed a question to Jin's grandparents for their input, they would generally describe not being concerned about his mental health. For example, Jin's grandfather asked at one point, "What is the problem if he is just a thinker and sensitive boy?"

Jin reported worries across several domains and endorsed worries about academics, his own and his family's safety, health, family finances, the future, perfectionism, little things that have happened, and issues going on in the world. His worries often involve information that he hears from the news and that triggers a wave of topical worries, which then seem to escalate over a short period of time and slowly dissipate "until the next worry." While he demonstrated insight into the level of his worry, he was less aware of how some of his behaviors served to maintain his worry, especially the reassurance seeking. Similarly, when asked about some of his behaviors like requesting a weather station for Christmas or watching the news, Jin noted that he likes to be prepared and indicated positive beliefs about the utility of his worry. Similarly, when asked about his frequent check-ins related to his family members' health, he reported it was his job to make sure they were caring for themselves and spoke openly about his father's death and his belief that he had to step up to help his family.

Jin met more than one of the physiological criteria related to GAD: having difficulty relaxing, experiencing muscle aches as well as headaches, and trouble falling asleep most nights. He described his difficulty unwinding before bedtime and "shutting off" his brain. When assessing the bedtime routine with both Jin and his mother, they acknowledged that it is often a drawn-out process that results in Jin frequently getting out of bed to ask his mother questions. Jin also described that he has begun to worry about his inability to sleep each night asking, "What if I can't fall asleep, then I won't be able to wake up on time for school or I'll be too sleepy at school to pay attention in class?" Jin's mother acknowledged that she has on occasion yelled at Jin for stalling or not being able to just go to sleep. This indicates increasing disruption in the family system.

Given Jin's closeness to his grandparents, the therapist made sure to assess how they could be incorporated into treatment. Jin spends a significant amount of time with his grandfather. During the intake, the grandfather expressed his belief that Jin's worry isn't pathological, but is consistent with his nature as a thinker and sensitive boy. It was necessary to validate the grandfather's experience of his grandson and monitor any messaging that may be dismissive of treatment and subvert treatment goals. Furthermore, the therapist needed to assess the extent to which Jin was getting access to news that was not developmentally appropriate, and how the grandfather was inadvertently reinforcing reassurance-seeking behaviors. The therapist was wise to engage the grandfather, as well as other family members. Also, it was important to assess how Jin's worry-related beliefs about his "job" in the family were related to collective views in *this* family system. While there are many known cultural references to collective responsibility in traditional Chinese families (see Hodges & Oei, 2007; Hwang, Wood, Lin, & Cheung, 2006), the therapist still wants to understand how Jin is going beyond expected roles for a 10-year-old, even within a family that values collectivist principles.

Other sources of diagnostic information are also useful in supporting the GAD and informing treatment planning (see Figure 10.1). First, Jin was referred to treatment by his pediatrician after presenting to her for headaches. After completing various medical follow-up testing, his pediatrician screened for anxiety and mood issues and concluded his headaches were related to chronic tension, anxiety, and stress. Two points are especially relevant here: (1) The headaches may speak to the severity of his tension and level of impairment, and (2) the therapist will likely want to secure consent to speak to his pediatrician and any other medical providers for collateral information and ongoing discussion regarding Jin's headaches.

Behavioral observation during the intake also yielded useful data. For example, although he separated easily from his family when it came time to enter the office, Jin hugged each of them and muttered, "Because you never know." Upon follow-up, the therapist noted that Jin always hugs his family upon any departure and clarified that such worry related to his fears of bad things happening. The therapist noted that some of Jin's behaviors could have a superstitious quality to them, and that it would be important to assess if these were developmentally transient or linked to an element of his worry. The therapist conducted assessment to rule out a diagnosis of

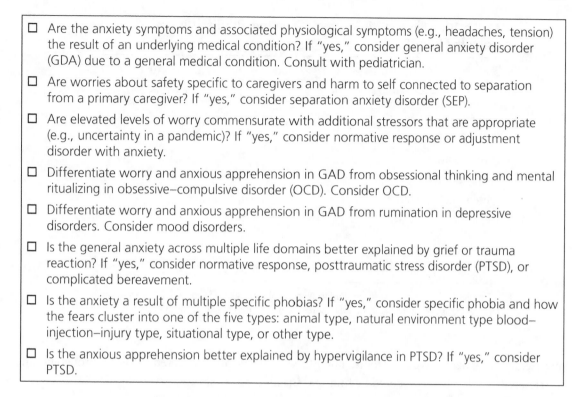

☐ Are the anxiety symptoms and associated physiological symptoms (e.g., headaches, tension) the result of an underlying medical condition? If "yes," consider general anxiety disorder (GDA) due to a general medical condition. Consult with pediatrician.

☐ Are worries about safety specific to caregivers and harm to self connected to separation from a primary caregiver? If "yes," consider separation anxiety disorder (SEP).

☐ Are elevated levels of worry commensurate with additional stressors that are appropriate (e.g., uncertainty in a pandemic)? If "yes," consider normative response or adjustment disorder with anxiety.

☐ Differentiate worry and anxious apprehension in GAD from obsessional thinking and mental ritualizing in obsessive–compulsive disorder (OCD). Consider OCD.

☐ Differentiate worry and anxious apprehension in GAD from rumination in depressive disorders. Consider mood disorders.

☐ Is the general anxiety across multiple life domains better explained by grief or trauma reaction? If "yes," consider normative response, posttraumatic stress disorder (PTSD), or complicated bereavement.

☐ Is the anxiety a result of multiple specific phobias? If "yes," consider specific phobia and how the fears cluster into one of the five types: animal type, natural environment type blood–injection–injury type, situational type, or other type.

☐ Is the anxious apprehension better explained by hypervigilance in PTSD? If "yes," consider PTSD.

FIGURE 10.1. Diagnostic clarification checklist: GAD.

obsessive–compulsive disorder (OCD), differentiating between worrying and intrusive obsessions. For example, the therapist could assess the nature of Jin's checking behaviors versus compulsive behaviors (see Comer et al., 2004). Typically, GAD-related intrusive thoughts reflect concerns rooted in real-world problems and events (the news, tasks, interpersonal interactions), even if those worries are excessive and repetitive (e.g., "My father died suddenly, so I always worry my mother will go, too, unless I watch after her"). In OCD, the intrusive obsessions do not have direct ties necessarily to logical realities; they can reference fantastical beliefs or cause–effect relationships that even the youth recognize as illogical (e.g., "My mother will die if I don't tell her I love her three times"). Furthermore, in OCD, intrusive thoughts are almost always routinely followed by repetitive and compulsive rituals. The ritual is usually the same action or sequences of actions (e.g., telling his mother he loved her three times). In GAD, youth often attempt many actions to relieve their worry; however, the attempts take varied forms (e.g., reassurance seeking, planning, overcompensating) and are less ritualistic. Jin did not appear to meet the criteria for OCD.

Additionally, Jin completed self-report assessments and his mother completed child-focused assessments, including the Revised Children's Anxiety and Depression Scale (RCADS). Both Jin and his mother's responses resulted in T scores in the clinical range for GAD, and the mother's report also indicated elevation in depressive symptoms (Table 10.1). Although Jin did not meet the criteria for major depressive disorder (MDD), persistent depressive disorder, or any mood-related disorders per the semi-structured assessments, Jin's mother did note and express her concerns that her son was a serious boy who had difficulty having fun. Given potential overlap between worry and the rumination associated with depressive states, the therapist should continue to monitor

TABLE 10.1. Jin and His Mother's Symptom Profile at Intake Using the RCADS

	Mother		Youth	
	Raw scores	T scores	Raw scores	T scores
Separation anxiety	13	> 80**	9	69*
Generalized anxiety	18	> 80**	16	> 80**
Panic disorder	6	74**	5	53
Social anxiety	19	79**	17	64
Obsessions/compulsions	6	67*	11	65
Depression	13	> 80**	7	50
Total anxiety	62	> 80**	58	71**
Total anxiety and depression	75**	> 80**	65	68*

*T scores higher than 65 indicate borderline clinical threshold. **Scores of 70 or higher indicate scores above clinical threshold. T scores are normalized based on youth's age and gender.

any escalation of depressive symptoms. The RCADS profile also indicated the extent to which Jin worries, with multiple items scored by him and his mother as "always."

Goal Setting and Defining Target Problems

Although assessment is always ongoing, the initial collection of diagnostic information gathered via semi-structured clinical interview, behavioral observation, self- and parent-report forms, and other collateral can be aggregated and reviewed with Jin and his mother. The therapist and mother agreed that his grandparents should be present and included from the outset. Providing a comprehensive explanation for a collection of symptoms and experiences in the feedback session, the therapist may be confirming what the patient and parent already know in some instances. Jin's mother was not surprised to hear about Jin meeting the criteria for GAD. The therapist also worked to normalize some of Jin's worry while explaining that many of his worries were interfering or "messing things up" for him in various ways. Since the feedback included Jin's grandparents given their daily presence in his life, the therapist was wise to acknowledge their perspective while providing psychoeducation on the potential negative effects on Jin's health and development the GAD was having.

It was important to work with Jin and his mother to set realistic goals since Jin's worries were many and pervasive. It was key to develop goals as specific and measurable as possible. While many worriers—adult and child—describe that others often offer advice such as "stop worrying," this is not useful or practical advice. Since Jin's academic performance had not yet been adversely impacted, it might have been difficult to tackle some of the academic-related worries head-on. Instead, it was important to understand how subtler areas of avoidance were interfering with academic performance. For example, his teachers noted that he would not take risks raising his hand if he was not 100% sure of an answer. His excessive preparation for fairly straightforward tests also connected to his worries about getting into a "good college." In Jin's case, parent, child, and therapist goals were devised as follows:

Parent's Goals

- Have more fun.
- Stop assuming the worst; worry less about everything.
- Decrease number of times he asks questions.
- Learn how not to yell at him or become so frustrated.
- Develop better sleep habits and go to bed on time.
- Watch less news.

Child's Goals

- "Shut off my brain."
- Learn how to get rid of the "worry zombies" and keep the "worry helper" thoughts.

Therapist's Goals

- Decrease reassurance-seeking behaviors (e.g., questions, conversations at bedtime, news checking).
- Increase use of coping behaviors to manage worry.
- Teach mother (and grandparents) skills to decrease reassurance-responding and accommodation behaviors.

Figure 10.2 is a completed Goals Tracker worksheet for Jin's target problems (a blank version is available as Worksheet 11 in Appendix A). When goal setting, the therapist worked with Jin to translate his first stated goal to "shut off my brain" into a more realistic goal. Despite our best efforts at times, shutting off our brains is not a realistic (or necessarily healthy) goal! When discussing this, Jin creatively described that sometimes it felt as if his worries were like zombies that relentlessly pursued him. The therapist worked with Jin to express his goal in this way: he could learn skills and strategies to "battle the worry zombies" while keeping near the "worry helper" thoughts (these are coping thoughts). Since Jin loved comic books, he used his own creative, visual language to describe his worries and establish goals. The language of this goal was then interwoven throughout treatment.

Also given Jin's age, treatment needed to involve his mother and grandparents. Understandably, Jin's mother worried about the negativity in his worries ("I wish he would stop assuming the worst, and there was less worry about everything") and his inability to have fun. The therapist worked with Jin's mother to make these goals *realistic* and operationalize them to determine indicators of progress. For example, "Less worry about everything" would be especially difficult at first, but therapist and mother worked to translate this goal into skills Jin could learn and practice. For example, the therapist could teach the mother to learn and practice coaching Jin to identify and challenge his catastrophic worry and inclination for assuming the worst. When goal setting. the therapist could work with Jin's mother to operationalize and specify less well-defined goals by asking, "How will we know he is having more fun?" or "How will we know if he has better sleep habits?" Lastly, for the parent-stated goal of decreasing the number of times Jin asks reassurance-seeking questions, there is a related goal for his mother (and perhaps grandparents): *how to* provide reassurance-type answers (or not).

WORKSHEET 11. Goals Tracker

Work with your therapist to brainstorm possible specific, meaningful, and achievable goals. Think through what outcomes you expect to see. And then, keep track of how your child does each week.

Parent Goals	Desired Outcomes	Week 1	Week 2	Week 3	Week 4	Week 5
Less worry about everything	Rate "worry zombies" (0–10); parents see child catching worry zombies (+). (Remember to praise!)	10; caught +2 times	10; caught +3 times	8.4; caught +5 times	7.2; caught +10 times	7.1; caught +7 times
Decrease reassurance-seeking questions.	Number of reassurance-seeking questions per day	Too many, lost count	Too many	M: 14 T: 13 W: 11 Th: 6 Fr: 6 Sa: 14 Su: 5	M: 11 T: 9 W: 7 Th: 7 Fr: 4 Sa: 5 Su: 5	M: 8 T: 6 W: 12 Th: 5 Fr: 3 Sa: 5 Su: 7
Improve sleep and go to bed on time.	Number of times he followed bedtime routine	0	1	2	4	4

Youth Goals	Desired Outcomes	Week 1	Week 2	Week 3	Week 4	Week 5
Shut off my brain.	Rate worry zombies (0–10).	10	10	8.4	7.2	7.1
Learn how to get rid of the "worry zombies."	Practice catching worry zombie traps; # of traps caught.	8	11	4	5	5
Practice worry helpers.	Mindfulness practice	1 time	0 times	3 times	3 times	4 times

FIGURE 10.2. Completed Goals Tracker worksheet for Jin.

264

CASE CONCEPTUALIZATION

CBT Model

Given the number of worry domains and relative ubiquity of Jin's worry, it can be overwhelming to aggregate the assessment materials into a cohesive formulation. Data across informants (child, caregiver, pediatrician, teacher, therapist) and across formats (semi-structured interview, self- and parent-report forms, behavioral observation) support a level of worry and concomitant symptomatology that are clinically significant and impairing. Accounting for development, it is clear that Jin worries *more* than other youth his age and *about more topics,* including those not typically considered at this stage of development.

Jin appears to have been temperamentally more anxious and more curious as a toddler, and the death of his father impacted his early development and, of course, his family system. The therapist understood Jin's GAD to have emerged from his cautious, apprehensive style, becoming associated with a worry process that focused on questions of safety, health, and perfectionism. Jin sought answers to provide certainty about feared outcomes. A what if worry triggered internal distress and usually additional what if worries and questions. As a coping strategy, he asked others to reassure him of positive outcomes. As their acquiescence brought temporary relief, thereby negatively reinforcing the questions, the more he repeated them. Given his father's death, his family naturally became more overprotective of him and his sister, and likely overattended to his inquiries. While this is understandable given the context, the family's concern reinforced the notion that issues of safety, health, and related topics were something to monitor closely and served a reasonable threat.

Relatedly, as Jin evidenced a bias toward negatively valenced information signaling possible threat or danger in his environment, he began to attend to these cues (e.g., in the news) and his worries absorbed the most current sources of threat. Normatively, future-oriented "worry" can aid in planning and problem solving and be effective to this end. Jin's worry behaviors are intermittently reinforced as his future-oriented worry and planning behaviors are associated with the non-occurrence of the feared negative catastrophic event (e.g., "If I get a weather station to track bad weather, I can stay safe from the hurricane"). Also, his negative future-oriented worry is reinforced both by the attention of those around him (e.g., mother's concerns and conversations with grandfather about the news) *and* at times, it changes their own observable behaviors (e.g., when he asks his mother if she took her vitamins and then she takes them). Like most problematic behaviors, Jin's worries were occasionally reinforced because they were artificially linked with desired outcomes. What distinguishes worry processes from other constructive planning and problem solving is the excessiveness of the worry and the lack of progress. One rule of thumb we like to use is the "5-minute rule." If a youth (or adult) has been thinking, planning, working on a problem for more than 5 minutes and they have not made any measurable progress on it (e.g., defined the problem better, brainstormed realistic solutions, attempted a solution), then the thinking can be considered "worry." If the thinking led to some kind of constructive end, it can be considered "planning" or "problem solving." In this way, deciding whether a youth is worrying or problem solving very much depends on the results: Did it help or is the youth stuck?

The example diagrammed in Figure 10.3 illustrates how Jin's worry is triggered by hearing about a neighbor who has cancer. He initially worries about getting cancer himself and then about his mother and grandparents "catching cancer." He has difficulty letting go of this worry. He asks his grandfather if he knows people with cancer and wants to use the family computer to

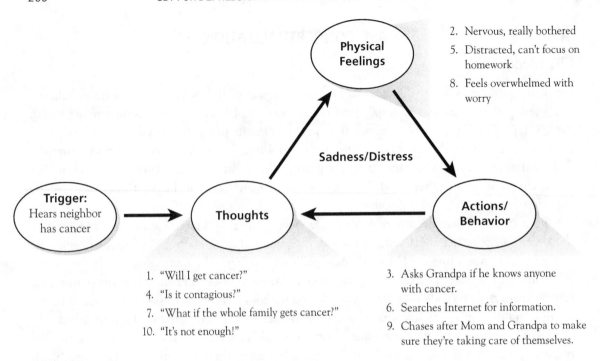

2. Nervous, really bothered
5. Distracted, can't focus on homework
8. Feels overwhelmed with worry

1. "Will I get cancer?"
4. "Is it contagious?"
7. "What if the whole family gets cancer?"
10. "It's not enough!"

3. Asks Grandpa if he knows anyone with cancer.
6. Searches Internet for information.
9. Chases after Mom and Grandpa to make sure they're taking care of themselves.

FIGURE 10.3. Individualized CBT conceptualization for Jin. His thoughts, feelings, and behavior cycle continuously in a downward spiral (follow the numbers in order: 1, 2, 3, etc. see how the thought–feeling–action cycle flows into another).

search online for more information. While he is doing his homework, he is distracted by thoughts of his grandparents and mother getting sick and he experiences tension as well. When his mother comes home from work, he immediately asks her about cancer and if she remembered to take her vitamins.

Teaching Jin and his mother to draw the CBT triangle and give examples allows the therapist to introduce the central aspects of the CBT model and the interplay among Jin's worried thoughts, somatic distress, and behaviors (and the behavioral responses from those around him). Jin can learn to identify his worry thoughts and recognize how they might become "worry zombies" ("Oh no, what if we get cancer? Then I'll miss school, too, and be so behind on work. What if grandpa gets cancer and then dies? Did Mom go to her doctor's appointment like she is supposed to?"). As one worry leads to the next about himself and his family, Jin becomes increasingly focused on his cognitions, which makes it difficult for him to concentrate on his homework, triggering anxiety about that: "I'm never gonna finish this homework"). He then experiences increasing physiological tension and irritability as he imagines his mother becoming sick. His behavioral responses include reassurance seeking from his grandfather, the TV, the computer, and his mother. The therapist can show Jin how one worry feeds another worry (worry zombies create other worry zombies, which can lead to a "zombie apocalypse" in his imaginings). All are focused on negative outcomes. When Jin gets some reassurance, he briefly feels better but he continues to worry and experience tension throughout the evening into bedtime. As he continues to worry, he will cope as he knows how—asking questions, making his mother "promise" to take her vitamins and go to the doctor. The goal here is to demonstrate how Jin's thoughts–feelings–behaviors continue to interact to create distress for him. It will be helpful to have Jin's mother review this CBT model worksheet with

Jin and ask her to complete her own. This will reveal her own patterns of responding, especially given her reported feelings of guilt and frustration in answering his questions and in yelling. These worksheets provide a preliminary layout for points of intervention.

Functional Assessment

Given that Jin's worry content runs across the domains of school, family, health, crime, and weather, functional assessments are especially useful for understanding the worry process and the factors that maintain it. See Figure 10.4 (a blank version is available as Worksheet 1 in Appendix A) for a sample of how his specific worries may be triggered, his emotional and behavioral responses, and the immediate and longer-term outcomes. By completing these worksheets with the youth (and their parents), patterns of antecedents and consequences invariably emerge and will guide needed interventions. As noted, it can be overwhelming to address the many worries in a youth who worries about everything. The functional assessment exercises assigned for home practice and completed in session highlight more manageable patterns of worry–response cycles. For Jin, when worries are triggered, they are emotionally distressing and difficult to interrupt, and this initiates a pattern of trying to manage them with pathological reassurance seeking as well as "planning research" and planned avoidance.

For example (Figure 10.4), when Jin learns about a possible thunderstorm at the end of the week that *may* coincide with his school field trip, he becomes immediately nervous and scared, and his behavioral responses include reassurance seeking from his grandfather, teacher, mother, and weather people. The minor reassurance he receives is insufficient, so he seeks out information from other sources (e.g., watching the weather channel) and planning (e.g., asking the teacher what the "plan" is for stormy weather the day of the field trip). He also preemptively seeks to avoid going on the trip by asking his mother if he can just stay home. Ultimately, his grandfather accommodates Jin's worry and "rescues" his grandson by allowing Jin to stay home with him. Typical of other youth with GAD, Jin enacts multiple "coping" strategies until one or more outcomes make him feel "safe."

The potential effects of this planned escape/avoidance/rescue on maintaining Jin's worry process can be seen graphically by reviewing the habituation curve (see Handout 23 in Appendix A). He has difficulty stopping himself from worrying and concentrating on other matters, and he experiences brief relief as he scans for weather information or has the hope of staying home with his grandfather. Notably as more functional assessments will elucidate, Jin's worry is not unique to thunderstorms (or a specific phobia); rather, his worry reflects a pattern of antecedent, response, and consequences with other weather-related events. These worries generalize to other worries of safety (e.g., "What if we lose power?" "What if there is flooding in the house?" "What if we have to evacuate?").

Whereas other classmates are excited for the school field trip, Jin's catastrophic worries interfere with his ability to expect favorable outcomes. In the days leading up to the trip, the teacher or peers reference the trip, and Jin becomes worried, experiences distress, and then engages in maladaptive coping and reassurance seeking. This worry–response cycle contributes to distress and family conflict in the immediate days leading up to the trip, and it may have intermediate and longer-term consequences that should be assessed. For example, Jin's preoccupation with worry and his inability to engage in affirmative conversations about the trip lead him to miss opportunities to socialize positively with his peers. If he is allowed to avoid the field trip, he misses out on the educational and normative social experiences from the trip itself. Completing the functional assessment

WORKSHEET 1. Trigger and Response

Tell us about your triggers and how you reacted. Describe your feelings, what you did (action), what happened right away (immediate outcome), and then what happened later (long-term outcome).

Antecedent → Behavioral and Emotional Response → Consequences

Trigger	Feeling (emotional response)	Action (behavioral response)	Immediate Results (What keeps it going?)	Long-Term Results (What gets you in trouble?)
My Mom is arguing with Grandpa for showing me the news.	Anxious, nervous.	Tried to ask if everyone is OK or if they are mad at me. Go to my room, worry about what will happen.	They keep shooing me off. I'm anxious, unable to concentrate on homework.	Have difficulty sleeping, can't eat dinner.
I have state tests coming up.	Very worried.	Ask teacher what I need to study.	Relieved because teacher said there are no tests to study for but then I got nervous again and thought I should review just in case.	Mom told me to put my books away to go to sleep. Mom annoyed I think.
Heard there may be a thunderstorm at the end of the week when we are supposed to go on our field trip to Fairy Tale Forest.	Nervous, scared.	Check the weather, ask Grandpa to check the weather, ask Mom about staying home, ask the teacher what the bad weather plan is.	Mom won't let me stay home. Teacher hasn't answered me. I want to check other weather sources. Grandpa said I could stay with him—so that was good.	Mom got annoyed with me. Classmate made fun of me for not wanting to go on trip.

FIGURE 10.4. Individualized functional assessment of worry and anxiety.

268

over time reveals the true impact of Jin's worry–response cycle. It becomes apparent that the costs of Jin's safety seeking may outweigh any presumed negative outcome from a potential storm.

TREATMENT PLANNING

How do you develop a treatment plan for someone who worries about everything? It can be initially overwhelming given the number of worries, and it can become clinically alluring to plan at the level of specific worry content. Based on the intake evaluation and ongoing functional assessments, treatment planning will include a roadmap for targeting areas of impairment based on the particular antecedent triggers, emotional and behavioral responses, and short- and longer-term consequences of the youth and family. To the extent that Jin's family is involved in his worry process and reinforcing his maladaptive coping, they must be included in the plan (see Tables 10.2 and 10.3).

Jin's pervasive and extensive worry and pattern of asking questions are impairing his own well-being and family functioning. Additional impairments may be emerging in his academic and social domains. The intervention process aims to provide Jin with the skills for identifying and coping with his worry, and defending against and slaying the worry zombies. Knowing the role of his family members in differentially reinforcing his worry process requires providing his mother and hopefully his grandfather with the skills for responding (or not) to his worry–distress–questions pattern. As is generally necessary in working with youth, the CB intervention process works from the *inside out*, working with the youth to develop skills, and from the *outside in*, to target the environmental elements that may be maintaining the anxious process.

(text resumes on page 274)

TABLE 10.2. Jin's Broad Treatment Plan for GAD

Treatment goals	Interventions
Decrease worry; have more fun.	Psychoeducation about GAD and worry, thought–action–mood tracking, progress monitoring
Increase coping with worry.	Identifying worries and cognitive distortions (worry zombies and traps); cognitive restructuring; mindfulness (practice keeping worry helpers); worry time; reward charts, problem solving; tolerating uncertainty; exposure
Decrease reassurance seeking.	Limit setting (questions, news scanning); reward chart; practice tolerating uncertainty; exposure
Improve caregiver coaching.	Coping coach strategies: empathize and encourage; catch the positive/specific labeled praise; reward chart; role-play limit setting; family communication practice
Improve sleep hygiene and regulate sleep cycle.	Worry coping/worry time; sleep hygiene; relaxation; mindfulness; reward charts

TABLE 10.3. Jin's Detailed Treatment Plan for Depression

Sessions 1–2

Assessment
- Assess presenting problems.
- Conduct diagnostic assessment with a focus on impairment (real-life functioning).
- Administer symptom profile measures (e.g., RCADS).
- Assess target problems and treatment goals, focusing on improving daily functioning.
- Assess caregiver/family–child interactions, including those with grandparents and sibling.
- Conduct collateral assessments as needed with the youth's school (e.g., counselor, teacher, school nurse); retrieve past psychological assessments (e.g., academic/learning assessments); request parents' complete release of information to speak to school contact(s).
- Evaluate co-occurring medical conditions; consult with pediatrician who referred Jin regarding headaches.
- Assess need for medication and psychiatric referral.

Psychoeducation
- Review assessment and generate target problems with youth and caregiver.
- Create idiographic target problems tracker.
- Collaborate on case conceptualization: CBT model and functional assessment with particular focus on role of reassurance-seeking behaviors.
- Provide caregiver and youth with information handouts on GAD and CBT.

Home practice
- Complete CBT model and functional assessment forms.

Sessions 3–4

Assessment
- Evaluate and discuss home practice.
- Complete target problems tracker.
- Direct youth and his mother to complete symptom tracker every fourth session (e.g., RCADS).

Interventions
- Implement in-session reward chart for home practice completion.
- Review and refine individual functional assessments.
- Practice identifying worry thoughts ("worry zombies"), feelings (e.g., tension, headaches), behaviors (e.g., avoidance, reassurance seeking), and cognitive distortions (e.g., thinking traps).
- Introduce cognitive restructuring (finding "worry helpers").
- Introduce mindfulness.

Home practice
- Complete thinking traps tracker.
- Complete coping thoughts tracker.
- Monitor reward program.

Sessions 5–6

Assessment
- As in Sessions 3–4

(continued)

TABLE 10.3. *(continued)*

Interventions
- Continue in-session reward chart for home practice completion.
- Continue to identify worries and thinking traps, and practice Socratic questioning and coping thoughts ("worry helpers").
- Practice mindfulness.
- Introduce and practice problem solving.
- Introduce "worry time."
- Instruct caregiver(s) (in separate sessions as needed) on psychoeducation review, coping coach skills, empathize and encourage, coach and approach, specific labeled praise and catch the positive, how to role-play limit setting on reassurance seeking.

Home practice
- Practice the development of coping thoughts with coping thoughts tracker.
- Track worry time.
- Practice mindfulness.
- Monitor reward plan.
- Ask parent to practice their coping coach skills.

Sessions 7–8

Assessment
- As in Sessions 3–4

Interventions
- Continue in-session reward chart for home practice completion.
- Continue coping thoughts and problem-solving practice.
- Continue mindfulness practice.
- Review worry time.
- Introduce formal in-office and at-home exposures.
- Introduce developmentally appropriate psychoeducation and sleep routine.
- Meet with caregiver(s) (in separate sessions as needed) to develop a home behavior plan and continue coping coach skills, empathize and encourage, coach and approach, specific labeled praise and catch the positive, role-play of limit setting on reassurance seeking.

Home practice
- Track worry time.
- Track at-home exposures.
- Monitor reward plans.

Sessions 9–10

Assessment
- As in Sessions 3–4

Interventions
- Continue in-session reward chart for home practice completion and in-office exposure efforts.
- Review at-home exposures.
- Review worry time.
- Conduct in-office worry-focused exposures.

(continued)

TABLE 10.3. *(continued)*

- Meet with caregiver(s) (in separate sessions as needed) to review and troubleshoot home behavior plan and continue coping coach skills, empathize and encourage, coach and approach, specific labeled praise and catch the positive.
- Follow up with collateral sources at school.
- Check in with referring physician.

Home practice
- Track worry time.
- Track at-home exposures.
- Monitor sleep routine and schedule.
- Monitor reward plans.

Sessions 11–12

Assessment
- As in Sessions 3–4

Interventions
- Continue in-session reward chart for home practice completion and in-office exposure efforts.
- Review at-home exposures.
- Continue in-office worry-focused exposures.
- Meet with caregiver(s) (in separate sessions as needed) to review and troubleshoot home behavior plan.
- Assess youth functioning across home/family, school/work, peer, and recreation domains.

Home practice
- Have youth refine steps of the exposure hierarchy.
- Complete at-home worry exposures.
- Monitor reward plans.

Sessions 13–14

Assessment
- As in Sessions 3–4

Interventions
- Continue in-session reward chart for home practice completion and in-office exposure efforts.
- Review at-home exposures.
- Continue in-office worry-focused exposures and practicing moderate to challenging exposures.
- Meet with caregiver(s) (in separate sessions as needed) to review and troubleshoot home behavior plan.
- Check in on sleep routine.
- Check in on caregiver/family interaction patterns during exposure phase.

Home practice
- Have youth continue practicing hierarchy challenges outside of session.
- Monitor use of coping skills and self-reward for successful attempts at challenges.
- Monitor reward plans.
- Sessions 15–16

Assessment
- As in Sessions 3–4

(continued)

TABLE 10.3. *(continued)*

Interventions
- Continue in-session reward chart for home practice completion and in-office exposure efforts.
- Continue practicing steps of exposure hierarchy, through exposures and behavioral challenges, focusing on the youth's core goals and any barriers.
- Discuss with Jin's mother the cultural and familial aspects of the death of Jin's father, the family's experience and expression of grief, their continued conversations around his death; plan for a family session with the patient.
- Hold family session(s) focused on a developmentally appropriate discussion of the father's death.

Home practice
- Have youth continue practicing hierarchy challenges outside of session.
- Monitor use of coping skills and self-reward for successful attempts at challenges.
- Monitor reward plans.

Sessions 16–20

Assessment
- As in Sessions 3–4

Interventions
- Continue in-session reward chart for home practice completion and in-office exposure efforts.
- Review at-home exposures and family discussion; review patient reactions.
- Practice challenging steps of exposure hierarchy, through exposures and behavioral challenges, focusing on the youth's core goals and any barriers.
- Review assessments and progress monitoring; introduce the option of tapering off sessions.

Home practice
- Have youth continue practicing hierarchy challenges outside of session.
- Monitor use of coping skills and self-reward for successful attempts at challenges.
- Monitor reward plans.

Sessions 21–25 (biweekly for maintenance)

Assessment
- As in Sessions 3–4

Psychoeducation
- Introduce relapse prevention phase.
- Review and discuss progress with youth and caregiver.
- Discuss termination.

Interventions
- Practice increasingly/difficult challenging steps of exposure hierarchy, through exposures and behavioral challenges, focusing on the youth's core goals and any barriers.

Home practice
- Have youth continue practicing hierarchy challenges outside of session.
- Monitor use of coping skills and self-reward for successful attempts at challenges.
- Monitor reward plan.

INTERVENTION COMPONENTS AND PROCESS

Psychoeducation

Psychoeducation is an essential aspect of treatment. Jin is a "worrier." He is also curious and a planner. Psychoeducation will include helping Jin and his family to recognize and retain the valued aspects of his curiosity and adaptive planning in differentiating the pathological aspects of his worry. Indeed, he demonstrates some insight by labeling his concerns as "worry zombies," but he is currently limited in how he copes with them. To the extent possible, it may be essential to engage Jin's grandparents to appreciate the grandfather's compassion ("He's just a sensitive child"), while also helping them understand how Jin's anxiety might be having a deleterious impact on his health and development. Psychoeducation teaches the CBT model for GAD, and the broad interplay among thoughts, feelings, and behaviors. Behaviors in this sense are not just what Jin does (asks questions) or does not do (go on field trips on stormy days), but also *how* these behaviors are reinforced and maintained. When discussing GAD or excessive worry with the youth or family, the therapist can provide Handouts 22, 23, and 24 to summarize this information (reproducible versions are available in Appendix A; see also Appendix B for a listing of additional reliable sources).

Like many anxious youth, Jin is not a squeaky wheel, but his excessive reassurance seeking is beginning to become disruptive. Throughout these chapters, we have reiterated that anxiety is *normal*; it's good for you. Worry can be a useful process. Concern and engagement around a problem are essential for problem solving and planning behaviors. Worry reflects the initial activation of anxiety that comes from a novel problem. As youth grow older, they advance in language and cognitive development, as well as increasing exposure to and awareness of potentially harmful elements in their immediate and broader environments (e.g., safety, failure, death). Some worry and curiosity are normative aspects of development, and most youth are able to effectively move beyond the worry process and engage in problem solving. For Jin and his family, it is important to highlight how he not only experiences his worry, but that it has become part of who he is—he *is* a worrier. His worry has taken over and is interfering with his ability to have fun, go to sleep, take trips, and have regular discourse with his mother. He is also worrying about issues that are not necessarily developmentally appropriate—being a "Little Man" is a role associated with his GAD. Importantly, psychoeducation should include: the likely influence of Jin's father's death on the family system in a global sense, Jin's perceived role as a worrier *about his family* members, and his family members' worry *about him* and his sensitivities. At this point in treatment, the specific impact of his father's death on his cognitive schema is unclear, but it is important to continue to work with the family to assess this factor.

A central aim of psychoeducation is to gather multiple examples to provide an understanding of the process of a triggered worry, usually about Jin's own or his family's health or well-being, some internal distress, and a sequence of reassurance-seeking behaviors, escape, or avoidance. Importantly, psychoeducation provides the opportunity to aid Jin in understanding how his worry is filled with perceptions about negative events happening. That is, he sees huge worry zombies everywhere; they are closer and more dangerous than they actually are, and he is on the lookout for worry zombies that have not even appeared yet. While worry can be natural, excessively worrying puts one at a disadvantage—worrying about everything is as useful as worrying about nothing.

Self-Talk and Cognitive Restructuring

As a worrier, the content of Jin's thoughts includes negative expectations about safety, health, academics, and the future. He has difficulty controlling anxious self-talk and the distress associated with it. Youth with GAD may get stuck in multiple thinking traps, for example: worry thoughts may focus on negative outcomes (looking for the negative) or anticipate future negative events (fortune-telling) or predict that something horrible may happen (catastrophizing) and they will be unable to handle it. These worries may become focused on consuming external reassurance for coping [what if (Tell me, Tell me)]. The worrier overestimates the bad outcome and its consequences and underestimates their ability to handle it.

As Jin completes the Thinking Traps Tracker worksheet (see Figure 10.5; a blank version is available as Worksheet 5 in Appendix A), he learns how to recognize his automatic negative thoughts, how they may be connected to his somatic experience, and then his pattern of getting stuck in particular thinking traps. Additionally, if Jin tracks these worries as they occur, he may be able to slow down the automatic nature of the worries triggering additional worries. Recall that generally what distinguishes GAD from non-GAD youth is the number, frequency, intensity, and controllability of worry. When teaching about the cognitions and the interplay of thoughts, feelings, and behaviors, the therapist can validate and normalize a given worry while teaching the youth to identify and attend to the distortions and strategies for cognitive restructuring (see Worksheet 5 and Handout 2 in Appendix A).

Jin's worry about the next school day's events often interferes with his ability to fall asleep. When he gets into bed, he begins worrying about the scheduled spelling test, which begins a cascade of worry and thinking traps. He experiences tension and nervousness in connection with his worries, which are, of course, not conducive to relaxation and sleep. His negative prediction "I won't remember all of [the spelling words]" is an example of negative *fortune-telling* and possibly *jumping to conclusions*. This worry then jumps to *what if* worries about not being able to fall asleep, which includes *jumping to conclusions* and *all-or-nothing thinking*. In Jin's worry cascade, this will result in his being the only person in the household who is awake and then failing the test, which for him is *catastrophic* thinking with worry zombies leading him to the *zombie apocalypse*. Given Jin's age, he may not be familiar with the terms "catastrophic" or "catastrophizing," so finding a reference he can understand aids in teaching him how to recognize this thinking trap (e.g., disaster, worst ever, zombie apocalypse). Another worry includes him becoming a *self-critic* as he thinks to himself, "I stink at sleeping." So many worries and thinking traps! In some youth with GAD who experience worries at bedtime, the worry can jump to worry about sleep itself, which may indeed ironically trigger the feared outcome (reduced sleep).

Initially, therapist and youth can work together to track worries, noticing and rating somatic experiences and automatic thoughts, and labeling associated thinking traps. Thus, for Jin, it makes sense that he is so tense and nervous when in bed given the nature and content of his thoughts. In the above example, Jin described that he got out of his bed 3 times to seek reassurance from his mother, which is one of his primary coping strategies. This resulted in a familiar pattern—his mother getting "mad at me."

Teaching GAD youth cognitive restructuring includes having them slow down and recognize their thinking traps and then become thought detectives and ask questions. For example:

"What are the chances you will forget all the words?"
"What usually happens during spelling tests?"
"How many spelling tests have you failed?"
"What's the worst that can happen if you forget one word or two words?"
"What's the worst that can happen if you fail the test? And what's the worst that can happen
  if that happens?"

WORKSHEET 5. Thinking Traps Tracker

What thinking traps do you fall into when feeling sad, anxious, or distressed? For each situation, describe and rate how you feel. Describe your automatic thought (the first thought that comes into your head). What thinking trap might you be falling into? How does that make you feel (the result)?

Trigger	Feeling (Rate 0–10: "not at all" to "excruciating")	Thought	Thinking Trap	Result?
Waiting for my sister to leave the house before school.	Stressed out, stomachache (7)	"I'm gonna miss the bus!" "I'm going to be late and the teacher will be mad." "I'll be sent to the principal." "I'll miss math period." "It will mess up my math grade."	Fortune-telling, catastrophizing, zombie apocalypse	Got cranky, yelled at her, felt guilty (10)
Heard about a school shooting on the news.	Really tense (8)	"Our school is next. I just know it." "My class is on the first floor so we will be shot first." "What if we are trapped?" "I stink at sleeping."	Catastrophizing, what if (Tell me, Tell me), zombie apocalypse, taking things too personally (The Self-Critic)	Started getting jittery, couldn't fall asleep, went looking for Mom at night (9)
Couldn't sleep because of spelling test.	Tense, nervous (8)	"I won't remember all of them." "What if I'm awake all night?" "What if I'm the only one in the house awake?" "I won't be able to concentrate for the test and I'll fail." "I'm going to be so sleepy tomorrow at school." "I stink at sleeping."	What if (Tell Me, Tell Me), fortune-telling, catastrophizing, zombie apocalypse, taking things too personally (The Self-Critic)	Got out of bed 3 times, went looking for Mom, she got mad at me the last time. Don't know what time I fell asleep (10)

FIGURE 10.5. Completed Thinking Traps Tracker worksheet for Jin.

"What can you do if you forget one word?"

"What happens if you can't fall asleep?"

"How many times have you stayed awake all night?"

"What's the worst that can happen if you stay awake all night?"

"Do you stink at all parts of sleeping?"

"Are you ever pretty good at sleeping?"

"Is it helpful to worry about failing or staying awake all night?"

"What are the worry zombies and what are the worry helpers here?"

As with being a good detective, the list of questions is endless. The goals are to help Jin channel his curiosity and challenge the automatic negative thoughts rather than accept them outright, recognize some of the thinking errors and the utility of some of the worries, and introduce some controllability. The goal is not to encourage positive thinking per se. After all, *if* he stays awake all night, he may indeed feel very tired and have difficulty concentrating in school the next day. Rather, it is the therapist's job to help Jin understand that his fatalistic assumptions hold him back more than the realistic picture. The therapist can start to help Jin identify personalized thinking traps and start labeling them, and then problem-solve so he will be able to recognize the worry helpers among the worry zombies and even convert the worry zombies into worry helpers. Here is how this looks:

THERAPIST: So, when was the last time you were awake all night?

JIN: I dunno. I don't remember it. Never really.

THERAPIST: OK, sounds like it's never happened that you were awake ALL night, but maybe it was harder for you to fall asleep when worry zombies about tests were attacking?

JIN: Yeah.

THERAPIST: This time it was spelling test zombies?

JIN: Yeah.

THERAPIST: OK, so let's say you did actually stay awake all night this time. What's the worst that can happen if you're awake all night?

JIN: I'll be super-sleepy at school tomorrow and mess up on my test.

THERAPIST: That's definitely happened to me when I've been super-sleepy coming to work sometimes. It's a stinky feeling. What does it feel like for you when you're super-sleepy?

JIN: I yawn a lot. And I have a headache sometimes.

THERAPIST: Oh man, that does stink. And what happens? And do you perform really badly on stuff at school?

JIN: Uh, no.

THERAPIST: So you haven't gotten a bad grade from being super-sleepy at school yet?

JIN: I don't think so.

THERAPIST: Let's say you did get a bad grade on your spelling test like the worry zombies are telling you? What kind of bad grade?

JIN: Like an 8 out of 10.

THERAPIST: And what happens if you get an 8.

JIN: It's a B, and it will mess up my whole grade.

THERAPIST: For the whole year?

JIN: Yeah.

THERAPIST: So one 8 will mess up the whole year? Can you tell what the worry zombies are trying to do here?

JIN: Zombie apocalypse?

THERAPIST: YES! As a zombie slayer, what can you say back?

JIN: Maybe an 8 won't mess up my WHOLE grade?

THERAPIST: Yes! Now back to being super-sleepy. Even if you're super-sleepy and you get an 8, it probably won't mess up your whole grade for the year. How can you challenge that worry zombie and make it a worry helper?

JIN: I'm going to try to sleep, but even if I don't sleep all night, it won't mess up my grade for the whole year.

The therapist continues to help Jin challenge the worry thoughts and recognize catastrophic thinking about the potential effects of not sleeping and not performing well on his test. Over time the therapist works with Jin to continue carrying his zombie apocalypse worries to their worst-case conclusions, asking for example: "What's the worst that can happen if you did get a lower grade in spelling for the year?" In this way, Jin learns to tolerate some uncertainty regarding the possibility of the feared outcome.

The therapist can also help Jin to recognize possible *positive* beliefs about his worry and associated worry-related behaviors. In helping Jin to track his worries and thinking traps and link them to his feelings, the therapist can also inquire about the meta-cognitive aspects of his worry. That is, what does Jin think about his worrying when he is worrying? It becomes clear that Jin believes it is important to worry in order to do well in school and to "make sure" his family is healthy and safe. The therapist can assist Jin in understanding that, in part, Jin continues to worry as much as he does *because he thinks it's good for him (and his family)*. A portion of the cognitive work can target these beliefs that may be reinforcing Jin's worry process. The idea is not to eliminate worry, but to disrupt its excessiveness. Here are two questions you can pose to him:

"How do you think worrying helps you?"
"What would happen if you didn't worry about grades (your family's health, safety, etc.)?"

Coping thoughts can target worry content as well as process and possible positive impressions about (excessive) worrying. The therapist helps Jin practice catching high levels of worry, labeling it, and then coping by disrupting the frequency, duration, and excessiveness of his assumptions (see Worksheet 16 and Handout 2; reproducible versions are available in Appendix A). For example:

"I know that just before bedtime is when I worry most, so I see you coming, worry zombies!"
"I changed that worry zombie about my test into a worry helper already. And I studied, so I don't have to worry anymore today!"

As the Thinking Traps Tracker worksheet reveals (see Figure 10.6; a blank version is available as Worksheet 16 in Appendix A), Jin's worry often results in his reassurance-seeking behaviors (e.g., looking for his mother). Part of the work here is to assist Jin in recognizing this pattern, and how he is trying to cope but is actually making the worry zombies stronger. This is a way of enlisting him in behavior change (and exposure, see below).

THERAPIST: The worry zombies get you so upset that you go to Mom at night and ask her some of the same questions over and over again.

JIN: Yeah, she tries to help me and then she gets annoyed.

THERAPIST: Yeah, she said that, too. Part of fighting the worry zombies is knowing that you <u>can</u> go to your mom BUT you don't *always* <u>have to</u> when you are feeling tense or stressed. We want to practice having you answer some of those worry zombies yourself because you can! I bet you can even say what your mom will tell you before she even says it.

JIN: Yeah. She says, "You'll be fine, Jin-Jin" or "Just try to sleep," but then if I come back, she gets mad.

THERAPIST: OK, so what if instead of going to Mom right away when you're worried at night, you waited and practiced some of your coping thoughts first?

Working with youth to slow down and utilize delay as a strategy may be effective on several interrelated levels. First, this strategy breaks the automaticity of worry triggers and immediate use of the usual maladaptive responding (going to Mom for reassurance). Second, and related, it creates the potential to practice new coping behaviors. Third, it creates the opportunity for habituation (perhaps the distress diminishes *without* going to Mom). Finally, it may allow for self-efficacy and mastery.

In the above example, the therapist is working with Jin to build his coping arsenal, disrupt the automaticity of reassurance seeking, and decrease attention to his worry process and escalations with his mother (see the functional assessment diagrammed in Figure 10.4). The therapist should prepare Jin's mother for this behavioral experiment when it comes time for exposures. The therapist can train his mother to give specific labeled praise for brave behaviors and develop a reward plan that reinforces him for increasing the amount of time he stays in his room at night and decreases his visits to her with worry-related questions. Another helpful strategy is to meet with the parent to develop a scripted response that mirrors the therapy work for when Jin comes to her with worry; the therapist and mother can role-play various scenarios. Jin's mother first can learn to empathize and encourage Jin to use his coping thoughts and skills, with later exposures removing much of her responding (see Chapter 5 for more examples).

Problem Solving and Mindfulness

As Jin completes various trackers, he and his caregivers learn that when faced with a "problem" that triggers stress, worry or anxiety, he "solves" it with excessive worrying, reassurance seeking, and in some cases, avoidance. While these efforts in coping may bring short-term relief via negative reinforcement, they also reinforce the worry process and often this results in additional distress. The therapist can engage Jin in evaluating the pros and cons of this approach. See Chapter 2 for examples of engaging traditional problem solving when the youth is anxious.

WORKSHEET 16. Coping Thoughts Tracker

Brainstorm coping thoughts that could respond to your thinking trap! Try and come up with coping statements that are more realistic and ask, "How am I not seeing the whole picture?"

Trigger	Thought	Thinking Trap	Coping Thought	Result?
Worry about spelling test before bedtime.	"I'm going to forget some words and totally blow it."	Fortune-telling, all-or-nothing thinking, zombie apocalypse	"I studied." "I never totally blew it before." "Worry zombies are trying to get me to freak out. I'm not going to let them!"	Felt calmer; stopped myself from leaving my room to ask Mom.
Teacher talked about climate change.	"There are going to be all of these horrible storms." "What if it happens tomorrow?" "The Earth is going to disappear."	Fortune-telling, zombie apocalypse	"Climate change is bad but it doesn't mean there is going to be a bad storm tomorrow." "I don't have to check the weather to feel better." "My worry helper will be to ask the teacher how I can help."	Felt good that I had a plan; really wanted to ask about the weather and if there would be a storm tomorrow but didn't.
Mom sounded sick.	"She's sick. What if she forgot to take her vitamin? What if she misses work?" "What if she dies?"	Zombie apocalypse	"Just because she gets sick doesn't mean she will die." "Mom is really good about taking care of herself. I don't need to remind her."	Felt less stressed; didn't ask her if she took her vitamin; Mom told me she was proud of me and we laughed.

FIGURE 10.6. Completed Coping Thoughts Tracker worksheet for Jin.

Another approach to addressing the frequent intrusive thoughts that worriers experience is to teach youth how to relate to their thoughts differently through mindfulness training. As noted in Chapter 2, mindfulness can serve as a complementary skill to cognitive restructuring and a strategy for helping Jin gain distance from his extensive worries. The goal is to teach Jin to recognize that his worries are thoughts, and just that, thoughts. He does not necessarily need to act (e.g., via reassurance seeking, checking the weather); rather, he can learn to simply observe and watch his thoughts. The therapist can teach mindfulness training to help with this point (for more information, see Chapter 2 and Handout 3 that offers a sample mindfulness script; a reproducible version of the latter is available in Appendix A). This skill may be particularly useful for Jin given his propensity for visual and imaginative thought, and can be adapted for the therapy language used already and for his younger age. For example, the therapist can work with Jin to imagine each "worry zombie" on a raft floating downstream or the "worry zombie" spinning on a merry-go-round. In this way, he can also learn to observe the worry and *tolerate* the associated distress while breaking a cycle of maladaptive coping.

Teaching mindfulness to younger worriers in this way may also afford the opportunity to introduce *humor* as a possible coping strategy. Observing worry zombies circling on a merry-go-round or watching as worry zombies float by on a raft or "fun pool noodle" without "fighting" them can take away some of their "power" and prove to be fun and funny.

Exposures

The very nature of GAD and its multiple domains may make the process of developing fear and avoidance hierarchies daunting. Some clinicians have discussed struggling to conceptualize and then operationalize exposures for worry and its anticipated outcomes (e.g., how do we create exposures targeting fear of getting an illness, death, not getting into college?). Worries are grounded in a semblance of reality and reflect scenarios with uncertain outcomes that may not come to fruition for many years. How does one "disprove" a worry for which the outcomes are unknown (e.g., developing cancer, getting into college)? As such, functional assessments of a youth's worry are central to exposure planning and design in GAD. "What is the function of the worry and associated beliefs about worry?" "What are the associated behaviors negatively reinforcing worry?" "What impact on developmental functioning can we observe right now?" Worry hierarchies can be constructed broadly or by domain of worry: academic, social, interpersonal, safety, family, health, community and world issues. For example, referring back to Jin's comprehensive assessment, he experiences significant worries about school performance and getting into college, his own and his family's health, safety in several situations including severe weather. He engages in several worry-related behaviors that reinforce and maintain his worrying and discomfort; importantly, his family members participate in many of these accommodating behaviors as well. The therapist will work with the family to recognize these, explain the rationale for exposures (see Chapter 2 for background and examples), and develop worry hierarchies that lay the groundwork for the exposure phase of treatment. The following are challenge hierarchies for three of Jin's worry domains:

Hierarchy Challenge A: Worrying about School

1. Raise my hand when I am 100% sure of the answer.
2. Raise my hand when I am less than 100% sure of the answer.

3. Plan to arrive at school 5 minutes late.
4. Ask teacher only one question about homework assignment.
5. Ask Mom only one question about homework assignment.
6. Ask teacher zero questions today about homework assignment.
7. Ask Mom zero questions today about homework assignment.
8. Get an answer wrong on the spelling test purposely.
9. Have 15 minutes of zombie apocalypse worry time (e.g., on failing all grades, not getting into college) with no worry behaviors (e.g., no checking of the online grade portal, asking reassurance-seeking questions of Mom or teacher).

Hierarchy Challenge B: Worrying about Illness/Safety

1. Check the weather forecast only 1 time per day.
2. Check the weather forecast 0 times per day.
3. Delay 1 hour before asking Mom or Grandpa weather-related questions.
4. Delay 2 hours before asking Mom or Grandpa weather-related questions.
5. Ask Mom or Grandpa 0 questions about the weather forecast.
6. Go on school field trip without checking the weather the day before the trip.
7. Look up weather reports from stormy areas (e.g., Caribbean during hurricane season) but do not check the weather forecast in your own area.
8. Look at pictures of sharks.
9. Talk about going in the ocean on the next family beach day.
10. Go to the beach and stand at the edge of the water for 20 minutes.
11. Go to the beach and stand and play in the surf for 20 minutes.
12. Talk about contracting measles.
13. Carry a laminated photo of what the measles looks like.
14. Have 15 minutes of zombie apocalypse worry time (e.g., on contracting measles, Zika virus) without engaging in the usual worry behaviors (e.g., not searching medical websites).

Hierarchy Challenge C: Worrying about Mother's Health

1. Delay 1 hour before asking Mom if she took her vitamins.
2. Delay 1 hour before asking Mom if she scheduled her doctor's appointment.
3. Delay 2 hours before asking Mom if she took her vitamins.
4. Delay 2 hours before asking Mom if she scheduled her doctor's appointment.
5. Have Mom respond only 1 time to my reassurance-seeking question.
6. Have Mom not respond to my reassurance-seeking question.
7. Ask Mom 0 questions about taking her vitamins.
8. Ask Mom 0 questions about getting her doctor's appointment.
9. Read websites on chronic illnesses without asking Mom about her health.
10. Discuss father's death.
11. Have 15 minutes of zombie apocalypse worry time (e.g., on Mom lying sick in bed) without engaging in the usual worry behaviors (e.g., not asking Mom how she is feeling, looking online for cancer information).

As can be seen in these sample hierarchies, the exposures target the range of Jin's worries and involve a combination of strategies that include: systematic delay and extinction of reassurance-seeking behaviors (i.e., across people and websites); associated reduction in accommodation behaviors by family members; imaginal exposures to feared situations and outcomes; increased flexibility in ambiguous and unplanned situations; and worry time without compensatory worry behaviors. Some of these exposures can be conducted in the therapist's office, and some are best planned for home or school. Some of these exposures can be designed for daily practice (e.g., zombie apocalypse worry time), some are lower frequency, naturally occurring events (e.g., school field trips), and some require additional family coordination (e.g., a family beach trip).

Given the significant amount of time Jin spends worrying about health topics generally, his mother's health specifically, and the crucial role of reassurance seeking, the treatment plan will include Jin's mother in exposures. These types of exposures can serve to disrupt the usual pattern of responding between Jin and his mother that has come to reinforce his worry about her. In the exposure to his worry thoughts about his mother's health, the therapist can have Jin identify his specific automatic thoughts and anticipated outcomes, his beliefs about the utility and effectiveness of his worry in keeping her healthy, and ultimately resist the "checking" behaviors of asking her about her health and health-related behaviors. Importantly, Jin can focus on continuing to engage in his present task (e.g., doing homework, watching TV, going to bed) while tolerating the distress of not asking his mother if she remembered to take her medicine or if she ate a healthy lunch while at work. When done in session, the therapist can serve as a coping coach to help the youth bear the distress (including using coping statements). When done at home, the caregiver is assigned that role.

For these exposures, the therapist will also want to work with Jin's mother to develop a new script for responding (or not) to Jin. Jin's mother can learn to empathize with and encourage him while also not giving in to the worry zombies (she can say something like "I appreciate your caring about me but I can take care of my own health"). Often, the therapist will want to work with parents to assess their own automatic thoughts regarding not responding to reassurance-seeking questioning by their anxious child. Also, since many of these exposures will—by default—be practiced at home, therapists might want to practice these via role play in session with the child and their parent(s).

Worry Time

Worry time is an assigned discrete amount of time that a youth can use for the express purpose of worrying. Assigning worry time can have both paradoxical and functional effects. One of the negatively reinforcing functions of excessive worry is that it gives the youth the illusion that they are working on the problem. Excessive worry about the future or situations out of our control is not constructive, and if the "problem" never gets solved, the youth continues to worry about the problem. Ceasing the worry would be tantamount to giving up on the problem. By assigning a designated worry time, the therapist is giving permission to the youth to put the problem aside and to come back to it at worry time. During that time, the youth is allowed to worry all they want! Paradoxically, most youth either forget about worry time or forget the specific worries they had, because they were either forgotten or resolved themselves. But promising a later worry time enables the youth to move on from the earlier stuck moment without becoming entrenched.

Worry time can play a functional role by encouraging skill building. By creating a daily intentional period for worry, for example, 15 to 20 minutes, youth can approach their worry with some agency (e.g., "I will worry about getting into college during my worry time"). At worry time, they promise to eliminate seeking reassurance or distracting themselves from the discomfort when it arises (i.e., "I'm not avoiding future-oriented worry about getting into college. I'm going to do it on purpose"). With worry time, youth (and depending on their age, their parents) are instructed to select a time each day to worry on purpose about all of their worries. During these 15 minutes, youth are encouraged to identify and express every one of their anxious automatic thoughts, what ifs, and negative predictions. They can say their worries aloud or write them down on a blank sheet of paper or designated journal. In this way, therapists are able to prescribe the symptom with an understanding of the *function* of the worry. When utilized as an exposure, worry time also functions to trigger the cognitive and physiological aspects of worry, while creating opportunities to resist accommodation behaviors and tolerate associated worry distress.

For Jin and his mother, daily worry time as exposure for the "zombie apocalypse" worries allows for the calling up of catastrophic, worst-case worries so that he may practice watching the worry zombies float by. He also practices tolerating the discomfort without engaging in reassurance-seeking behaviors. When Jin tracks his worries, the therapist notes the leap from his automatic thought to catastrophic thinking trap. His worry zombies regarding his mother taking her vitamins become a catastrophic zombie apocalypse belief that if his mother does not take her vitamins, she will get very sick and die.

As is evident throughout this book, where there is avoidance in a system in which anxiety exists, there is likely a target for intervention (i.e., approach and exposures). Although not explicitly stated, understanding Jin's worry about his mother's health may connect to his father's death when he was younger. Because of his family's worry about Jin as a sensitive child and worrier, they avoided discussing his father's death with him. While it might have been developmentally appropriate to withhold certain details, the family system appeared to overprotect Jin as well. When carrying forward his worry through Socratic questioning, Jin's worry about his mother becoming ill was connected to concern for her, as well as fear of catastrophic outcomes connected to illness as they were with his father (i.e., death). As a result of the ongoing secrecy and avoidance surrounding the illness and death of Jin's father, the therapist worked with both Jin and his mother to add this to the worry hierarchy because it was clear he was thinking about the topic anyway. This illustrates an important point in working with youth and families generally: often parents worry about discussing a certain issue, while youth may already be thinking and worrying about that very topic. As in this case with Jin, the therapist can work with his mother and grandparents to have an age-appropriate discussion with him about what happened to his father and answer questions about his illness and death.

As Jin progresses through these exposures and decreases reassurance-seeking behaviors, the therapist works with him on developing a set of self-praise statements when he delays or altogether resists asking his mother a reassurance-related question (see Figure 10.7; a blank version is available as Worksheet 6 in Appendix A). For example:

THERAPIST: So, it looks like at school you again heard about people not getting the measles vaccine and you felt really worried about Mom?

JIN: Yeah.

THERAPIST: And what were the worry zombies trying to get you to do?

JIN: Ask her if she got her shot for it.

WORKSHEET 6. *In Vivo* Exposure/Behavioral Experiment

Complete this worksheet with the youth as you are preparing for a behavioral experiment.

1. Situation (What's the situation?):

At school, people are talking about the measles, and I wanted to ask Mom if she got her shot.

2. Feelings: **Distress Rating:** ___80___

Worried, scared, tense

3. Anxious/Negative Thoughts:	**Thinking Traps (See list below.)**
"Measles are gross." "Maybe Mom will get measles." "I never heard her talk about getting a measles shot." "What if she gets the measles?" "She probably didn't get her shot." "Do people die from the measles?"	Jumping to conclusions, catastrophizing, zombie apocalypse

Thinking Traps: mind reading, fortune-telling, catastrophizing, jumping to conclusions, what if's, discounting the positives, looking for the negatives, overgeneralizing, all-or-nothing thinking, should statements, taking things too personally, blaming.

4. Coping Thoughts (How do you respond to your anxious thoughts?):

"The worry zombies are at it again."
"I don't have to ask Mom if she got her measles shot."

Challenge Questions: Do I know for certain that _____? Am I 100% sure that _____? What evidence do I have that _____? What is the worst that could happen? How bad is that? Do I have a crystal ball?

5. Achievable Behavioral Goals (What do you want to accomplish?):

Goal	Accomplished?
a. Don't ask Mom even though I really really wanted to.	Yes
b. Watch the worry zombie float down the river.	Yes
c.	

6. Rewards:

Reward	Earned?
a. I told myself, "Good job, you did better than the worry zombies."	
b.	
c.	

FIGURE 10.7. Exposure worksheet addressing health worries.

THERAPIST: It looks like it made you pretty uncomfortable?

JIN: Yeah. Measles looks gross, and I didn't want her to get it.

THERAPIST: Just that they're gross? Or, that you didn't want her to die from it.

JIN: Yeah, that she'd die, I guess.

THERAPIST: That's scary to worry about your Mom getting sick from the measles and dying! It makes sense that you'd be pretty uncomfortable at an 80 [distress rating] if you were having those worries, right?

JIN: Yeah.

THERAPIST: And for the thinking traps, that seems like jumping to conclusions and catastrophizing and zombie apocalypse to me, too! Now it's true that measles are gross and people do get sick and die from it, and it looks like you were able to recognize your worries and challenge them and watch them float away WITHOUT having to ask your Mom for reassurance! Way to go!

JIN: Thanks. I did it. I guess.

THERAPIST: No guessing! You did it. You were able to tolerate your worry and handle it without asking Mom questions that we know feeds the worry zombies! And I really like how you told yourself that you did a good job. That's important when we do brave things like standing up to the worry zombies. Are you prepared if they come back?

JIN: I think so.

THERAPIST: Because they might STILL want you to ask your Mom about the measles.

JIN: Probably.

THERAPIST: What can you do if you have measles worry again?

JIN: Tell myself I don't have to ask Mom. She can take care of herself.

THERAPIST: Yes! And what else?

JIN: Watch the worry zombie thought float away again?

THERAPIST: Yep! On a fun pool noodle? Or, a kayak?

JIN: (*laughs*) Fun pool noodle.

THERAPIST: Solid choice. I'm so proud of you for using your skills, doing this exposure homework, and standing up to the worry zombies!

The therapist also can capitalize on themes that arise from the home practice exposures to create exposures that allow the youth to experience the anxiety associated with their worry in session and to use their skills. Though Jin's worry is triggered by the measles in this instance, he broadly worries about illness befalling himself or his family; like other youth with GAD, this particular worry is reflective of zeitgeist news coverage. To expand his exposure hierarchy and stay with the measles theme, for example, the therapist and Jin can collaboratively agree to exposures that include having a discussion about the measles, imagining his mother getting the measles, looking at microscopic images of the measles or Ebola virus, and even printing a picture of the Ebola virus to carry around with him every day. Who doesn't love carrying around a laminated picture of a virus? These last examples are creative ways for therapists and youth to intentionally call up worry topics and have youth tolerate the distress provoked, habituate, and break the pattern of reinforcing behaviors. As discussed, exposures are rooted in the functional assessment of a youth's patterns of worry combined with problem solving and creativity in targeting those patterns.

IDENTIFYING PARENT–CHILD INTERACTION PATTERNS

The nature of Jin's worries as well as his age will require significant involvement from Jin's mother, and if willing, his grandparents. Jin's worry includes multiple interactions with his mother and family members, and many of these patterns serve to reinforce his worries and worry behaviors. As above, the therapist will work with the youth to teach skills to cope with worry, tolerate distress, and resist reassurance seeking; also, the therapist will want to be sure to work with the caregivers by providing psychoeducation, helping them to identify their own anxious thoughts and then coping self-talk, and practice scripts for how to empathize and encourage youth to practice their coping skills when they become anxious.

For Jin's exposures, his mother will need to become more involved to better understand how to respond (and not respond) when he comes to her repeatedly for reassurance. In collaborating with Jin on devising the exposure hierarchies, his family opts to vary his reassurance seeking in terms of delaying his asking as well as how many times his mother will respond. This means that his mother will need to be included in the planning of these exposure practices at home, and in-session exposures will need to include Jin's mother at various points. See Chapter 5 for further examples of assessing parent–child interaction patterns.

Empathize and Encourage: Coach and Approach

Youth anxieties and worries can be overwhelming. Therefore, therapists will want to model empathizing with the parents' distress, anxiety, frustration, and even annoyance. Having a child repeat the same question over and over again can indeed be annoying. Parents may be tired and have their own worries. Not responding to your anxious child's questions may seem counterintuitive. Working with parents requires they understand the functional assessment exercises and therefore the rationale for exposures. It may be more straightforward for caregivers to understand how avoiding a school trip or a family day at the beach may reinforce worry and anxiety. Understanding functionally how answering reassurance-seeking questions or checking behaviors reinforces worry may be trickier for some caregivers. The therapist can share Handout 11, previously described in Chapter 5. and use Worksheet 9 (both available as reproducible forms in Appendix A) to help Jin's mother understand where she might be falling into common parent traps (Figure 10.8). Consider the following exchange and where Jin's mother could use guidance in identifying how she could respond more helpfully:

JIN'S MOTHER: I'm supposed to ignore him when he asks me a question?

THERAPIST: Not quite. First you want to empathize with his worry and how he is feeling. For example, "I know you really care about me and that you worry about my health." Or, "It looks like the worry zombies are really making you worry about the weather right now." And then you would encourage him to use a skill.

WORKSHEET 9. Parent–Child Chain Analysis

Conduct your own analysis of challenging interactions. Can you identify any parenting traps? What alternatives could you try?

	Action/Response	Parenting Trap	Potential Solution or Skills to Use?
Prompting Event:	Jin is worried about my health as his mom.		
Child Action:	Jin asks me if I've gotten the flu shot.		
Parent Response:	I try to ignore him; tell him "I'm not answering you anymore."	Unplanned ignoring; Aggressive–Coercive	Empathize and encourage; show I understand.
Child Reaction:	He kept following me, crying, telling me to answer him.		
Parent Response:	I tell him I've gotten all my shots, and he doesn't have to worry.	Accommodation	Empathize and encourage; prompt mindfulness.
Conflict/Problem Behavior:	He settles down and goes away.		
Outcome 1 (What happened)?	He was fine for a while.		
Outcome 2:	He came back later and asked the same question again and again.		
Outcome 3:			

FIGURE 10.8. Chain analysis of caregiver–child interactions in Jin's case.

JIN'S MOTHER: Which skill?

THERAPIST: You can remind him to label the worry zombie or the thinking trap. Or, remind him that he can use his distress tolerance skill of watching the worry float away. Remind him to use one of his worry helper coping thoughts, or that he and the whole family are practicing what happens when he does not ask a worry question over and over again.

JIN'S MOTHER: What if he keeps asking?

THERAPIST: The goal is for you to coach Jin through these worry periods without necessarily giving him "the answer" or "certainty." First validate and then model problem solving and approach behaviors.

To get Jin's buy-in, early exposures may focus on his mother practicing to delay reassurance-seeking questioning and to limit rather than eliminate responding. The goal is for both the youth and parent to be able to recognize the pattern of anxiety and accommodating and begin to introduce new skills and responding, while learning to tolerate the distress that will be provoked. It may be helpful for the therapist and parent to role-play different scripts for different scenarios. See Chapter 5 for more examples of empathize and encourage for youth with anxiety and depression.

At times, parents in a family may differentially respond to a youth's worries. It will be important for the therapist to assess this over the course of treatment. In Jin's case, Jin's grandfather appears to be a central figure to include. Generally, and with cultural humility, the therapist will also want to be sensitive to his beliefs about Jin. The therapist can also provide education on how overidentifying or accommodating Jin's avoidance may be maintaining Jin's anxieties. The therapist and grandfather can discuss alternative ways to respond, and one goal might be for Jin to teach his grandfather the coping skills he is learning in treatment and to have his grandfather participate in-session and at-home exposures. Furthermore, given the functional role of Jin's grandfather, it may be especially helpful for the therapist and grandfather to collaboratively brainstorm activities other than news watching that they can share.

Reward Charts and Contingency Management

The therapist and Jin agreed on an in-session reward chart that focused on home practice completion of the various worksheets over the different phases of treatment. Initially, Jin's mother expressed doubts that she would be able to maintain an at-home chart, so only an in-session chart was developed for the initial phase. However, the therapist emphasized and modeled specific labeled praise for her and assigned home practice for her to monitor her own automatic thoughts and reactions when Jin approached her with reassurance-seeking questioning. Although starting with a chart at home may have been ideal, the therapist did not wish to risk inconsistent implementation if a plan was pushed through. The therapist prioritized the in-session chart during the early phase and mother's straightforward home practice in service of functional assessment.

Later in treatment, the therapist and mother agreed on a simple reward chart connected to home exposure practice (see Figure 10.9; a blank version is available as Worksheet 14 in Appendix A). Also see Chapter 5 for more reward system examples. Jin was able to earn points for specific at-home exposures from the agreed-upon fear and avoidance hierarchy (see earlier). Jin's mother was also coached to use "bonus points" paired with specific labeled praise and "catch the positive" whenever she caught Jin being brave and using skills in naturally occurring situations (e.g., "I

WORKSHEET 14. Goals and Rewards Chart

Whenever we're trying new skills, we should reward ourselves for making the effort. First, brainstorm achievable, meaningful goals. Then, pick how you would reward yourself for each accomplishment.

Goals I Can Match Myself	Reward	M	T	W	TR	F	Sat	Sun	# of Days Achieved
Asking teacher only one question about homework	Get ice cream at Penguin's ice cream if I do this 4 times/wk.	Y	Y	Y	Y	N	—	—	4
Checking weather only 1 time a day	Get to watch anime show every day I do this.	N	N	Y	N	Y	N	Y	3

Goals My Parents Can Reward Me For	Reward	M	T	W	TR	F	Sat	Sun	# of Days Achieved
Don't ask Mom about vitamins.	Comic book if I do this 3 times a week	Y	N	Y	N	Y	N	—	3

FIGURE 10.9. Goals and rewards chart for Jin.

noticed you didn't ask me if I took my vitamins today. I'm so proud of you for that, so I'm going to give you a bonus point on your chart!"). Jin could then exchange his points for small prizes (e.g., comic books, going for ice cream).

The reward chart should be selected carefully and in discussion with caregivers. The reward targets need to be potent and meaningful to the youth; however, the therapist will want to be careful to not select items that might inadvertently (or advertently!) reinforce anxiety. For example, Jin wanted to "save up my points for a weather station." Of course, this is not to say that he can never own a weather station; however, given his current worry behaviors associated with checking the weather out of fear for safety, this was not deemed a suitable reward during the treatment phase.

Collaborating with the School and Other Providers

Like other youth, Jin may not present with in-school behavioral challenges or be bothersome to his teachers, and his worries may be connected to his fairly solid level of academic functioning. As such, it may be easy to overlook collaboration with the school for these youth. Again, the decision to collaborate with a school or designated school personnel should be based on a functional assessment of the youth's anxiety. For Jin, he had received some feedback from teachers that he could and should participate more. Given his worries about getting an answer wrong and wanting to be "100% sure" of an answer, he is not an academic risk-taker and he asks his teacher several reassurance-related questions. Therefore, it may be prudent for the therapist to engage his teacher to: (1) provide psychoeducation on the treatment model and the nature of his extensive worrying and associated behaviors, (2) discuss strategies for positively reinforcing his hand-raising and risk-taking behaviors, (3) limit answers to his separate reassurance seeking and identify a viable script if needed, and (4) address opportunities for the teacher's involvement in school exposures as appropriate. For instance, "On Tuesday, his target is to raise his hand during reading without being 100% sure he knows all of the words in the passage to be read." In this example, the teacher can work with the therapist to devise the exposure and be prepared to encourage, coach, and, it is hoped, positively reinforce Jin's effort to raise his hand (see Chapter 11 for additional examples of school collaboration.).

In addition to the school, it is helpful for the therapist to collaborate with Jin's pediatrician over the course of treatment and provide updates on his progress. Since she made the initial referral and it was connected to Jin's physiological experiences of tension and headaches, monitoring these over the course of treatment will also be key.

Progress Monitoring

Jin's mother noted a spike in his worry-related behaviors when she first started limiting her responses to his reassurance-seeking questions and utilizing the empathize and encourage script; fortunately, the therapist had informed her of this possibility in advance during the early phase of psychoeducation. However, after some practice, she observed a decrease in these behaviors, especially at nighttime and an increase in his use of coping strategies. The home practice tracking evidenced improvements in his sleep routine, as did earlier bedtimes (one of his mother's main goals for him).

Jin and his mother "gamified" his reward chart, and it started with her careful tracking of the number of questions asked at bedtime. Starting at 21 questions per night, she challenged (and rewarded) Jin both for decreasing the number of repeated questions each night AND for utilizing coping statements (e.g., especially about "blasting worry zombies") and worry time. Jin even started to include his grandfather in his worry time practice. Over the course of a few weeks, his reassurance-seeking questions decreased to three to four per night. His mother reported tracking her own frustration and decreases in her yelling behaviors in the evening.

A brief glance at Jin's item responses on the RCADS at Week 12 revealed that he now rated several items as "sometimes" (1) or "often" (2), rather than always. Although he still met criteria for clinical levels of GAD according to his and his mother's report, this indicates measurable progress (see Table 10.4), including lower scores across other anxiety- and depression-related domains.

Jin also demonstrated an improved ability to tolerate uncertainty regarding future negative events. He also denied having any headaches for several months.

TERMINATION AND RELAPSE PREVENTION

Jin continued to worry across a multitude of topics; however, he demonstrated acquisition of cognitive coping skills, especially "playing detective" toward his thoughts, catching the zombie apocalypse (catastrophizing), and mindfully watching his worry thoughts float away (usually on a fun pool noodle). As noted, the frequency of his worrying decreased.

Jin practiced daily worry time that effectively contained and redirected his worry from other times of the day, and he delayed and caught much of his reassurance-seeking questions and checking behaviors. His mother also praised and reinforced him more for his coping than his worrying, which resulted in significant decreases in family conflicts. As a result, the therapist and family began discussing tapering sessions to biweekly as part of a termination plan with ongoing exposures and relapse prevention. The latter included identifying potential antecedents to spikes in worry and planning ahead for skill use. Antecedents included any family health issues, large weather events over the upcoming seasons (e.g., superstorms, heatwaves, blizzards), and standardized state tests later in the school year. The therapist and Jin developed a list of his "worry helpers"

TABLE 10.4. Jin's Symptom Profile at Week 12 Using the RCADS

	Mother		Youth	
	Raw scores	T scores	Raw scores	T scores
Separation anxiety	7	78**	5	60
Generalized anxiety	10	73**	12	67*
Panic disorder	3	53	4	51
Social anxiety	14	63	13	53
Obsessions/compulsions	6	61	5	51
Depression	8	58	6	46
Total anxiety	40	70*	39	57
Total anxiety and depression	48	69*	45	55

*T scores higher than 65 indicate borderline clinical threshold. **Scores of 70 or higher indicate scores above clinical threshold. T scores are normalized based on youth's age and gender.

that could always be called on to "blast the worry zombies." Relapse prevention for this family also included addressing the timeline and parameters for Jin's earning a cell phone and monitoring use of the phone's potential for excessive reassurance seeking (e.g., texting Mom questions) and checking behaviors (e.g., weather apps).

Prognosis and Follow–Up

Jin's young age and pervasiveness of worry presented a challenge for the therapist to creatively introduce cognitive coping skills and behavioral skills practice. Jin's mother also acknowledged at times "giving in," especially and understandably when she was fatigued. That said, Jin demonstrated creative skill use, increasing humor and confidence, as did his mother, which are prognostically encouraging. His anxious temperament and sensitivities, level of worry, and beliefs about the function of worry will require that he and his family continue to practice skill use.

Challenges in This Case

Jin's case was selected for its challenges. He is a young worrier in a multigenerational household with a single parent whose partner died several years ago and who is exhausted much of the time and doing her best. The extensive levels of Jin's worries can feel overwhelming to a therapist. There are also cultural values and prior family-based communication decisions regarding Jin's father's death (e.g., with respect to grief, expressiveness around death) that the therapist will want to navigate with the family in future sessions as they progress through treatment to assist Jin with healthier coping of his worries. These family-based discussions may serve as exposures for addressing previously avoided anxiety-provoking topics as well as opportunities to provide psychoeducation to normalize grief and honor cultural traditions. It became apparent that multiple members of the family held positive attributes to worry, considering it essential for good performance and connected family care. The therapist made sure to assess for these beliefs about worry in all family members, provide education, and involve others in exposures as needed. Since Jin is fairly young, some degree of asking questions out of curiosity is natural and normative. A key target for limiting reassurance seeking is to learn to distinguish which questions to answer because they are necessary for providing corrective information and those that have been asked and answered previously. Relatedly, therapists must account for a given youth's cognitive development level more than a specific age.

SUMMARY AND KEY POINTS

Worry is often confused for constructive problem solving, but in the context of GAD, worry is nonproductive, excessive, and uncontrollable. With a solid CBT conceptualization that incorporates key family members, cultural values, and history, problematic behaviors and functional impairments associated with worry can be ameliorated. Also:

- A youth's positive beliefs about worry and its function (e.g., "It helps me prepare for tests") can be a barrier to constructive thinking.
- Cognitive distortions for youth with GAD may include negative future-oriented, all-or-

nothing, and catastrophic thinking that can be targeted with cognitive coping skills, mindfulness, therapist modeling use of Socratic questioning, and joining with the youth in collaborative empiricism.

- The therapist should target somatic symptoms associated with worry.
- Worry time can be utilized to delay and disrupt worry immediacy and to practice coping skills.
- Caregivers likely need to practice scripts for limited responding to, and setting limits on, reassurance-seeking behaviors.
- When designing exposures for worries, the therapist can target feared outcomes or exposure to stimuli that trigger worry. If concrete fears are testable, those can serve as a valuable target. If fears are untestable or ambiguous (e.g., "I will never get into college"), the therapist develops exposures designed to trigger those fears and help the youth tolerate the uncertainty of outcomes.

CHAPTER 11

School Refusal
and Problematic Attendance

School absence has become an increasing problem, such that 14% of middle schoolers and 21% of high schoolers are missing 10% or more of school days a year in America (U.S. Department of Education, 2019). Problematic absenteeism occurs for multiple reasons (Heyne, Gren-Landell, Melvin, & Gentle-Genitty, 2019). It can occur because parents withdraw a student from school to meet some need at home (e.g., to provide child care, to earn income). It can occur because of student behavioral problems that lead the school to exclude the child from attending (e.g., disciplinary action, at-home suspensions). And it can occur because the child elects to skip or leave school to pursue more desired activities (i.e., truancy). School refusal (SR) is the type of attendance problem that is most associated with anxiety and depression in youth (Heyne et al., 2019; Kearney, 2008). SR is characterized by (1) poor attendance and/or disruption to the school day, (2) significant distress associated with entry to, or remaining in, school, and (3) parent awareness of the youth's absenteeism (Berg, 2002). The youth does not demonstrate notable conduct problems other than poor attendance, and the caregivers will have made a good faith effort to try and return the student to school (Heyne et al., 2019).

School-refusing youth will often show mood and behavioral disruption throughout the day; having difficulty waking from bed; participating in the morning routine; getting to the bus, train, or car to drive to school; making their way into the school building; and staying in class throughout the day. School-refusing youth can be seen making repeated requests to go to the counselor's or nurse's office or making requests for the caregiver to pick them up from school. After-school activities may bring a short reprieve, but homework often results in frustrations and bedtime conjures dread at the thought of a new day. The youth has restless sleep that contributes to increasing fatigue, leading to increased difficulty waking in the morning, and starting the cycle again. As a result, SR leads to a significant number of partial or whole-day absences, tardiness, missed class time (e.g., nurse or counselor visits), and other disruptions to the youth's routine that affect attendance (e.g., morning tantrums, sleep difficulties, somatic complaints). Caregivers may have initially done battle with the student each morning to cajole, push, or incentivize the student to go to school. Increasing tension, conflict, and resistance typically lead to increasing concessions and accommodation by the caregivers, including their own tardiness or reduced hours at work. Many families will have sought individualized education or 504 plans to seek accommodations at school, and many will have considered switching their child's school placement.

The short- and long-term effects of SR behavior are dramatic and include poor academic performance, social alienation, family conflict, and potential child maltreatment from lack of supervision (Last & Straus, 1990; Kearney & Albano, 2007; King & Bernstein, 2001; King, Tonge, Heyne, & Ollendick, 2000). Continued absenteeism is associated with legal troubles, financial distress, and increased rates of high-risk behaviors (e.g., alcohol and drug use, risky sexual behavior), and ultimately can be associated with poor long-term occupational and social functioning (Kearney, 2008; King & Bernstein, 2001). Moreover, SR can be a costly burden to the education system in terms of professional time (guidance counselors, teachers, principals, social workers, etc.) as well as the expense of alternative schools for children who are terminated from the public school system for SR behavior (Chu, Guarino, Mele, O'Connell, & Coto, 2019).

Despite the visible nature of these disruptions, there is often a substantial lag time between the onset of SR problems and a family seeking help. Findings from a New Zealand specialty clinic found that 80% of families waited up to 2 years to seek treatment after the initial problems began (McShane, Walter, & Rey, 2001). Unfortunately, once absenteeism reaches chronic status, intervention becomes more intensive and challenging (Kearney & Graczyk, 2014) and outcomes less certain (Okuyama, Okada, Kuribayashi, & Kaneko, 1999). Flexible and robust intervention is required for school-refusing youth that entails coordinated interventions with youth, family, and the school system.

PSYCHOSOCIAL AND CONTEXTUAL CORRELATES OF SR

Families often present for treatment frustrated by attempts to identify the original source of the youth's SR problems; however, research suggests that triggering events and circumstances are diverse and multifactorial. In one sample of New Zealand treatment-seekers (McShane et al., 2001), multiple triggers were reported as primarily accounting for SR episodes, including: conflict at home (in 43% of families); conflict with peers (34%); academic difficulties (31%), family separation (21%); changing school or moving homes (25%); and physical illness (20%). Bullying was identifiable in 14% of cases. More than half (54%) lived in intact families and 39% in single-parent homes. Psychiatric illness was reported in 53% and 34% in maternal and paternal medical histories, respectively. This list covers every major domain of youth life (family, peers, academics, health); no single risk factor was associated with more than 40% of cases, with the possible exception of maternal psychiatric illness. Because families often come to therapy wanting to identify the "root cause" of SR in order to address that specific problem, therapists need to be prepared to educate families about the multifactorial nature of SR and to refocus them on more immediate functional assessments rather than historical examinations. As one analogy goes, when the house is on fire, we focus on ways to get everyone out of the house, and then we may try to understand the original cause or causes of the fire. If a youth is school-refusing and absent consistently, the house is on fire and we need to address the immediate "danger" and factors maintaining the fire.

Psychosocial Correlates

Significant cognitive, emotional, and behavioral dysregulation has been associated with SR behavior. Clinically, youth with SR present with a high degree of somatic symptoms (e.g., sickness, panic attacks, muscle tension, stomachaches, sleep disturbances, migraines and headaches); behavioral dysregulation (e.g., clinging, freezing, reassurance seeking, escape, oppositionality, and defiance); and catastrophic thinking (e.g., "I can't handle it," "I can't make it through the day," "School's too hard"). In community samples (Egger, Costello, & Angold, 2003), anxiety-based SR has been reliably associated with greater worries related to separation (e.g., "fear of what will happen at home while at school," "worry of harm befalling parent") and fears specific to school. However, only 5–35% of youth reported these fears; thus, SR should not be seen as synonymous with separation anxiety or fear of school-specific events or triggers. Eight to 32% of youth refusing school also reported significant sleep difficulties related to separation ("rises to check on family during the night," "reluctant to sleep alone") and depression (fatigue, insomnia). Somatic complaints were also common, with over a quarter of youth reporting headaches and stomachaches, and youth with SR also appear to have consistent difficulty in peer relationships (Egger et al., 2003). They were significantly more shy than youth with other school attendance problems (e.g., truancy), more likely to experience bullying or teasing, and had difficulty making friends due to both withdrawal and increased aggression and conflict with peers.

Research supports the notion that school refusers rely on nonpreferred emotion regulation strategies. In a comparison of nonclinical community youth and youth seeking treatment for SR, youth with SR reported using more expressive suppression and less cognitive reappraisal than nonclinical youth when coping with emotions (Hughes, Gullone, Dudley, & Tonge, 2010). In general, reappraisal (thinking about the situation differently) is considered a healthier coping strategy as it is employed prior to the generation of an emotional reaction and requires one to mobilize higher-order thinking to change emotional impact. On the other hand, expressive suppression (controlling outward expressions of emotions, like one's facial response), is a response-focused strategy that follows the emotional reaction and entails suppression, which prioritizes short-term emotional relief over long-term change. Thus, SR youth may require emotions education and skills to help cope with stress without suppression.

Family Correlates

Examinations of anxiety and depression rates in parents of SR youth indicate higher rates than community samples (Martin, Cabrol, Bouvard, Lepine, & Mouren-Simeoni, 1999); 50% of mothers and 20% of fathers met criteria for a depressive disorder; 80% of mothers and 50% of fathers met criteria for an anxiety disorder. This indicates links between certain types of parent disorders and youth expression of SR.

Family environment (e.g., organization, conflict, enmeshment, attitudes toward education and culture), limited financial and instrumental resources (e.g., transportation, child care), and parent distress are also linked to problematic attendance issues (Kearney & Silverman, 1995; Havik, Bru, & Ertasvåg, 2015; McShane et al., 2001; Reid, 2005). Increased levels of general family enmeshment, increased conflict (coercive processes, blame, resentment), detachment of individuals within the family (lack of engagement), disrupted communication and affective expression, and isolation of the family from other social contacts have all been tied to SR (Kearney & Silverman, 1995). Mothers and fathers of SR youth rated their own family as performing poorly in accomplishing basic family roles and low in cohesion and adaptability (rigidity) compared to their "ideal" family (Bernstein, Garfinkel, & Borchardt, 1990). Other research has identified par-

298 CBT FOR DEPRESSION AND ANXIETY DISORDERS IN YOUTH

ent discipline, reported by youth, as lax and inconsistent with increased parent attempts to exert control (Corville-Smith, Ryan, Adams, & Dalicandro, 1998). Family therapy to improve cohesion and flexibility seems important to improving depression and somatic symptoms.

School and Peer Correlates

It is often presumed that SR is the result of a poor match between student and school setting. As a result, most SR youth experience multiple transfers across schools in an attempt to find the right "match" (McShane et al., 2001). Indeed, school attendance problems and ultimate school dropout have been associated with school climate, school policies, and student engagement at school (Brookmeyer, Fanti, & Henrich, 2006). Perceptions of school safety, organization, teacher and peer support, feelings of community, and having clear, consistent disciplinary and attendance policies impact attendance rates (Hendron & Kearney, 2016; Kearney, 2008; Maynard, Salas-Wright, Vaughn, & Peters, 2012). Likewise, having solid peer networks in and out of school is associated with attendance (e.g., Baly, Cornell, & Lovegrove, 2014; Glew, Fan, Katon, Rivara, & Kernic, 2005). Anxious poor attenders tend to report social anxiety, low quantity and quality of friendships, bullying victimization, and social isolation (Egger et al., 2003). Still, school and peer factors are individual and difficult to fix immediately (Wilkins, 2008). Changing schools is not an easy process and families often find similar problems follow the student to the next institution. Nevertheless, close work with schools to problem-solve accommodations can be helpful to aid school reentry and retention.

CBT MODEL OF SR

The cognitive-behavioral therapy (CBT) model (Chapter 1) helps to tease out the multiple intrapersonal and interpersonal processes maintaining SR in youth. The prospect of going to school any given day can trigger individual youth thoughts (e.g., "I can't keep up at school") and emotions (e.g., dread, anxiety, defeat) that prompt the initial urge to stay in bed. Parents can inadvertently reinforce the behavior through accommodations (e.g., allowing a delayed start) or criticizing the wrong behaviors (e.g., criticizing a youth's late start when the youth is still attempting to go). In this complex set of mood dysregulation and interpersonal interactions, the CBT therapist uses all of their skills to assess individual strengths and limitations, conduct functional assessment, and teach proactive skills.

To address these needs, a collection of medical and cognitive-behavioral interventions has been examined and received empirical support. Early clinical trials suggest tricyclic antidepressants (TCAs, such as imipramine) plus 8 weeks of CBT resulted in superior outcomes to CBT plus pill placebo (Bernstein et al., 2000), creating stark improvement (mean school attendance was 70%) over the control group (mean attendance was 28%). However, most doctors are reluctant to prescribe tricyclic medications to youth due to their risky side effect profile. More recent trials of selective serotonin reuptake inhibitors (SSRIs, such as fluoxetine) have failed to replicate these kinds of additive benefit (Melvin & Gordon, 2019). In two recent trials, a combination of CBT with fluoxetine did not improve attendance outcomes over CBT alone. In contrast, CBT alone improved mean attendance from < 50% to 72% (Wu et al., 2013) and 15% to 55% (Melvin et al., 2017) over the prior 4 weeks. These results support previous research that suggested CBT is effective for improving returning students to school (Heyne et al., 2002; King et al., 1998; Last, Hansen, & Franco, 1998; Maynard et al., 2015).

One approach that matches well to the functional assessment approach espoused in this book is the prescriptive CBT approach (Chorpita, Albano, & Barlow, 1996; Kearney & Albano, 2007; Kearney & Silverman, 1990, 1999). This approach is based on research by Kearney (2007) who established that youth attribute their SR behaviors to one of four functions: (1) avoidance of school-related stimuli that provoke negative affect (e.g., fear of experiencing panic attacks); (2) escape from aversive social or evaluative situations (e.g., a test or presentation, bullying); (3) pursuit of attention from significant others (e.g., getting sympathy or support from parents and teachers); and (4) pursuit of tangible rewards outside of school (e.g., screen time and games when at home). After conducting a functional assessment, appropriate and tailored interventions can then be applied. Investigators have argued that such an approach helps address issues related to the diagnostic complexity of SR youth, irrespective of clinical diagnosis. Furthermore, a functional assessment provides more direct information that can be used to select interventions based on specific triggers and reinforcers.

CASE VIGNETTE: RICK

This case demonstrates how CB assessment and interventions can be applied to cases where SR is a primary referral question. Rick is a 13-year-old Indian American cisgender boy in the eighth grade who was referred to an outpatient clinic after having missed 25 days of the current school year and 15 consecutive days following winter break. Starting in kindergarten, Rick developed difficulty waking in the morning, and his tardiness escalated. On average, Rick has missed about 10 days of school each year, mostly after transitions and vacations. Rick was also very attached to his older brother and sister who lived away at college. The episode leading up to his referral began after his siblings had come home for winter break and then returned to college. The parents cited school warnings about attendance and grades as a principal reason for seeking treatment, plus a more general concern regarding Rick's diminishing social activities.

Other than Rick's poor school attendance, he was an otherwise healthy teen who had met all expected developmental milestones on time. He generally maintained good grades (mostly A's with 1–2 B's), which had begun to decline. Peers generally found him likable, and Rick had little problem making friends, but friendships would often wane over time as Rick committed minimal effort to maintain them. He was intermittently involved in extracurricular activities, like hockey and band; however, his participation waivered during periods of poor school attendance. Rick lived with his mother, father, and maternal grandmother. He had two older brothers, 18 and 20, who lived away at college and with whom Rick was very close.

To encourage school attendance, the family tried comforting him by giving him rewards like video games and sending him to therapists. Rick was taking 50 mg of sertraline daily to help with school attendance. In the past week, the parents had tried locking the playroom during school hours so that Rick did not have access to video games, and the mother found this action helpful. Rick's mother reported that his SR interfered with family functioning, such as spending time consulting with school counselors, needing to go to work late or leave work early to accommodate Rick's refusal, and committing a significant amount of time and effort implementing interventions.

ASSESSMENT OF SR

At intake (Sessions 1–2), the therapist separately completed the Anxiety Disorders Interview Schedule (ADIS) with Rick and his parents. He met the criteria for social anxiety disorder (SAD) and panic disorder (PD); major depression disorder (MDD) was ruled out. Rick's SAD centered around a fear of embarrassment by peers and being the center of attention. His parents described Rick as being "anxious his whole life." Rick reported significant fears of answering questions in class, giving oral reports, reading aloud, asking a teacher for help, writing on the chalkboard, attending band and lacrosse practice, performing as a lacrosse goalie, inviting new friends to get together, speaking to unfamiliar people, attending parties, and being assertive. For instance, he fell on the playground and scraped his knee and would not go to the nurse for fear of drawing attention to himself. One time he saw a fellow student's lunch bag break at school and everyone laughed. After that, Rick refused to carry his own lunch in a bag out of fear of embarrassment. As a result, Rick has eliminated nearly all social scenarios outside of school and home. He declines most social invitations unless his older brothers are attending.

Rick also met the criteria for panic disorder as he reported that he was "always panicky" when he was at school, always worried about the next panic attack. He experiences panic attacks daily during school. His major symptoms included trembling, hyperventilation, tension, accelerated heartbeat, sweaty palms, stiff neck, and headaches. Although his mother did not believe that he feared these physical sensations per se, she reported that Rick often worries about having future panic attacks. She also confirmed his report that the panic attacks can happen anywhere (school, home, at the mall), but they were most impairing at school because Rick felt trapped there. He experienced about five panic attacks a week, each lasting about 10 minutes, but residual physical symptoms remained throughout the day. His teacher would often send him to the school counselor due to the severity of his trembling. Some days, his parents would pick him up from school when the trembling would not abate, and on particularly bad days, Rick would stay home from school. As a result, Rick would miss other enjoyable activities, like band practice, because of fears of school and panic attacks. Rick denied that the panic attacks were due to social fears, except for the secondary fear of being embarrassed after having an attack.

As a result of Rick's chronic panic attacks and social anxiety, Rick expressed discouragement and difficulty motivating himself to engage in activities he used to enjoy. He enjoyed lacrosse, both because he liked his teammates and because he liked working at a skill he could improve. He left the team because of school stress and because the coach said that school absences would affect his eligibility. He also used to play drums in the band but now rarely practices and has routinely missed practice. Recently, Rick reported to his mother that he wondered if it would be easier to just quit everything than to keep trying. During a risk assessment, the child denied wanting to die or having any interest in hurting himself, but he admitted feeling hopeless about his situation. Despite endorsing anhedonia (disinterest in activities), hopelessness, and avolition, he did not report enough symptoms to meet criteria for MDD.

Although SR does not qualify as a formal diagnosis, his poor attendance called for specific assessment. Rick and his parents attributed Rick's poor attendance to his anxiety and the belief that he feels more comfortable at home. When asked what made school difficult for Rick, his mother indicated that fear of embarrassment (e.g., answering questions in class) and attention (e.g., being up at bat in gym class) were his prime concerns. Worry about panic attacks exacerbated his concerns: he worried about feeling out of control and being judged by peers for having panic attacks. When Rick did stay home, he played video games and searched gaming blogs and websites.

Several questions help clarify the nature of SR and identify key targets of treatment (see Figure 11.1). Parent awareness is the primary factor that distinguishes distress-based school SR from truancy (Heyne et al., 2019). Rick's parents were aware of his absences and spent the majority of mornings trying to coax him to go to school. Rick's mother was primarily responsible for morning routines, which were characterized by alternating cycles of accommodation and criticism. Evidence of truancy would indicate multisystemic interventions that typically involve social services, child welfare, or juvenile justice systems (Maynard, McCrea, Pigott, & Kelly, 2012; Sutphen, Ford, & Flaherty, 2010). Absences related to peer victimization or bullying call for adult intervention (a parent or school official) involving peer mediation and intervention with the alleged bully. Identify any parent-initiated absences that occur due to limited availability of child care and other resources (e.g., single-parent households where parents work multiple jobs; parents asking teens to stay home to care for younger siblings or accompany medically ill or non-English-speaking family members to appointments). Such concerns would trigger resource interventions.

Acute or chronic medical illnesses in youth are commonly identified as a cause or trigger of school absences (Kearney, 2008), and the challenge is determining what level of attendance is suitable for the given medical condition. Absences that start with legitimate medical illnesses can be followed by extended missed days. Youth with a history of SR often miss days after long

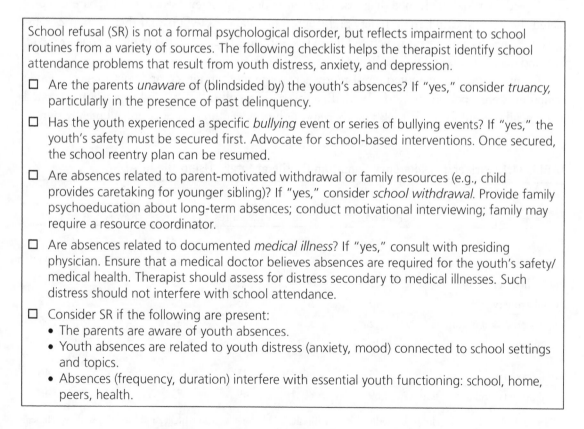

School refusal (SR) is not a formal psychological disorder, but reflects impairment to school routines from a variety of sources. The following checklist helps the therapist identify school attendance problems that result from youth distress, anxiety, and depression.

☐ Are the parents *unaware* of (blindsided by) the youth's absences? If "yes," consider *truancy,* particularly in the presence of past delinquency.

☐ Has the youth experienced a specific *bullying* event or series of bullying events? If "yes," the youth's safety must be secured first. Advocate for school-based interventions. Once secured, the school reentry plan can be resumed.

☐ Are absences related to parent-motivated withdrawal or family resources (e.g., child provides caretaking for younger sibling)? If "yes," consider *school withdrawal.* Provide family psychoeducation about long-term absences; conduct motivational interviewing; family may require a resource coordinator.

☐ Are absences related to documented *medical illness*? If "yes," consult with presiding physician. Ensure that a medical doctor believes absences are required for the youth's safety/medical health. Therapist should assess for distress secondary to medical illnesses. Such distress should not interfere with school attendance.

☐ Consider SR if the following are present:
  • The parents are aware of youth absences.
  • Youth absences are related to youth distress (anxiety, mood) connected to school settings and topics.
  • Absences (frequency, duration) interfere with essential youth functioning: school, home, peers, health.

FIGURE 11.1. Diagnostic clarification checklist: SR.

weekends, holidays, and interruption to the school routine due to a cold or flu. It is also common for school avoiders to experience significant somatic symptoms when it is time to go to school. Headaches, stomachaches, muscle aches, hyperventilation, and nausea are frequent symptoms reported by youth who struggle to get to school. This phenomenon is amplified in youth who have diagnosed medical conditions (e.g., migraines, asthma, gastrointestinal disorders, audio-sensory disorders, etc.). Ultimately, it is important to consult with the youth's pediatrician or specialist (e.g., neurologist) to help determine the youth's fitness to attend school regularly. Often, it is difficult for school-refusing youth to distinguish medical illness from emotional or physical discomfort. Once a medical professional indicates that a youth can return to school without further injury or exacerbating the medical condition, the therapist's job is to help the client tolerate any remaining discomfort that occasionally comes from going to school. During early assessment, assess for chronic and acute medical conditions and their potential role in school attendance problems.

Rick's presentation indicates his attendance problems qualify for distress-based SR, as his absences followed a consistent pattern that was obvious to his parents. Rick experienced the most difficultly returning to school after summer break and holiday vacations, particularly after he had spent a lot of time with his older siblings. His parents were aware of his absenteeism and knew when he was staying home. He had not reported any bullying or victimization, and his absenteeism was not related to intentional parent school withdrawal. Rick noted numerous physical symptoms associated with his panic attacks and believed that it would be dangerous if he had an attack at school.

Objective measures helped diagnose Rick's attendance problems. Rick and his parents completed the Revised Children's Anxiety and Depression Scale (RCADS), and their responses reinforced the results of the semi-structured interview, showing T scores in the clinical range for SAD, PD, and depression (see Table 11.1).

Common themes presented consistently across the mother, father, and youth reports. Panic symptoms were reported above the borderline threshold for all reporters, and depression was rated as clinically severe for both Rick's mother and father. Social anxiety was only clinically signifi-

TABLE 11.1. Rick and His Parents' Symptom Profile at Intake Using the RCADS

	Mother		Father		Youth	
	Raw scores	T scores	Raw scores	T scores	Raw scores	T scores
Separation anxiety	6	68*	5	64	2	49
Generalized anxiety	5	57	2	45	1	33
Panic disorder	12	>80**	4	65	9	66*
Social anxiety	16	70	13	63	12	52
Obsessions/compulsions	2	52	1	47	0	35
Depression	16	>80**	11	>80**	9	56
Total anxiety	49	>80**	33	67*	24	46
Total anxiety and depression	69	>80**	49	75**	33	48

*T scores higher than 65 indicate borderline clinical threshold. **Scores of 70 or higher indicate scores above clinical threshold. T scores are normalized based on youth's age and gender.

cant in the mother's report, but the youth and his father reported elevated symptoms as well. Disagreement between parents and youth regarding anxiety and other problem areas is common (Choudhury, Pimentel, & Kendall, 2003; De Los Reyes & Kazdin, 2005), and each report provides a unique perspective. A therapist might use this assessment to prioritize symptom areas where agreement is most evident (e.g., panic attacks, physical symptoms) or where the greatest intensity resides (e.g., depression). At the least, symptom profiles can help initiate a discussion with the family to identify top concerns, provide psychoeducation, and collaborate on goals.

In addition to symptom profiles, assessing the functions that SR plays for the youth can help direct treatment. Rick and his mother completed the School Refusal Assessment Scale—Revised (SRAS-R; available from Kearney, 2002), and the summary scores indicated that Rick was primarily concerned with fear of negative evaluation and avoidance of negative affect, consistent with his panic disorder profile. This additional assessment helped confirm that a main target of therapy should include teaching Rick ways to manage somatic symptoms and expectations for panic when he approaches school. Furthermore, youth with SR who meet criteria for anxiety or depression disorders typically present with significant emotion dysregulation and behavioral dyscontrol. During assessment, the therapist should consider making a referral to a child psychiatrist to consider appropriateness for medication (see Chapter 4 for recommendations on introducing this possibility to youth and caregivers).

In summary, semi-structured interviewing and evidence-based parent- and youth-report questionnaires support a diagnostic picture that includes SAD and PD. The primary treatment targets focus on Rick's discomfort with the negative affect he feels in school settings (e.g., panic attacks) and fear of social evaluation and embarrassment. In addition, it would be worthwhile to monitor Rick's subclinical depressive symptoms.

Goal Setting and Defining Target Problems

As the therapist provided a thorough review of her diagnostic assessment to Rick and his parents (Sessions 3–4), she initiated a collaborative discussion to identify concrete treatment objectives. To generate treatment goals, the therapist helped the parents and Rick identify changes they would like to see in meaningful life domains (school, peers, family, health). As always, the therapist helped Rick and his parents stay specific, concrete, and goal-oriented.

Parents' Goals

- Go to school more often (increasing number of partial days Rick attended, followed by increasing number of full days of attendance).
- Make more friends and participate in social activities more frequently.
- Decrease frequency of panic attacks.
- Reduce family conflict around school routine.

Child's Goals

- Decrease feeling nervous about going to school.
- Reduce frequency of panic attacks.
- Improve energy to do things I used to like to do.

Therapist's Goals

- Increase school attendance (increasing partial attendance and then full attendance).
- Increase tolerance of distress when panic attacks occur.
- Reduce family conflict around school routine.
- Increase social contact with friends and participation in extracurricular activities.
- Reduce fears of negative social evaluation.
- Improve interest, energy, and mood while engaging daily activities.

To help monitor progress in goals, therapists can convert treatment goals into an idiographic outcome measure that focuses on individualized functional outcomes and is easy to monitor weekly (Weisz et al., 2011). The value of such personalized measures has become increasingly recognized in the field. Figure 11.2 (a blank version is available as Worksheet 11 in Appendix A) illustrates Rick's goals in a target problems worksheet, organized by parent and youth goals. It is essential to define goals in concrete and measurable terms that can be assessed on a weekly basis. One can define them in terms of event frequency, dimensional ratings of distress, or any number of ways. The key feature is that the target problems tracker provides a consistent way to note therapy progress. In this case, Rick and his parents had slightly different goals that are reflected in the tracker. Set expectations that progress is not anticipated for every goal at the same time. Expecting change across all dimensions would be unrealistic and overwhelming. Instead, laying out goals in this way helps everyone keep an eye on the ultimate prize, even as the group makes choices about which goals to prioritize.

Motivational Interviewing

One of the hallmarks of SR is the avolition that comes from the youth's inability to manage their distress when approaching school. The school setting has become such an emotionally punishing context that the youth commonly displays ambivalent feelings, at best, about returning to school. In these cases, the therapist makes use of a change plan worksheet (a blank version is available as Worksheet 3 in Appendix A) to understand the barriers to reentry and possible facilitators; see Chapter 2 for a more in-depth description. The therapist can also perform a decision matrix exercise with the youth and caregivers to make these issues concrete (Figure 11.3). Here, the therapist attends to both the pros of returning to school (to identify incentives) and cons of not returning (to help the youth recognize realistic potential consequences). Likewise, the therapist reviews the pros of not returning to detect any unrealistic fantasies (e.g., "Maybe I don't have to make up the work"), and cons of returning to problem-solve the barriers to reentry. Together, the therapist, youth, and caregivers use the decision matrix to gain a realistic picture of the challenges ahead of them as they commit to change.

CASE CONCEPTUALIZATION

CBT Model

As can be seen above, Rick's SR is represented by a complex, heterogeneous set of symptoms, characterized by social anxiety, panic attacks, and depressed mood. His poor school attendance stems from his inability to manage the distress triggered in school throughout the day. Diagram-

WORKSHEET 11. Goals Tracker

Work with your therapist to brainstorm possible specific, meaningful, and achievable goals. Think through what outcomes you expect to see. And then, keep track of how your child does each week.

Parent Goals	Desired Outcomes	Week 1	Week 2	Week 3	Week 4	Week 5
Go to school more often.	Count number of days attended.	3	4	3	4	5
Make more friends; increase social interactions.	Count number of social events.	0	0	1	0	1
Decrease panic attacks.	Count number and rate intensity of panic attacks (0 "none" to 10 "out of control").	2 attacks (intensity 8)	3 (7)	2 (7)	0	2 (5)
Reduce family conflict.	Count number and intensity of arguments (0 "none" to 10 "destructive").	4 fights (intensity 10)	4 (5)	2 (6)	1 (7)	1 (4)

Youth Goals	Desired Outcomes	Week 1	Week 2	Week 3	Week 4	Week 5
Decrease nervous feelings around school.	Rate anxiety in going to school on 0 (none) to 10 (extreme).	9	8	10	7	7
Reduce frequency of panic attacks.	Count number and rate intensity of panic attacks (0 "none" to 10 "out of control").	2 attacks (intensity 7)	2 (6)	3 (10)	1 (3)	1 (4)
Improve energy in things I used to like.	Rate energy over week on 0 (no energy) to 10 (great energy).	4	4	5	5	6

FIGURE 11.2. Early Goals Tracker worksheet for Rick.

305

Decision to Make: Returning to School

	Pros	Cons
Going Back	• See my friends. • Maybe feel more energy. • Feel better about myself.	• Feel awful, have panic attacks. • Have to answer teachers and kids about where I've been.
Not Going Back	• Easier—don't have to face my problems. • Maybe I don't have to make up my work.	• I'll only get worse. • I probably will have to make up the work. • I might have to go to summer school or repeat a grade. • My friends will get even more suspicious.

FIGURE 11.3. Using a decision matrix to clarify the pros and cons of school reentry for Rick.

ming Rick's reaction to school triggers within the CBT model can help clarify the process for clients, parents, and therapist (see Figure 11.4).

Rick's first trigger in the morning is the ringing of his alarm clock. He has the thought "I forgot that math homework" (1). He immediately feels butterflies in his stomach (2), which leads him to hit the snooze button (3), giving him temporary relief and reprieve. When the alarm wakes him again, he thinks, "I'm feeling sick" (4), leading to a headache (5), and pulling the

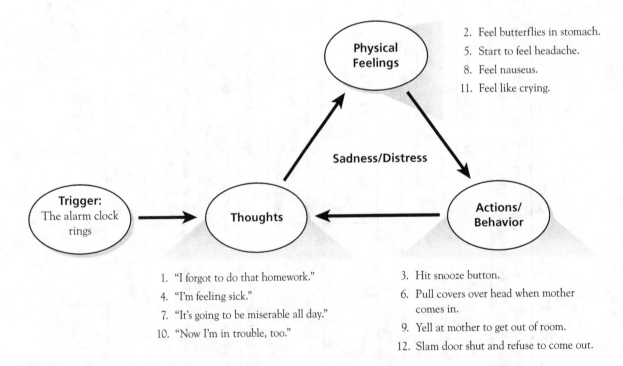

2. Feel butterflies in stomach.
5. Start to feel headache.
8. Feel nauseus.
11. Feel like crying.

1. "I forgot to do that homework."
4. "I'm feeling sick."
7. "It's going to be miserable all day."
10. "Now I'm in trouble, too."

3. Hit snooze button.
6. Pull covers over head when mother comes in.
9. Yell at mother to get out of room.
12. Slam door shut and refuse to come out.

FIGURE 11.4. Individualized CBT conceptualization for a school avoiding episode.

sheets over his head (6). This sequence of increasingly panicked thoughts, somatic symptoms, and actions intensifies in a downward spiral until Rick experiences a full panic attack and is arguing with his mother. The episode only ends when Rick barricades the door and the mother leaves him alone.

The utility of this case conceptualization is that it can demystify an overwhelming scenario for the parent and youth and illustrate where a challenging episode begins. When providing psychoeducation, the therapist can illustrate the CBT model to parents and youth to help understand their own downward spirals and gain insight into their own process. In addition, details about specific thoughts, somatic symptoms, and actions offer targets at which to direct therapy interventions.

Functional Assessment

A second step to formalizing one's case formulation is to conduct a functional assessment to identify the patterns that maintain the youth's avoidance behaviors. Figure 11.5 (a blank version is available as Worksheet 1 in Appendix A) gives examples of antecedent triggers, emotional and behavioral response, and the consequences that ultimately reinforce fearful and oppositional reactions. This worksheet can be completed in session with a youth or can be assigned as home practice. Notice that the three triggers elicit three different types of emotions (panic, anxiety, sadness), but the function that is maintaining the escape behavior is the youth's ability to avoid distress. Unplugging the alarm clock and pulling the sheets over his head allows Rick to put off getting up for another few minutes. Hiding in the bathroom helps Rick escape awkward interactions or possible evaluation by other kids, and going to the nurse's office helps distract him from thoughts about his academic underperformance. Still, each comes with likely longer-term consequences: increasing tardiness and absences or loss of class credit. In each instance, Rick is prioritizing short-term relief at the sacrifice of long-term costs because his distress is so palpable. The role of the functional assessment is to help make these choices clearer to the youth and parents.

When completing a functional assessment with the youth, several points are worth emphasizing (see Chapter 1 for a full review). First, we encourage the youth to identify their initial emotional response to the trigger, because we conceptualize the subsequent behaviors as maladaptive (un-useful) attempts to cope with initial distress. For example, the youth unplugs the alarm clock and pulls the cover over his head because it is so difficult for him to tolerate the fear and panic he is feeling when the alarm clock rings.

Next, highlight what happens when the youth unplugs the alarm clock, including the immediate results and long-term consequences. The immediate result is that the youth feels better. Check this against your own experience. When you hear the alarm clock blare after a night of far-too-little sleep, don't you wish that alarm clock would shut up? And when you press the snooze button, how do you feel? Immediate relief, right? It is the same experience for a school-refusing youth, but intensified. It is this immediate relief that increases the chances (reinforces the likelihood) that the youth will unplug the clock again and again. The more intense the initial panic, the more likely that unplugging the alarm clock will be reinforced. This functional assessment identifies the moment-to-moment experience and why maladaptive coping strategies continue.

Every action has consequences. So, even though unplugging the alarm "worked" in the short term (it relieves the panic), it also comes with secondary, long-term consequences. In this example,

WORKSHEET 1. Trigger and Response

Tell us about your triggers and how you reacted. Describe your feelings, what you did (action), what happened right away (immediate outcome), and then what happened later (long-term outcome).

```
┌──────────────┐      ┌──────────────────────┐      ┌──────────────┐
│  Antecedent  │ ───▶ │    Behavioral and    │ ───▶ │ Consequences │
└──────────────┘      │  Emotional Response  │      └──────────────┘
                      └──────────────────────┘
```

Trigger	Feeling (emotional response)	Action (behavioral response)	Immediate Results (What keeps it going?)	Long-Term Results (What gets you in trouble?)
I hear the alarm go off on the day of a big test.	Fear, panic	Unplug alarm clock, pull covers over my head.	Feel better; skip test.	Get another absence, maybe get grade deduction, parents will be angry.
I see those kids that bug me in the hallway.	Anxious	Duck into the bathroom, wait it out.	Relief, safe	Late for class; get another tardy.
I think about how I'm failing classes.	Depressed, discouraged	Put head down, ask to go to nurse.	Escape class that's bringing me down.	Maybe lose credit for class.

FIGURE 11.5. Individualized functional assessment of SR behavior.

the youth gets another absence on his record, he fails to get credit for the required assignment, and his parents become increasingly frustrated with him and disheartened in their parenting efficacy. Unfortunately, it is difficult for anyone struggling with emotion regulation to keep these long-term consequences in mind when they are feeling initial panic. And so, unplugging the alarm seems to be the best answer, because it "solves" the problem immediately. Prioritizing short-term relief at the expense of long-term consequences is common among youth diagnosed with SR and other anxiety and mood disorders.

TREATMENT PLANNING

Armed with a diagnosis, case conceptualization, and list of target problems, the therapist can then plan an outline of interventions to address the youth's concerns. Tables 11.2 and 11.3 are designed to help in writing managed care treatment plans and reports. Table 11.2 lists sample treatment goals and appropriate interventions that match Rick's case. Table 11.3 shows the sequence of interventions for a 25-session course of treatment for SR. Notice that much of the plan adapts interventions used for other disorders (e.g., PD, depression, social anxiety). This reflects the multidimensional nature of emotional distress experienced by youth with SR behaviors.

In keeping with the current evidence base, multiple cognitive-behavioral strategies are used to address this multifaceted problem. Psychoeducation for both youth and parents, rewards management, behavioral activation and activity monitoring, cognitive restructuring, and exposure exercises are all common interventions for SR. The detailed treatment plan emphasizes strategies specific to panic, social anxiety, and depressed mood, consistent with Rick's presentation.

TABLE 11.2. Rick's Broad Treatment Plan for School Refusal

Treatment goals	Interventions
Increase school attendance.	Psychoeducation about SR and relation to distress as an avoidance of negative affect; reward plans; strategies to address panic and social anxiety
Increase distress tolerance related to panic attacks.	Psychoeducation about panic attacks, interoceptive and *in vivo* exposures
Reduce family conflict around school routine.	Psychoeducation about family interaction patterns, communication analysis, reward plans
Increase social contact with friends and activities, secondary to discouragement and depressed mood.	Behavioral activation to social situations, exposures to support seeking
Reduce fears of negative social evaluation.	*In vivo* exposures, cognitive restructuring
Improve interest, energy, and mood in daily activities.	Psychoeducation about depression, thought–action–mood tracking, behavioral activation

TABLE 11.3. Rick's Detailed Treatment Plan for SR

Sessions 1–2

Assessment
- Assess presenting problems.
- Conduct diagnostic assessment with a focus on impairment (real-life functioning).
- Administer symptom profile measures (e.g., RCADS).
- Assess target problems and treatment goals, focusing on improving daily functioning.
- Assess past attempts (including past treatment) to address problem.
- Assess caregiver–child interactions.
- Conduct collateral assessments as needed with the youth's school (e.g., counselor, teacher, school nurse); retrieve past psychological assessments (e.g., academic/learning assessments); request parents' complete release of information to speak to school contact(s).
- Evaluate co-occurring medical conditions; consult with pediatrician or specialist (e.g., gastroenterologist) as indicated.
- Assess need for medication and psychiatric referral.

Psychoeducation
- Review assessment and generate target problems with youth and parents.
- Create idiographic target problems tracker.
- Collaborate on case conceptualization: CBT model and functional assessment.
- Provide parents and youth with fact sheet on SR and CBT.
- Identify school liaison and obtain appropriate consents to coordinate with school.
- Educate parents about the potential benefits of medication.

Home practice
- Monitor attendance and triggers for attendance problems: CBT model and functional assessment.
- Have youth track their reactions to distress and short- and long-term outcomes (functional assessment) in relation to school routines.
- Have parents track caregiver–youth interactions around school routines.

Sessions 3–4

Assessment
- Evaluate and discuss home practice.
- Complete target problems tracker.
- Complete symptom tracker every fourth session (e.g., RCADS).

Interventions
- Present model of SR as avoidance of distress; reinforce with examples from functional assessment.
- Conduct motivational interviewing to highlight the trade-off between short-term gains and long-term consequences.
- Review caregiver–youth interaction patterns. Identify the key patterns.
- Implement daily renewable reward program for youth with caregiver cooperation to encourage graded school attendance in exchange for valued rewards.
- Establish joint youth, family, and school meeting to identify common goals and roles.

Home practice
- Monitor school reentry within daily renewable reward charts.
- Monitor caregiver–youth interaction tracker.
- Monitor functional assessments, helping youth to distinguish short- and long-term consequences.

(continued)

TABLE 11.3. *(continued)*

Sessions 5–6

Assessment
- As in Sessions 3–4

Interventions
- Review daily renewable rewards program. Continue to improve the plan by reinforcing success and problem-solving barriers. Modify goals and rewards as youth succeeds or experiences setbacks.
- Review and refine individual functional assessments to see where youth is falling into behavioral traps.
- Introduce communication analysis and family problem solving to help caregivers use empathize and encourage and deescalation techniques.
- Collaborate with school liaison to bridge reward programs with incentives at school. Create ongoing feedback system.

Home practice
- Monitor school reentry within daily renewable reward charts.
- Monitor caregiver–youth interaction tracker.
- Monitor functional assessments, helping youth to distinguish short- and long-term consequences.

Sessions 7–8

Assessment
- As in Sessions 3–4

Interventions
- Provide psychoeducation around good sleep hygiene, emphasizing routine regulation. Discuss developmental expectations around sleep routines.
- Teach relaxation exercises to use at sleep time.
- Obtain update in any medication treatment the youth is receiving; consult with presiding psychiatrist.
- Obtain feedback at school.

Home practice
- Monitor sleep changes.
- Monitor use of relaxation exercises.

Sessions 9–10

Assessment
- As in Sessions 3–4

Interventions
- Exposures and behavioral challenges: Build challenge hierarchy or hierarchies, focusing on social evaluation and panic symptoms. Situations will help the youth practice skills to overcome barriers they normally face.
- Practice first steps of hierarchy in session.
- Obtain feedback from school and caregivers on attendance and reward plans.

Home practice
- Youth refines steps of challenge hierarchy.
- Youth attempts first steps of hierarchy outside of session.

(continued)

TABLE 11.3. *(continued)*

Sessions 11–12

Assessment
- As in Sessions 3–4

Interventions
- Monitor self-talk: Teach youth the link between their thoughts and school, anxiety, and distress.
- Teach youth to identify thinking traps through cognitive restructuring and challenge unrealistically negative thoughts with more realistic coping thoughts.
- Conduct ongoing behavioral experiments/exposures on social and panic targets.
- Obtain feedback from school and caregivers on attendance and reward plans.

Home practice
- Monitor thoughts–action–feelings tracker.
- Monitor thinking traps tracker.
- Practice exposure exercises outside of session.

Sessions 13–14

Assessment
- As in Sessions 3–4

Interventions
- Exposures and behavioral experiments: Practice moderately challenging situations, focusing on the core challenges related to SR in different situations: before, during, after school; social and extracurricular activities, nighttime/morning routines.
- Monitor thinking traps and practice cognitive restructuring.
- Assess youth activity levels and determine the need for behavioral activation, as school attendance reestablishes. Incorporate meaningful activities to reinforce attendance at school.

Home practice
- Direct youth to continue practicing hierarchy challenges outside of session.
- Monitor use of coping skills and self-reward for successful attempts at challenges.

Sessions 15–16

Assessment
- As in Sessions 3–4

Interventions
- Exposures and behavioral challenges: Continue practicing moderately challenging steps of challenge hierarchy, focusing on youth's core goals and barriers.
- Monitor thinking traps and practice cognitive restructuring.
- Obtain feedback from school and caregivers on attendance and reward plans.
- Check in with caregivers about interaction patterns with youth.

Home practice
- Direct youth to continue practicing hierarchy challenges outside of session.
- Monitor use of coping skills and self-reward for successful attempts at challenges.

(continued)

TABLE 11.3. *(continued)*

Sessions 16–20

Assessment
• As in Sessions 3–4

Interventions
• Exposures and behavioral challenges: Practice increasingly/difficult challenging steps of challenge hierarchy, focusing on youth's core goals and barriers.
• Check in about activity scheduling and balance of youth attendance, academics, and activities.

Home practice
• Direct youth to continue practicing hierarchy challenges outside of session.
• Monitor use of coping skills and self-reward for successful attempts at challenges.

Sessions 21–25 (biweekly for maintenance)

Assessment
• As in Sessions 3–4

Psychoeducation
• Introduce relapse prevention phase.
• Discuss termination.

Interventions
• Establish routine regulation around bedtime, wake time, attendance, and daily activities. Make school a natural habit of daily routine.
• Exposures and behavioral challenges: Practice increasingly/difficult challenging steps of challenge hierarchy, focusing on youth's core goals and barriers.
• Monitor activity scheduling and balance of youth attendance, academics, and activities.
• Monitor caregiver–youth interactions to encourage maintenance of caregiver encouragement strategies.

Home practice
• Direct youth to continue practicing hierarchy challenges outside of session.
• Monitor use of coping skills and self-reward for successful attempts at challenges.

INTERVENTION COMPONENTS AND PROCESS

Psychoeducation

After developing a joint case conceptualization and treatment plan with the youth and parents, the therapist will educate the clients on the nature of SR, the cognitive-behavioral conceptualization of the problem, the rationale for the various interventions, and treatment options (including medication). It is critical to use examples from the youth's own experience to illustrate how their problem is triggered and maintained. The therapist can use Handouts 25 and 26 (reproducible versions are available in Appendix A) to help provide education about several key issues in managing SR: (1) the importance of school attendance, (2) how a fear of negative affect leads to ineffective escape patterns, (3) how to distinguish medical illnesses from emotional distress, and (4) how parent–child interactive patterns perpetuate SR.

Avoiding and Escaping from Negative Affect

As discussed in Chapter 1, the habituation curve provides a useful visual to explain how escape can reinforce the belief that avoiding feared situations is the only way to manage them. Handout 27 (a reproducible version is available in Appendix A) can be used to illustrate this concept with the youth and their caregivers. In this case, Rick would begin to feel a stomachache, dread, and a headache as soon as his mother would prompt him to prepare for school. Complaints and resistance increased during bathroom time, breakfast, the car ride to school, and finally school and classroom entry. A number of times Rick would choose to escape as his distress increased. He could resist rising from bed, refuse to get in the car, or refuse to enter the school building. Choosing to escape had two effects. First, his distress would immediately drop. Resisting his mom's prompts to rise from bed until she stopped led to instantaneous relief ("I get to stay home!"). Over time, even if not explicitly stated, Rick came to understand this: "Escaping a distressing situation makes me feel better."

Of course, escape also deprived Rick of the opportunity to learn that things often get better over time (e.g., he may habituate to the distress) or that he could handle things if he continued to feel distressed (e.g., tolerated the distress or gained a sense of self-efficacy). Likewise, if Rick escapes from school, he is deprived of all the potentially positive things that may happen at school (e.g., seeing friends, learning something interesting, participating in extracurricular activities). For all these reasons, Rick suffers longer-term deficits to achieve short-term relief. We want to communicate to parents and youth that pushing to get "over the hump" is essential and worth the effort, because the longer-term consequences far outweigh the benefits of feeling better in the moment.

Distinguishing "Legitimate" Medical Illnesses from Somatic Symptoms

Numerous physical complaints are common among youth with SR, including headaches, stomachaches, muscle tension, nausea, and fatigue (Kearney, 2008). Youth will protest attendance due to physical symptoms and illnesses, citing the likelihood that catastrophic outcomes will occur at school (e.g., they will vomit in class, have uncontrollable hyperventilation) or that attendance is fruitless (e.g., the parents will have to pick them up before the school day ends). The timing and consistency of the link between school and symptom onsets often lead parents to suspect the youth is trying to intentionally manipulate them.

In these cases, we communicate simple rules for parents to follow. Medical doctors we have worked with have suggested that staying home from school is only justified in the presence of (1) a fever, (2) uncontrolled diarrhea, or (3) uncontrolled vomiting. If any of these conditions exist, the child should be in the doctor's office or emergency room. One episode of vomiting in the morning is not sufficient to stay home. When the child exhibits chronic somatic symptoms, it always helps to consult with the child's pediatrician or specialist to assess the extent, cause, and consequences of medical illnesses. As behaviorists, we are most interested to learn if there is any medical reason the youth should not attend school (e.g., the youth would put other youth at risk for a contagious disease, attendance would put the youth at greater medical risk).

Medical evaluations of youth with SR typically reveal two findings. One kind of medical consult will determine that "anxiety" is the primary reason for poor school attendance. In these cases, physicians will share their impressions that they can find no medical explanation for the youth's somatic symptoms. The second kind of medical consult will confirm some chronic medical condition (e.g., migraines, digestive disorder, musculature disorder) that contributes to pain or discomfort, but the physician provides reassurance that *school attendance will not further harm* the youth or exacerbate the youth's medical condition. We consider getting either kind of consult as having received *medical clearance* to encourage school attendance.

In either case, we start from the premise that the youth's pain, discomfort, and anxiety are real. We assume that the youth wishes to return to school and is not leveraging their pain to gain some instrumental outcome (e.g., skip homework). Armed with a medical consult, we can more confidently say, "You have received medical clearance to go back to school. While your pain is real, going to school won't make your medical condition any worse. So, let's figure out how to help you manage that discomfort even as you go to school."

A sports analogy may help. Athletes often suffer physical injuries that continue to impact performance even after medical treatment and rehabilitation have been completed. For example, a soccer player may tear her anterior cruciate ligament (ACL), which challenges her ability to cut and turn quickly. After surgery and several months of rehabilitation, the medical team will give her "medical clearance" to return to the soccer pitch. Even then, the player may be tentative in her play because she is worried about suffering further injury. We respect the fact that this player may still experience pain and perform tentatively, but the medical clearance reassures her that the playing itself will not further injure the ACL. Likewise, a teen with migraines may experience discomfort and disorientation, but the act of going to school is not expected to make the underlying condition any worse.

In Rick's case, he often reported generalized physical symptoms (e.g., headache, upset stomach, lightheadedness) that he interpreted as signs of sickness or of future panic attacks. His therapist provided psychoeducation that these symptoms were common in panic disorder and that having a panic attack was different from contracting a medical illness. She then taught Rick to use a feelings thermometer to rate the intensity of his physical symptoms (see Figure 2.3 and Worksheet 4 in Appendix A). With youth who complain of physical symptoms, it is critical to help them see that physical pain and illness exist on a continuum, rather than an all-or-nothing scale. The therapist helps him honestly identify a critical threshold that both parents and youth agree is too painful to go to school (say, a "7" on a 10-point scale). However, anything below this threshold indicates that the youth could attend school, even if they might genuinely experience discomfort. Although families initially fear this approach will justify the youth reporting scores above the critical threshold each day, we have found that, paradoxically, youth find it liberating to have a way to honestly report pain and receive validation for it (see the "Affective Education" section in Chapter 2 for details about developing a feelings thermometer). Finally, the therapist used cognitive restructuring to challenge catastrophic thinking and fortune-telling thinking traps. For example, she reminded Rick that having some physical symptoms does not necessitate having a full-blown panic attack. She also helped him recall times when he had experienced panic attacks during the school day and survived them.

SLEEP HYGIENE EDUCATION

Poor sleep routines and dysregulation are often found in youth with SR and can be mistaken for other medical conditions. However, limited and disrupted sleep routines are frequently the result of anxiety and worry that accumulate by the end of the day and lead to sleep resistance. At bedtime and through the night, worries about unfinished schoolwork and the next school day hinder the youth's ability to settle down. Chapter 2 describes an approach the therapist can take to assess sleep hygiene quality and problem-solve issues that prevent a youth from regulating sleep and wake time. Teaching the youth relaxation skills (Chapter 2) can help them both achieve a more restful sleep and restore a sense of calm when challenges emerge.

Stressing Parent and School Involvement

Early in therapy, it is helpful to inform the parents of the vital role they play in sending the right messages to youth. Chapter 5 describes common parent–child interaction patterns that impair functioning in anxious and depressed youth. These are also explained later in this chapter and comprise an important part of treating SR in youth. Active collaboration among the family, therapist, and school is critical to success. Communicate that schools are not the enemy, despite potentially prior antagonistic interactions. Schools often have flexibility in schedules, accommodations, and criteria for advancement that can be useful in creating stepped re-entry to school. School personnel can also act as in-school behavioral coaches who can generalize lessons into the school day. We discuss specific school–parent collaboration below.

Self-Talk and Cognitive Restructuring

Common thinking traps for youth with SR include *catastrophizing, fortune-telling, discounting the positives,* and *looking for the negatives* (see Handout 2 in Appendix A). Examples of fortune-telling and catastrophizing include fears/assumptions that negative events will happen (e.g., getting sick at school, vomiting in front of other people, having a surprise quiz, getting teased by other kids) and that the outcomes will be far worse than is likely (e.g., you will be unable to get medical help, need to go to the hospital and be embarrassed, fail an assignment, lose all your friends). While some of these events may happen, the youth overestimates their chances of happening and exaggerates the magnitude of their consequences. Figure 11.6 (a blank version is available as Worksheet 5 in Appendix A) is a sample Thinking Traps Tracker worksheet for Rick. For example, Rick thinks, "I'm not ready for the test" upon waking up, and further ruminates: "This will kill my grade!" The first thought may reflect fortune-telling (overestimating the likelihood that he is not ready) and the second thought may reflect catastrophizing (overestimating the impact one bad grade will have on his overall grade).

Examples of discounting the positives typically center on doubts about the child's ability to handle untoward events or that others will not be available or willing to help, even when doubts do not reflect reality. These thinking traps reflect a dismissal of positive events that buffer the youth from negative events. For example, Rick might focus on the last time he had a panic attack in school ("The last time, I froze in the hall and then ran to the nurse's office"), while forgetting that he was able to use his relaxation and cognitive restructuring to help calm himself after the panic attack (discounting the positives). He might also focus on the lack of support at school ("Nobody at the school understands") even though the school nurse helped him practice his coping skills before returning to class (again discounting the positives). Instead, Rick chooses to focus on the nurse's initial skepticism when he first arrived at her office (looking for the negatives).

WORKSHEET 5. Thinking Traps Tracker

What thinking traps do you fall into when feeling sad, anxious, or distressed? For each situation, describe and rate how you feel. Describe your automatic thought (the first thought that comes into your head). What thinking trap might you be falling into? How does that make you feel (the result)?

Trigger	Feeling (Rate 0–10: "not at all" to "excruciating")	Thought	Thinking Trap	Result?
I hear the alarm go off on the day of a big test.	Fear, panic (7)	"I'm not ready for the test!" "This will kill my grade!"	Fortune-telling, catastrophizing	Felt worse (9).
I see those kids that bug me in the hallway.	Anxious (9)	"They want to kill me!" "They think I'm such a loser."	Catastrophizing, mind reading	Felt petrified (9).
My teacher is going around the room asking questions.	Sick to my stomach, depressed (7)	"Why bother; I can't do this." "My teacher will know how stupid I am."	Looking for the negatives, mind reading	Felt hopeless (10), refused to talk the rest of class.

FIGURE 11.6. Completed Thinking Traps Tracker for Rick.

317

WORKSHEET 16. Coping Thoughts Tracker

Brainstorm coping thoughts that could answer your thinking trap! Try and come up with coping statements that are more realistic and ask, "How am I not seeing the whole picture?"

Trigger	Thought	Thinking Trap	Coping Thought	Result?
I hear the alarm go off on the day of a big test.	"I'm not ready for the test!" "This will kill my grade!"	Fortune-telling Catastrophizing	"I didn't study as much as I wanted, but can still get some questions right." "The teacher throws out the lowest grade of the quarter."	Anxious (5) Calm (5)
Had a panic attack in the hallway.	"Last time, I totally froze." "No one would help." "The nurse didn't believe I was panicking."	Discounting the positives Looking for the negatives	"I was able to seek help even though I was panicking." "The nurse did eventually help me."	Nervous (4) Confident (3)

FIGURE 11.7. Completed Coping Thoughts Tracker for Rick.

In helping Rick challenge his thinking traps, the therapist worked with him to remember all the circumstances of his feared events (see Figure 11.7; a blank version is available as Worksheet 16 in Appendix A). For example, when Rick had a panic attack in the hallway, he recalled that he "totally froze" and that "no one was willing to help." The therapist asked for all the details of this event ("Can you tell me what happened after you froze in the hallway?"), and Rick revealed that he tried to stop two or three kids for help before he took a couple of deep breaths, put his head below his knees, and then proceeded to the nurse's office to take a break. The therapist noted that Rick may have frozen momentarily but that he collected himself and made it to the nurse's office. Given that, Rick had to acknowledge that his original thought (i.e., "totally froze") represented a thinking trap (discounting the positives) and deserved a more complete coping thought, such as "I only freaked out for a little," "Nobody noticed my panicking," and "I was able to seek help even though I was panicking." Rick chose the last thought because it helped him feel confident in his abilities to handle future attacks.

Effective coping thoughts do not sell fake optimism. They do not have to convince the youth that "everything will be all right." They should give the teen a reason to pause, consider alternatives, and instill some confidence in them to move forward. Any coping thought that is unrealistically optimistic (e.g., "I won't have any panic attacks in the future," "Everyone is always understanding when you have a panic attack") will likely be disproven and thus be ineffective.

Activity Monitoring and Behavioral Activation

Activity monitoring is an essential intervention when working with youth with SR (see Figure 11.8; a blank version is available as Worksheet 12 in Appendix A). Much like working with depressed youth, you need to identify (1) events that trigger changes in mood (both positive and negative) and (2) fluctuations in mood within and across days. Tracking activities and mood helps one identify the people, places, things, and events that are naturally reinforcing or naturally discouraging for the youth. Youth with SR are discouraged about the future and feel little incentive to try. Activity monitoring can demonstrate that the youth may still find enjoyment in several aspects of life, which yield goals to work toward.

In Rick's case, socializing with friends (whether in person or via text) and practicing lacrosse were linked with elevated moods. Homework and arguments were associated with negative moods. Also notice how events could change Rick's mood over the course of the day. On Monday, Rick was relaxed and calm while leisurely watching TV. Once his mother returned, they got into an argument, he skipped his tutoring session, and his mood declined. His mood remained low as Rick stayed in his room. Likewise, Rick started Thursday off like most days, having difficulty getting up and missing his two friends at lunch. Once he was given an opportunity to go to lacrosse practice, his mood elevated. It remained high as he hung out with friends and completed tutoring. Thus, positive or negative events and activities can shift a mood in the opposite direction. Observing patterns like this can help Rick identify the activities that lead to and maintain better moods.

When SR is the issue, activity monitoring can also help identify natural reinforcers that make it comfortable for the child to stay at home. Does the youth remain in bed asleep the whole time? Do they use electronic devices, watch TV, or entertain themself with other appealing activities? Are they interactive with other people inside or outside the house (e.g., siblings, parents, friends)? This information can then be used to devise incentives when developing contingency manage-

WORKSHEET 12. Activity Tracker

Sometimes we don't even know when we're getting stuck. Over the next week, track your activities, mood, and important events that happen each day! Then rate your mood from 0 to 10:

0 = "The worst mood I've ever felt."   **5** = "I'm feeling OK but not great."   **10** = "The best I've ever felt."

Example:

Looked after my little sister.		10

	Monday	Tuesday	Wednesday	Thursday	Friday	Saturday	Sunday
Morning	Couldn't get out of bed. Thought of all work I didn't do; Mom went to work. — 2	Woke up on time; couldn't get into bathroom; lay in bed; Mom went to work. — 4	Mom started yelling at me at 6:00; got to bathroom and breakfast. — 3	Mom started yelling at me to get up; got to bathroom and breakfast. — 3	Mom got me up, but I was late; skipped breakfast. — 3	Slept in. — 1	Slept in. — 1
Lunch	Slept in through lunch. — 6	Checked Instagram on phone. Ate lunch. — 5	Got to school late, but sat with Jake and Brian at lunch. — 7	Made 2 morning classes. Sat alone at lunch (friends were out sick). — 4	Made 1 morning class. Sat with Jake and Brian at lunch. — 7	Met up with lacrosse friends. Practiced. — 7	Did some math and English homework. Ate lunch. — 4
Afternoon	Watched TV; ate lunch. — 6	Texted friends; did some math homework. — 7	Sat through math, science, and language arts. No one bothered me. — 6	Lacrosse coach said I could come to practice if I went to classes. I went to all! — 8	Math teacher criticized me in class—said I wasn't doing work. — 2	Mom told me to do homework. We got into fight. — 4	Practiced lacrosse with friends. — 6
After school/late afternoon	Mom came back and got mad because I missed school. Skipped tutor. — 3	Met with tutor; got frustrated. — 4	Met with tutor. Did math. Made plans for the weekend with Jake and Brian. — 7	Lacrosse practice. Hung out with team after. Met tutor after. — 8	Lacrosse practice. Hung out with team after. Met with tutor after. — 6	Punished because I hadn't done enough homework. Couldn't go to movies with friends. — 3	Texted with friends. — 6
Evening	Stayed in room all night; didn't do work; Dad also yelled at me when he got home. — 2	Ate dinner; got help on math from Mom. — 6	Ate dinner; watched favorite TV show. — 8	No time for homework. Went to bed. — 7	Did math homework. Went to bed. — 7	Stayed in room; stared at ceiling. — 2	Did some social studies homework; went to bed. — 7

FIGURE 11.8. Tracking activities and mood to identify stressful triggers for Rick.

ment. Rick's dependence on devices suggested that these could be used as rewards. It also helps identify factors that make the home environment reinforcing or comfortable for the youth. This information can be used to guide parent strategies, such as restructuring morning activities to reduce the youth's comfort level at home.

Rick had access to the TV and his phone when he stayed home. The therapist worked with the parents to remove these as automatic rights and to instead install them as privileges to be earned. For example, if Rick did not rise from bed by the time his parents left for work, he was required to forfeit his phone, and the TV and video game power plugs were stored away.

Exposures and Behavioral Experiments

Based on the family's treatment goals and the therapist's case conceptualization, the therapist generated (with the family) three challenge hierarchies focused on school reentry and routine regulation, fear of social embarrassment, and panic-like symptoms. The hierarchies were designed to proceed from easiest to hardest, allowing Rick to build confidence and practice his skills along the way. It is not required to proceed in a lock-step manner, however. If Rick were to show good progress at a lower level, the therapist might choose to skip several levels to provide a tougher challenge. Likewise, there is no shame in returning to an easier level to help reinforce lessons the client appeared to master earlier. Recent research suggests that purposeful jumping around the hierarchy is useful to help the youth tolerate distress better and break unrealistic expectations of negative outcomes (Craske et al., 2014). Also, when multiple treatment goals call for multiple hierarchies, the therapist and client can focus on the target problem that requires the most immediate attention. However, switching between hierarchies can be useful when the youth appears to be stuck at one level.

Challenge Hierarchy A focuses on routine regulation and reentry to school and mostly takes the form of behavioral challenges. Each item in the hierarchy sets an incremental goal for Rick, going from easier to harder, that will help him practice his coping skills in increasingly challenging scenarios. The therapist and family brainstormed this list after identifying which incremental steps seemed achievable. They also identified the challenges that Rick would face (e.g., negative thinking and panic-like symptoms) and the coping skills (e.g., coping thoughts, incentives) that would help Rick push through the challenges.

Challenge Hierarchy A: Routine Regulation and Returning to School

1. Regulate morning routine (get up, eat breakfast, get dressed).
2. Drive to school; park in parking lot for a half-hour.
3. Go to school during off hours.
4. Go to school for morning; sit in counselor's office.
5. Cooperate with favorite home tutor.
6. Go to school for morning; sit in library for independent study (complete one homework assignment).
7. Cooperate with "less favored" home tutor.
8. Go to school for morning; independent study. Picked up for lunch, return for 1 P.M. class.
9. Go to one class, spend rest of morning in library.
10. Go to selected classes; return to library when needed.

11. Go to library, eat with friends in cafeteria.
12. Integrate more classes and natural reinforcers.

At the same stage of therapy, the therapist and family drafted Challenge Hierarchy B to address Rick's fear of embarrassment in social situations. This hierarchy reflects iterative exposures (from easier to harder) to social interactions that would challenge Rick's expectations about outcomes and people's impressions. When executing these exposures, the therapist would design each scenario to push Rick to interact increasingly with others, to allow him to expose himself more, and to highlight realistic outcomes (along the range of positive and negative). The goal of each exposure would be to help Rick arrive at a more balanced view of his own abilities and others' reactions.

Challenge Hierarchy B: Fear of Embarrassment

1. Present oral report aloud to therapist.
2. Present oral report with therapist and one other supportive audience member.
3. Present oral report to small audience of rowdy audience members.
4. Present oral report to small audience and purposely make mistakes.
   [Conduct above with varying levels of supports (notes, scripts, easy and difficult questions).]
5. Text friends from session; monitor hesitation, avoidance, and barriers.
6. Call friends from session; monitor hesitation, avoidance, and barriers.
7. Call and invite friends to hang out.
8. Arrange a social gathering with same-age peers (either with other clients at clinic or somewhere nearby). Practice introducing himself.
9. Go where people are (school yard, park, local stores, college campus) and practice introducing himself.
10. Repeat above while practicing asking multiple questions.
11. Repeat above while asking silly questions.

To address panic symptoms, the therapist laid out a series of interoceptive exposures (Challenge Hierarchy C following) designed to expose Rick to a variety of internal symptoms. The intention was to stimulate the very physical symptoms that Rick feared and to help him both tolerate these symptoms and overcome unrealistic expectations about their meaning (e.g., "I'm out of control," "I'll fall apart").

Challenge Hierarchy C: Panic Symptoms

1. Do calisthenics to activate physical symptoms (e.g., jumping jacks, push-ups, sit-ups, running upstairs).
2. Hyperventilate.
3. Spin around in circles or spin around with head positioned on whiffle ball bat.
4. Position yourself 6 feet from blank wall and stare to create disorientation and tension.

Before conducting each exposure, the therapist planned the exposure with the youth and parents to identify the goals, challenges, and coping efforts that would be required. Figure 11.9 (a

WORKSHEET 6. *In Vivo* Exposure/Behavioral Experiment

Complete this worksheet with the youth as you are preparing for a behavioral experiment.

1. Situation (What's the situation?):

Learning to tolerate sitting in the school parking lot for a half-hour

2. Feelings: **Distress Rating:** _95_

Panic, tightness in chest, sweating, headaches

3. Anxious/Negative Thoughts:	**Thinking Traps (See list below.)**
a. "I'm going to throw up."	a. Fortune- telling/catastrophizing
b. "Everyone will see me and think I'm stupid."	b. Mind reading
c. "If I can't get to class, why bother??"	c. All-or-nothing thinking
d. "I'm going to be miserable and I can't handle it!"	d. Catastrophizing

Thinking Traps: mind reading, fortune-telling, catastrophizing, jumping to conclusions, what if's, discounting the positives, looking for the negatives, overgeneralizing, all-or-nothing thinking, should statements, taking things too personally, blaming.

4. Coping Thoughts (How do you respond to your anxious thoughts?):

"I rarely throw up." "Even if I throw up, I can get past it."
"Everyone's too busy to notice—they're just running into school."
"Every step is a helpful step."
"It may be uncomfortable, but I can handle it."

Challenge Questions: Do I know for certain that _____? Am I 100% sure that _____? What evidence do I have that _____? What is the worst that could happen? How bad is that? Do I have a crystal ball?

5. Achievable Behavioral Goals (What do you want to accomplish?):

Goal	Accomplished?
a. Last 30 min	
b. Stay in the car the whole time.	
c. Read 3 ESPN articles on phone.	

6. Rewards:

Reward	Earned?
a. Get to go home afterward.	
b. Get online time until tutor comes.	
c.	

FIGURE 11.9. Exposure worksheet addressing school reentry.

blank version is available as Worksheet 6 in Appendix A) is an exposure worksheet the therapist helped Rick fill out in anticipation of completing Step 2 of the Returning to School hierarchy. The goal for this challenge was to get Rick to accept a drive to school in his mother's car and to sit in the school parking lot for a half-hour. Rick identified feelings of panic, tightness in his chest, and other somatic symptoms as he thought about getting in the car. He acknowledged unrealistically negative thoughts, too, such as "I'm going to throw up" and "If I can't get to class, why bother?" The therapist helped Rick identify potential thinking traps and generate coping thoughts. Next, it was important to identify concrete achievable goals that Rick could measure his success against. These goals should be challenging but achievable. This helps give the youth goals to aim for, and to feel a sense of accomplishment after reaching them. Of course, success is not an all-or-nothing endeavor, and rewards should be given based primarily on efforts to cope (see Chapter 2 for more details on executing and reviewing exposure exercises).

IDENTIFYING PARENT–CHILD INTERACTION PATTERNS

Functional assessment can be used to help understand how different members of a family influence each other reciprocally. For youth with SR, the therapist highlights several common family patterns described in Chapter 5 (using Handouts 8, 9, 10, and 11 in Appendix A): the *Accommodation Spiral* (parents respond to child distress by accommodating or facilitating avoidance), the *Passivity–Discouragement Spiral* (parents respond to youth fatigue, avolition, or hopelessness with a passive mentality that reinforces the youth's lack of efficacy), and the *Aggressive–Coercive Spiral* (parents respond to oppositional behavior with anger and criticism, leading to escalated aggression). The therapist introduces a worksheet to help Rick's mother keep track of their parent–child interaction patterns every week (see Figure 11.10; a blank version is available as Worksheet 24 in Appendix A).

By completing the tracker for a week, Rick and his mother noticed several patterns. First, the mother often accommodated Rick's upset by allowing him to cancel or avoid stressful situations, like meeting with his math tutor on Monday. By canceling the tutor, his mother successfully stopped Rick's protests for the day, but he continued to complain over the next couple of days. Negotiating in the middle of an argument also had its shortfalls. On Wednesday, Rick begged his mother to let him watch his favorite TV show before he met with the tutor. His mother conceded. After his show, Rick refused to meet with the tutor and locked himself in his room. This kind of pretask reward did not reinforce his meeting with the tutor and increased Rick's attempts to negotiate over the next few days.

Sometimes, drilling down on one sequence of events can be helpful to understand points for intervention. Figure 11.11 (a blank version is available as Worksheet 9 in Appendix A; see also Handout 11) illustrates a chain analysis of parent–child interaction. At each step, the mother falls into a different parenting trap because Rick is motivated to escape from his math assignments. By negotiating and accommodating, his mother is just postponing Rick's ultimate refusal. By the time she insists, Rick has learned that he can escape tutoring if his complaints escalate. At this point, it is much harder to avoid arguments and the two fall into a coercive–aggressive cycle. Using *empathize and encourage* and sticking to the prearranged reward plan are the recommended approaches to use here. When that fails, planned ignoring helps avoid escalation of conflict and removes any unwanted reinforcement of Rick's protests (e.g., distraction, interpersonal attention).

WORKSHEET 24. Weekly Parent–Child Interaction Patterns

Track your interactions with your child over the week and try to identify any parenting traps you fall into. What happened right away (immediate outcome) and then what happened later (long-term outcome)?

Day	Event	Child's Action	Parent's Response	Parent Pattern?	Immediate Result? Did behavior get better or worse right away?	Long-term Result? What happened over the next couple of days?
Example: Monday	Math tutor scheduled for next day.	Upset—Rick says he's overwhelmed.	Talked with him; canceled math tutor.	Accommodation	It stopped the complaining.	He continued protesting the next couple of days.
Wednesday	Tutor came to provide instruction.	Agreed to work with tutor if he could watch TV.	Agreed to let him watch TV even though he hadn't earned device time yet.	Accommodation (negotiation).	He would not work with tutor when she came. Became angry, yelling, and throwing headset. Once he calmed down, I explained this is why we can't deviate from contract.	He kept trying to bargain the next couple of days.
Thursday	Friends stopped over (unplanned) as the tutor was on her way.	He asked if I could call and cancel the tutor.	I told him it was too late. I told him, "I know it's hard with all the excitement, but he could do it."	Empathize and encourage.	He agreed to work with tutor and then I drove him over to one of their houses after.	He got his homework done that day.
Monday	Getting frustrated working with tutor after he had missed a couple of days.	He said he didn't like the tutor and refused to complete assignment.	I told him he had to work with tutor. Said, "I know it's difficult getting started again, but you can make it 45 minutes, and then you'll get computer time."	Empathize and encourage and follow through on contingency plans.	He begrudgingly agreed, but he pushed himself through. He said he was happy he did after.	Was happy the next morning because he had done his homework.

FIGURE 11.10. Weekly worksheet to track parent–child interaction patterns—in Rick's case, his school-refusing behaviors.

WORKSHEET 9. Parent–Child Chain Analysis

Can you identify any parenting traps? What alternatives could you try?			

	Action/Response	Parenting Trap	Potential Solution or Skills to Use?
Prompting Event:	Tutor came for math instruction.		
Child Action:	Rick agreed to work with tutor if he could watch TV.		
Parent Response:	I (Mom) agreed to let him watch TV even if he hadn't earned device time yet.	Accommodation (negotiation)	Empathize and encourage; remind child of reward plan.
Child Reaction:	Rick refused to meet with tutor when she came.		
Parent Response:	I insisted. Threatened to take away device time tomorrow.	Coercive–aggressive	Empathize and encourage; planned ignoring.
Conflict/Problem Behavior:	Rick threw his headset and started to curse at me.		
Outcome 1 (What happened)?	Rick didn't get any instruction time today.		
Outcome 2:	We ended up in a big fight.		
Outcome 3:	I ended up taking away his device time tomorrow.		

FIGURE 11.11. Chain analysis of parent–child interactions in Rick's case.

Empathize and Encourage

After seeing where caregivers fall into parenting traps, they should be encouraged to incorporate the dialectical parenting technique of "empathize and encourage," as discussed in Chapter 5. In this technique, parents acknowledge their youth's distress while also encouraging them to approach their fears and challenges. Encouraging active approach helps counter parenting traps (accommodation, discouragement, coercive–aggressive cycles). Recall the steps to empathize and encourage: (1) Empathize (actively listen to child's expressed emotions and label accurately),

(2) encourage (provide calm encouragement for approach behaviors), and (3) stop! (after repeating empathize and encouragement three times). Consider this typical escalation of conflict as Rick protests his mother's effort to encourage school attendance:

RICK: Mom, I'm not feeling good today; can I go in later?

MOTHER: I know Mondays are difficult, but we know you have to go to school.

RICK: But Mom, I think that hamburger I ate yesterday really made my stomach hurt.

MOTHER: Rick, I know that happens sometimes, but we can't keep missing school.

RICK: But Mom, this is different; I think I have food poisoning.

MOTHER: You know if you keep missing school, you're going to start losing credit.

RICK: I don't care; I won't be able to concentrate if I'm in pain all day.

[*This type of exchange continues for minutes, until frustration grows. . . .*]

MOTHER: Look, Rick, we've been here before and you know you have to go.

RICK: There's no point in going to school!

MOTHER: If you don't go today, we'll be taking away your Xbox the rest of the week!

RICK: I don't care—take it all away; just leave me alone!

MOTHER: It's an attitude like this that will never get you anywhere! Do you want to fail out of school?!

RICK: I don't care—leave me alone!

MOTHER: Fine, be a failure for all I care!

This kind of exchange is a sadly common scenario for many of the families we have worked with and reflects the increasing frustration and helplessness that Rick and his mother feel in the situation. In reviewing the exchange, one can see that the mother was not far off from our recommended strategy at the beginning of the exchange. She acknowledged Rick's challenge in getting to school and encouraged him to go to school. We can haggle over specific words, but the sentiment was on target. Unfortunately (and as one would expect), the interaction does not stop there. Rick protests, and instead of simply reinforcing empathize and encourage, the mother escalates her attempts to convince Rick that he should go to school. Unfortunately, attempts to negotiate typically do not convince the youth that school is desirable. Instead, conflict escalates and the mother resorts to shaming and critical statements. In this case, Rick is no closer to getting to school, and the last thing that Rick hears is that he will be a failure.

As we previously suggested, parents should limit themselves to three empathize and encourage statements. This sends the message the parents want while preventing escalation. After the third statement, walking away is essential even though it is one of the most challenging skills a parent can master. Consider this alternative scenario, emphasizing empathize and encourage statements:

RICK: Mom, I'm not feeling good today; can I go in later?

MOTHER: I know Monday's are difficulty [empathize], and we know you have to go to school [encourage].

RICK: But Mom, I think that hamburger I ate yesterday really made my stomach hurt.

MOTHER: Having a sick stomach can be really painful [empathize], and I want you to try getting into the bathroom [encourage].

RICK: I'm ready to vomit everywhere!

MOTHER: It's an awful feeling to feel sick [empathize], and I believe you have the ability to take the first steps today [encourage].

RICK: Mom! You're not listening!

[Mom gets up from the bedside and walks out of the room.]

In this exchange, Rick may still not get to school, but at least this approach avoids the escalating conflict (with the associated power struggles that entrench both parties). And the last thing (in fact, the only thing) that Rick hears is "I understand, and I still think you can get to school." This approach will not necessarily have immediate results in terms of increasing school attendance. However, if delivered consistently, it begins to communicate a changing mentality in the family that the parents can both honor the youth's pain and distress while also encouraging and expecting the youth to push through painful challenges. In other words, if the parents are consistently limiting their responses to empathize and encourage statements, there is less room for any of the other problematic parent–youth spirals.

As the parents improve at using empathize and encourage statements consistently and faithfully, the therapist can add in one additional intervention: to remind the youth of rewards and contingencies. Ultimately, it is the effective use of contingency management that will encourage increased attendance in school. That exchange would sound like this:

RICK: Mom, I'm not feeling good today; can I go in later?

MOTHER: I know Monday's are difficulty, and we know you have to go to school.

RICK: But Mom, I think that hamburger I ate yesterday really made my stomach hurt.

MOTHER: Having a sick stomach can be painful; try getting into the bathroom [reminder of rewards]. Remember, if you get into the bathroom by 7:00 and down to breakfast by 7:30, you'll earn your full hours of Xbox today!

RICK: I'm ready to vomit everywhere!

MOTHER: It's awful to feel sick, and I believe you can take these steps [reminder of rewards]. I really want you to earn all of your Xbox time today, so please try to get into the bathroom by 7:00.

RICK: Mom! You're not listening!

[Mom gets up from the bedside and walks out of the room.]

Reward Charts and Contingency Management

To facilitate behavioral change via extrinsic motivators (to start with), a comprehensive rewards program is often essential. As described in Chapter 5, a good contingency management approach includes: (1) defining concrete and achievable goals, (2) establishing meaningful rewards, (3) observing carefully ("Catch them being good"), and (4) rewarding promptly and consistently.

Below we describe the family's implementation of a reward plan for Rick (see Figure 11.12; a blank version is available as Worksheet 10 in Appendix A).

Step 1: Define Goals ("What do we want?")

Rick and his parents primarily wanted to improve on-time school attendance. Rick was already regularly attending school in the afternoons, but morning wake-time and routines proved the most difficult. It is key to start with a small set of focused goals or one risks overwhelming the system and failing at multiple goals at once. It is more effective to give the youth small successes before adding new goals. For example, after Rick showed reliable on-time attendance, the parents and therapist shifted to improving his use of in-home tutoring. This was critical to prevent him from falling further behind in math, making it more difficult for Rick to maintain attendance. Notice the goals are framed as goals to accomplish, rather than behaviors to extinguish (e.g., not "Don't fight back when Mom wakes you up"). This helps keep the focus on encouraging behaviors instead of having to punish undesirable behaviors.

Step 2: Establish Reward ("What's in it for me?")

The therapist helps the family set up a daily renewable reward chart (see Chapter 5) to encourage healthy morning routines. Access to the phone was chosen as the reward because it satisfied multiple desirable functions for Rick: keeping in touch with friends, playing games, accessing the Internet. Although Rick had previously been granted unfettered access to his phone, his parents explained that access to the phone was a privilege that needed to be earned. When Rick was routinely going to school, this "contract" didn't require specific explication. Now that Rick's attendance was inconsistent, the contract had to be spelled out concretely.

Rewards were frontloaded to provide the greatest reward for early waking and on-time school arrival. The reward was delayed for late morning arrivals and delayed further for afternoon arrivals. Providing some reward at levels the youth is already accomplishing is an effective practice to minimize discouragement and to continue reintroducing the youth to the reinforcing qualities of the reward (i.e., if a youth never gets their phone, they may learn to live without it and effectively eliminate a potential reinforcer). No reward was given if Rick did not attend school at all.

Step 3: Observe Carefully ("Catch them being good.")

Rick was praised instantly upon making it to school, and the parents used an online calendar to keep track of his arrival time. This way, both parents could keep abreast of his attendance and send encouraging text messages to Rick when he succeeded. It also kept both parents informed of what rewards Rick had earned that day.

Step 4: Reward on Time and Consistently ("Don't skimp on the payday.")

As part of the deal, Rick was allowed to use his phone for any duration after school as long as he accomplished his attendance goals. It was important for the parents to stick to the deal. Midway through the initiation of this plan, the parents noticed that Rick was not allotting sufficient time to complete his homework. While this might have been a reasonable expectation, the matter was

WORKSHEET 10. Daily Renewable Rewards Chart

Brainstorm step-by-step goals and rewards to go with each level. Then track success!

Theme: *School Attendance*

Goals (incremental levels)	Reward (incremental levels)	Sun	Mon	Tue	Wed.	Thu	Fri	Sat	# of Days Achieved
Get up by 6:30 A.M.	*Get phone to play music in bathroom.*	–	N	N	N	N	✓	–	1
Get to breakfast by 7:00 A.M.	*Get phone at breakfast table.*	–	N	N	N	N	✓	–	1
Get on bus by 7:30 A.M.	*Get phone when leaving house. Keep all day.*	–	N	N	N	✓	✓	–	2
Mom/Dad drive to school by 10:00 A.M.	*Pick up your phone at counselor's at lunchtime.*	–	N	✓	N	–	–	–	1
Get to school by lunchtime (noon).	*Get your phone when you arrive home after last school period.*	–	✓	–	N	–	–	–	1
Don't get to school at all.	*No phone*	–	–	–	✓	–	–	–	1

FIGURE 11.12. Daily renewable rewards chart for Rick.

330

NOT negotiated at the time of the original plan. Thus, Rick was in his rights to object the first time his parents demanded that he complete his math homework before using his phone. This change reflected an additional demand that Rick had not expected. This discouraged Rick, and he protested by going to school late the next day. This conflict could have been avoided by sticking to the plan. At worst, Rick would have missed a partial week's worth of schoolwork. The family can renegotiate the reward structure in subsequent sessions. Even as the parents ask for more, they will be coming to the bargaining table after earning credibility for holding to the original deal. We encourage families to stick with the original plan between therapy sessions so they can fully evaluate the pros and cons of the negotiated reward plan. For this reason, the early phase of working with youth with SR and their families may necessitate between-session check-ins to aid in coaching parents as they grapple with the likely scenarios or loopholes that may emerge.

Extinguishing Defiant and Destructive Behavior

For many youth with SR, opposition and defiance are not uncommon. Defiance during morning routines or protests when refusing tasks (e.g., homework) can escalate into conflict quickly. In these cases, both minor house rules (e.g., task refusal, arguments, name calling) and major ones (e.g., breaking property, physical aggression) can be broken. When such circumstances arise, put in place clearly defined rules with specific and limited consequences. Allowing youth to be aggressive toward caregivers or siblings or to destroy property can undermine the caregiver–youth relationship and reduce caregiver willingness to reward positive behaviors. The following steps can help the family plan specific, timely, and focused consequences for misbehavior.

Step 1: Establish House Rules

Rick's parents were amenable to learning communication techniques like "empathize and encourage" and were willing to ignore Rick's complaints and refusals. However, Rick would occasionally escalate his complaints to the level of verbal aggression and property destruction when his mother withheld access to his video game console to incentivize work with his home tutor. Rick would curse at both his mother and the instructor, calling them both names and telling them to "F-—off." He would then isolate himself in his room and throw things at the wall, breaking his possessions and creating holes in the wall. Rick's parents could tolerate anger and frustration, but personal attacks and property destruction were off limits.

Step 2: Define Consequences

The therapist helped the parents define the specific house rules they wanted to set and paired them with specific consequences. A therapist will also want to work with parents to name the value or reason for the house rules, for example, "We respect each other and our property even if we are upset" or "I want to be able to express my feelings more effectively and without verbal or physical aggression." Examples are given in Table 11.4.

After initial brainstorming with parents, the therapist and parents jointly described the risk of escalating aggression to Rick and spelled out the plan going forward. Rick protested by claiming that without his Xbox, he would refuse to attend school. The therapist reminded Rick that he could still gain access to his smartphone (his most preferred privilege) if he attended school—this

TABLE 11.4. Consequences of Breaking House Rules

House rules (off limits)	Consequence
Calling Mom or the home tutor a "b----" or similar disrespectful name	Loss of game time (Xbox) for 1 day
Verbally aggressing against anyone in the family, such as "F--- off" or "Go f--- yourself"	Loss of game time (Xbox) for 2 days
Damaging any personal items intentionally or causing damage to any property (house, car)	Loss of WiFi access for 1 day

would not be affected by acts of aggression. Thus, it was left up to Rick to decide if he wanted to still work toward phone access after he had lost Xbox access. Rick conceded to the plan, agreeing with the value and reasons for the rules, but was skeptical that he would be able to control himself.

Step 3: Be Consistent, Specific, and Punctual with Consequences

In the first week of implementation, Rick cursed at his mother and the home tutor once. The mother called the therapist for advice. The therapist reminded her to remind Rick of the house rules and to promptly take possession of the power cord for the Xbox. Rick protested, but his mother was able to procure the cord and restrict access for the day. Afterward, Rick apologized and asked for the cord back. The mother resisted and reminded Rick of the house rules. The next day, Rick participated in home instruction without incident. After 24 hours had passed, the mother reconnected the power cord to the Xbox. As the parents executed this plan consistently, Rick began to accept that his parents would act swiftly and consistently.

Collaborating with the School and Other Providers

Establishing a strong collaboration with the youth's school is essential to successful reintegration into school, to generalize therapy skills across contexts, and to optimizing the necessary supports the family needs to succeed. To this end, it is important to identify a school liaison and establish a system for ongoing feedback among key stakeholders. Below are suggested steps to develop a collaborative relationship with the youth's school. The therapist may use a worksheet to help guide collaborative discussions; Figure 11.13 (a blank version is available as Worksheet 25 in Appendix A) is one example of how to divide roles among key stakeholders at home and school.

1. **Get consent from parents to contact the school and for release of information.** The first step, critically, is to communicate your intentions to consult with the youth's school and to obtain caregiver consent that identifies the specific content to be exchanged with which individuals.

2. **Identify a school liaison.** Identify the school staff member who will serve as the main contact for the family and who can problem-solve with the therapist as necessary. It could be the school counselor, school social worker or psychologist, academic teacher, or administrator (e.g., vice principal, director of special services). This person should be familiar with the school reentry

WORKSHEET 25. School–Family Coordination Plan: Role Assignments

Brainstorm with student, parents, teachers, and school liaisons what each person can do to help accomplish the goals of the school reentry plan.

Situation	Child Role	Parent Role	School Role
1. Morning routine	a. Drag myself out of bed. b. Get ready. c.	a. Use empathize and encourage. b. Make bedroom aversive. c.	a. Potentially send attendance officer? b. c.
2. School arrival	a. Use relaxation. b. Use coping thoughts. c. Remember "stress hill."	a. Use empathize and encourage. b. Be directive but don't solve problems. c. Remind youth of rewards.	a. Can allow friend/other student/school staff to meet child. b. Allow for graded hierarchy for attendance/tardiness. c.
3. During school day	a. Apply graded reduction of nurse visits, etc. b. Use coping skills. c. Reward oneself for sticking in there!	a. Remove contact during day. b. Utilize graded reduction of contact if cold turkey not possible. c. Reward!	a. Provide reasonable accommodations. b. Adopt empathize and encourage approach. c. Provide encouragement but don't overaccommodate.
4. Departure/ after school	a. Take a break—you've earned it! b. Do homework in small chunks; figure out a plan with parents and teachers. c.	a. Call to reinforce successes. b. Encourage homework in small chunks. c.	a. Arrange needed tutoring. b. Collaborate on manageable homework plan. c.

FIGURE 11.13. A school–family coordination plan that assigns roles to maximize engagement and collaboration among caregivers, school professionals, and youth.

333

goals and plan, and willing to educate other school personnel about the plan (i.e. serve as a "local champion" for the family's therapeutic approach). For example, if the school counselor serves as the liaison, it may be necessary for them to approach the youth's general education teachers and explain the plan, negotiate homework completion, and arrange for graded reentry. This school liaison can also be the person responsible for returning feedback to the parents from teachers when the youth has begun reattending school. This liaison might also update administrative officials about the youth's progress in the plan.

3. **Schedule an initial meeting.** At a minimum, the therapist, the parent(s), and the school liaison should be present at this session. It would also be ideal to have the youth available, even if they do not participate in the entire meeting. Other key stakeholders could include members of the child study team, general education teachers who know the student well, or administrators who influence school policy (e.g., vice principal, director of special services). These meetings often take place at the school to facilitate as much school participation as possible and to give the therapist an opportunity to visit the school grounds to be able to visualize them in future sessions with the youth.

4. **Exchange information about youth's in-school and out-of-school behavior.** The most basic function of the school meeting is to encourage an equal exchange of information from multiple perspectives. Often, the parents come to this meeting with preconceived notions of school attitudes, assuming that the school blames the parent for the student's failures or that it is looking to withdraw whatever accommodations they have already made. Likewise, the school may arrive at the meeting assuming the parent has taken an antagonistic viewpoint toward the school. The therapist's role is to achieve common ground by giving the school and parents equal opportunity to outline the efforts each party has made to help the youth. Frequently, this discussion will communicate to the school how challenging it has been to encourage attendance, and (hopefully) it will communicate how invested the school is in the youth's well-being. Furthermore, this exchange of information can help identify key triggers, youth reactions, and adult responses that perpetuate poor attendance. This shared information can improve existing conceptualizations and functional assessments.

5. **Identify and agree on goals.** Just as all good problem solving starts with defining concrete, achievable goals, so does a good collaboration. In this case, the key is to help parents and school personnel come to an agreement on realistic goals to which each party can consent. The youth and family's needs should be met while also taking into account the limitations and restrictions of the school. The therapist's role is to help both parents and school identify common goals and values and then stay firm in outlining first steps. In the case of SR, school reentry ought to be a focus, but it will likely require smaller steps than the school anticipated, and there will no doubt be starts and stops and successes and setbacks. Once goals have been agreed to, the therapist can guide the team in outlining specific concrete steps designed to achieve goals. (A review of problem-solving skills might be helpful here; see Chapter 2.)

6. **Identify the school's limits and resources available to the family.** As steps are being outlined, identify concretely any resources the school has to aid school reentry and to communicate the school's limits. School resources include knowing which staff members are available to help and what flexibility exists in school policies. Is there a staff member who could help meet the youth at the school's front door? Do they have available independent study rooms or libraries where the youth could complete independent study instead of being in class? Can the youth stay

in the attendance office, counselor's office, or nurse's room if not comfortable going to class? Can the therapist, nurse, and team agree on a plan and consistent script to handle the student's pleas to go home? How flexible are the school's attendance policies? Is a tardy considered an absence? Can a student attend some class periods but not others? How flexible is the absence limit before the student fails?

Schools may also have reasonable limits or state and district rules that restrict their flexibility. Some schools may have rules about when a child is allowed to enter the school premises (or be locked out), the maximum number of absences before requiring a repeat of grade, individual teacher's rules about attendance and homework completion, state testing requirements, and the like. Certain schools and states also may have mandates regarding contacting state child protective services for "educational neglect" following a specific number of child absences. Knowing these limits helps you guide the procedures through realistic goal setting.

7. **Establish rewards both inside and outside of school.** Are there activities or rewards in the school that the youth values? For example, would the youth be motivated by certain extracurricular activities? What if these were normally reserved for students who fully attended, but this student could gain access to the privilege if they attended three periods? Some schools may have point systems that can be exchanged for goods or privileges. Establishing intrinsic and extrinsic rewards in school can help tilt the experience the youth has of a typical school day.

8. **Brainstorm ways to practice skills inside and outside of school (*in vivo* exposure).** Practice and homework are not just for after-school hours. While family members are often responsible for graded exposures that lead up to school reentry, the school can also help once the student arrives. Coordination across the entire continuum of school reentry is essential. For example, brainstorm with the school how and when the therapist and family can practice being on the school grounds. Is it OK for the parents to drive the youth to the parking lot and sit there for 2 hours? Would it be OK if they "loitered" outside the front steps? Once in school, can the counselor schedule regular meeting times to practice in-school exposures? Can teachers be instructed to look for opportunities to practice in class? When should accommodation be given (e.g., trips to the nurse)? These kinds of questions are important to have answered in advance with the school as there often may be strict rules about a student's presence both on and around school property.

9. **Establish ways to track accomplishments and reward success.** The therapist helps school personnel establish some kind of monitoring system that provides feedback to the parent and therapist, and immediate recognition of accomplishment to the youth. The same principles apply for home- and school-based reward systems. Be clear about rewards and how the youth earns them. When rewardable behavior is noticed, make sure the youth is recognized in a timely and consistent way, and follow through with the promised rewards.

10. **Establish roles for the youth, parent, school, and outside clinic.** Once goals, concrete steps, and a reward plan are designed, each member of the team identifies what roles they can play in executing the plan. In an attempt to think holistically about the youth's day and all its integrated parts, we recommend scheduling the challenges that can be expected across the whole school day. This increases awareness of the essential roles and steps that need to be accomplished in order to handle seamless transitions from morning through the school day to after school.

Notice that the youth, parent, and school can be assigned a role at each major transition point in the day (morning routine, school arrival, during the school day). In a tabular format, one could add additional roles for other team members (e.g., the outside therapist, a family friend, general education teacher). The purpose of such a table is to make concrete what is expected from each team member and which goals/steps should draw each person's attention.

It can be tempting to overcommit to roles. We would encourage each person to be realistic in committing to what is feasible. It is better to attend to some steps well than to spread oneself out over many steps. This is true even if some important roles are left unassigned. Treat the roles-assignment exercise as an *aspirational* to-do list. Prioritize the roles (and accompanying steps) that need to be assigned immediately and postpone the roles and steps that can be accomplished after initial goals are achieved.

In Rick's case, the school and his parents had been working together on school attendance for some time, given his longstanding pattern of missed days. Throughout grade school, Rick would miss about 10 days per year with a handful of tardies; holidays and breaks typically served as triggers for missed days. Entry into middle school the prior year produced several absences at the beginning of the school year, so Rick's parents had already met with the school counselor several times to alert her to his patterns and to generate a plan. Together, they arranged Rick's class schedule in seventh and eighth grades to start the day with what were more enjoyable classes for him (science and history) and to offer Rick extra instruction time (after school) in subjects where he struggled (math and English). These accommodations appeared to help Rick settle into the seventh grade, and his team crafted similar plans to transition to eighth grade when he again missed about six days of school to start the school year.

Both counselor and family were surprised when Rick would not return to school after the winter break. Even though breaks were always difficult, Rick would usually return full time after a day or two of partial absences. After a full week of absences, the family sought care at the clinic and enlisted the services of the outpatient therapist. By the time the intake was completed, Rick had missed 15 consecutive days of school following the break. One of the first interventions the therapist recommended was to schedule a joint school–family meeting. At this meeting, the parents, school counselor, and Rick's English teacher were present. The meeting was helpful in conveying to school staff the degree to which panic symptoms and social anxiety contributed to Rick's reluctance to attend school. It also conveyed how conflict escalated when Rick was pushed with criticism. The therapist illustrated Rick's typical behavioral triggers and reactions by sharing some of the functional assessment worksheets completed by the family. As a result, school staff agreed that they wanted to find approaches that encouraged attendance without increased conflict and aggression. Likewise, the school was able to describe the number of ways they tried to accommodate Rick's anxiety (e.g., altering his school schedule). Together, the information exchange provided impetus for encouraging approach through concrete goals, incentives, and stepwise practice.

Consistent with the goals established for him at home (Figure 11.13), the school agreed to graded reentry, allowing Rick to earn credit for days that he got to school by the fifth period, right after lunch. The school agreed to this plan based on the understanding that the goals would advance over time (i.e., he would come to school one period earlier each week). In addition, the school wanted to set home instruction as a concrete goal. Success would be rated by number of tutor sessions attended each week, and his effort by the home instructor on a 0–10 scale, with a 7 reflecting a minimally acceptable effort. It was made clear that progress would not proceed in a strictly linear pattern: there would be starts and stops, but as long as Rick was demonstrating effort to arrive, the school would permit flexibility. The daily renewable reward the school offered was to make band and lacrosse practice available on days he reached his benchmarks. Rick chose to be rewarded with band practice, because he felt he could sit in on practice and not perform while still seeing his friends. He reported feeling insecure about his physical fitness and so wanted to build up to the reward of attending lacrosse.

For accommodations, the school offered to continue Rick's home instruction for math and English. They were comfortable with Rick and his parents sitting in the parking lot until he was ready to enter the building, and they offered a "transition period" where he could sit in the counselor's office if he were to come before fifth period. At the same time, it was unlikely that the counselor would be able to sit with Rick for any length of time, so the school asked that Rick use any transition period as "independent study" time where he would work on homework from home instruction. Designating this as independent study permitted the school to leave Rick unattended in a staff member's office or counseling suite. In addition, the therapist agreed to provide an in-service presentation for the general education, counseling, and nursing staff about panic attacks in the youth. The school found this to be a great benefit to their staff, enabling them to better understand how to approach Rick and other students experiencing panic.

Progress Monitoring

After 20 weeks of therapy, Rick experienced improvement over several domains and achieved gains in important goals. School attendance was tracked daily in a de-identified Google spreadsheet that was visible to his parents, therapist, and school liaison. Rick and his parents completed an RCADS monthly to track broad symptom severity. Figure 11.14 shows his progress in panic symptoms across 20 weeks of therapy. The reports from both his mother and father demonstrated a fairly linear decline in panic symptoms after the initial 4 weeks. Rick reported a spike in panic attacks and panic symptoms during the first 4 weeks, but then rapid improvement thereafter.

Rick's reduction in panic attacks paralleled improved school attendance, with him steadily attending 3–4 days a week through the first month before increasing to 4–5 days per week during Weeks 4–12, and finally settling at full attendance (with occasional tardiness) by Week 20. As important were Rick's incorporation of social events and extracurricular activities, as reflected in his Goal (see Figure 11.15; a blank version is available as Worksheet 11). The school's cooperation

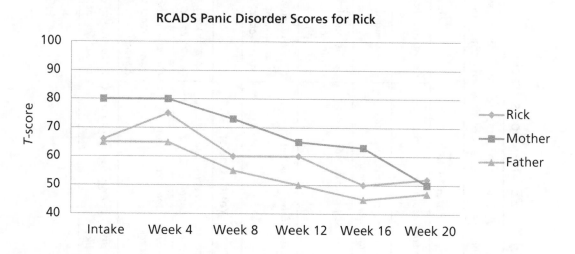

FIGURE 11.14. Symptom outcomes during therapy using the RCADS.

WORKSHEET 11. Goals Tracker

Work with your therapist to brainstorm possible specific, meaningful, and achievable goals. Think through what outcomes you expect to see. And then, keep track of how your child does each week.

Parent Goals:

	Desired Outcomes	Week 1	Week 2	Week 3	Weeks 4–19	Week 20
Go to school more often.	Count number of days attended.	3	4	3	…	5
Make more friends; increase social interactions.	Count number of social events.	0	0	1	…	2
Decrease panic attacks.	Count number and rate intensity of panic attacks (0 "none" to 10 "out of control").	2 attacks (intensity 8)	3 (7)	2 (7)	…	0
Reduce family conflict.	Count number and intensity of arguments (0 "none" to 10 "destructive").	4 fights (intensity 10)	4 (5)	2 (6)	…	0

Youth Goals:

	Outcome?	Week 1	Week 2	Week 3	Weeks 4–19	Week 20
Decrease nervous feelings around school.	Rate anxiety in going to school on 0 (none) to 10 (extreme).	9	8	10	…	4
Reduce frequency of panic attacks.	Count number and rate intensity of panic attacks (0 "none" to 10 "out of control").	2 attacks (intensity 7)	2 (6)	3 (10)	…	1 (4)
Improve energy in things I used to like.	Rate energy over week on 0 (no energy) to 10 (great energy).	4	4	5	…	7

FIGURE 11.15. Rick's Goals Tracker worksheet at termination.

in permitting Rick's involvement in band class for partial attendance was key in helping to motivate his attendance, and scheduling social activities was essential for countering Rick's assumptions that his friends were judging his absences. Both served to improve Rick's depressed mood and increase his energy.

TERMINATION AND RELAPSE PREVENTION

Success rates vary considerably for school-refusing youth (Maynard, Brendel, et al., 2015; Maynard, Heyne, et al., 2018), with initial success possible with early intervention. However, extended treatment with boosters can be expected to help youth continue to practice skills after the acute phase is finished. After Rick's steady school attendance was established, goals began to focus on the skills deficits that were the underpinnings of the refusal behavior. Attention was focused on activity scheduling and social activation. Cognitive techniques were used to challenge misinterpretations of panic symptoms and social evaluation. Parent management techniques and reward structures helped the family learn to support Rick in meeting his goals. As Session 20 approached, Rick's attendance had remained stable and his functioning in social and family domains had improved. The family and therapist decided to phase out therapy with biweekly sessions for 2–3 months before reevaluating (see Chapter 3). The family then anticipated moving to a monthly check-in schedule to review ongoing practice of skills, particularly focusing on routine maintenance and family interactions. At critical school transitions (returns from summer break and holidays), the family also anticipated reconnecting with the therapist to receive extra support. Using booster sessions in this way acknowledges the often chronic nature of SR and sets expectations appropriately for the parents and youth to anticipate ongoing management of symptoms into the future.

SUMMARY AND KEY POINTS

Like many youth with SR, Rick came to therapy with a chronic history of intermittent attendance problems and an acute episode that required immediate attention. The poor attendance can be attributed to multiple symptom domains (e.g., panic, social anxiety, depression) and problematic family interaction patterns (e.g., accommodation, aggressive–coercive cycle). Coordination with Rick's school also proved essential. Here are the key take-away points from the work with Rick:

- Psychoeducation is critical to help caregivers and school personnel understand SR as a function of avoidance of negative affect and less as a function of defiance.
- Family interaction patterns play a key role in maintaining SR behavior as families can fall into multiple traps, including the Accommodation Spiral and Aggressive–Coercive Spiral.
- Assessments should include idiographic target goals in addition to diagnostic and symptom information to ensure that therapy is working toward meaningful objectives that can be observed.
- Coordination with the youth's school is essential. As soon as possible, the therapist should identify a school liaison and help organize a joint meeting involving school, family, and therapist.

- Work with the youth is necessarily multimodal in that the youth will likely express multiple skill deficits in maladaptive thinking, activity selection, and emotion dysregulation.
- External rewards in the form of reward plans and contingency management can incentivize the effort to practice skills and boost attempts at school reentry until intrinsic motivation catches up.
- Caregiver communication styles likely need fine-tuning to bring them more in line with behavioral principles (i.e., praising desired behaviors and ignoring undesired behaviors).
- The treatment course may require extended booster sessions following an acute phase of therapy to help youth and families practice skills and maintain attendance.

Handouts and Worksheets

HANDOUT 1. General Cognitive–Behavioral Model

Notice how each of our emotions can be described by our thoughts, actions, and physical feelings and how they interact with each other.

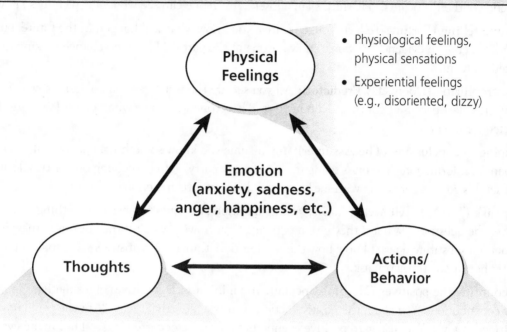

- Content of thoughts, self-statements
- Interpretations, attitudes, beliefs
- Information processing

- Observable actions
- Covert actions
- Cognitive behaviors (e.g., worry, rumination)

HANDOUT 2. Common Thinking Traps That Get Us Stuck

1. **Mind reading (Mind Reader):** You assume you know what other people think without sufficient evidence of their thoughts. "He thinks I'm a loser." "Everyone can see what cheap clothes I'm wearing."

2. **Fortune-telling (Fortune-Teller):** You're positive you know what will happen in the future, but you don't have enough evidence! "I won't know anyone at the party." "I have no chance making the basketball team."

3. **Catastrophizing (Doomsday Predictor):** All you see are the worst-case outcomes! "Now I'm going to fail this class because I got this 'B' on my test." "Everyone will know what a loser I am after I got rejected for the prom."

4. **Jumping to conclusions (The Assumer):** You assume you know something, but you only have a little amount of information. "No one's going to show for my party" (after receiving one or two declines). "My boyfriend is going to break up with me" (after he does not return a phone call).

5. **What if's (Tell Me, Tell Me):** You keep asking question after question because nothing seems to answer the question. "What if they give a pop quiz tomorrow?" "What if they test us on new material?" "What if a substitute doesn't know how the teacher does things?" No answers seem to reassure you, no matter how many times you ask.

6. **Discounting the positives (Nothing Special):** You minimize the positives of a situation or minimize your contributions. You claim the positive actions you take are trivial (e.g., "Anyone could have helped my friend study"). You disregard positive events that may have occurred (e.g., "They invite everyone who's in the honor society to that dinner").

7. **Looking for the negatives (Walking with Blinders On):** All you can see are the negative things happening around you. You can't see the positives. "I couldn't even find anything fun to do while my friend was here." "School is nothing but fake people."

8. **Overgeneralizing (The Big Snowball):** One bad thing happens, and everything will turn out the same. "See? Other kids don't give you a chance to be yourself." "I'm not very good at school—I don't think I have much to look forward to."

9. **All-or-nothing thinking (Black-and-White):** Everything's either all good or all bad. All perfect or all a failure. "If I don't get an 'A,' I'm a failure." "If you miss one party, people will forget about you."

10. **Should statements (Must/Has to Be):** You see events in terms of how things should be, rather than simply focusing on how they are. "I should ace all my exams." "I need to be available to my friends all the time." "My parents don't care about me if they make me go to school [my parents ought to let me stay home]."

11. **Taking things too personally (The Self-Critic):** If something goes wrong, it must be your fault. "We lost the game because of me." "I'll never get better." If someone says anything a little bit negative, it feels like the world is crashing.

12. **Blaming (Hot Potato):** You focus on the other person as the source of your negative feelings, because it is too difficult to take responsibility. "Why won't you let me stay home from school?" "Why is everyone against me?"

HANDOUT 3. "Luggage on a Conveyor Belt" Mindfulness Script

This script is to be used by the therapist to help practice mindfulness with their teen client.

For the next several minutes, we're going to be trying something. It may seem a little different, or even unnatural, but I want you to give it a try. Sometimes, our thoughts get the better of us, and today, we're going to try and just let go of them a little bit.

For this exercise, I'm going to ask you to simply notice your thoughts as they naturally come. The aim will be to watch any thoughts—whatever they may be—come into our mind, notice that they're there, but then allow them to pass through you without a fight. We will try to "accept" your thoughts for what they are, just thoughts. Sometimes, the more we fight our thoughts, the stronger they become.

So, for the next several minutes, I'd like you to imagine a conveyor belt in front of you; just like one you'd see at an airport. Think about how a conveyor belt works—luggage comes down a chute, lies down on the conveyor belt, and then circles around and around. Each piece of luggage gently slides down the chute and then begins its trip around the belt. If you just watched from afar, you'd see that if nobody came to pick up the luggage, the luggage would just go around in circles . . . coming around the front end, circling around, and disappearing around the back end. As you wait, you see the same luggage going around the front end and then back around the back end, slowly but surely circling around.

Well now, as you think of the luggage on this belt, I'd like you to start putting each thought that comes into your head onto a piece of luggage. Just like a label that gets stuck on the luggage. Each thought: gently stick it on the luggage and watch as the thought just stays on the belt, circling around and around. You may feel the urge to do something with the luggage or the thought. You may want to pick it up, put it down on the ground, stop it from circling around and around. You may feel the urge to turn away or distract yourself, to get bored by the circling luggage. When you notice this happening, just turn your attention back to the thought and just appreciate that it is circling gently on the belt in front of you. Sometimes, thoughts will suddenly disappear from the belt. When this happens, simply let them go. No reason to keep a thought on a belt when it doesn't want to be there.

You can either then observe silence as your client practices this, or you can facilitate by asking the client to describe their thought and helping them envision placing it on the luggage and circling around.

Now keep going. I will let you know when to stop. It may seem like a long time, but just allow your thoughts to come as they do.

HANDOUT 4. Facts about Sleep Hygiene

What is sleep hygiene?

Sleep hygiene is a variety of different practices and habits that are necessary to have good nighttime sleep quality and full daytime alertness.

Why is it important to practice good sleep hygiene?

Obtaining healthy sleep is important for both physical and mental health. It can also improve productivity and overall quality of life. Everyone, from children to older adults, can benefit from practicing good sleep habits.

How can I improve my sleep hygiene?

One of the most important sleep hygiene practices is to spend the appropriate amount of time asleep in bed, not too little or too excessive. To help set up good sleep hygiene practices, follow some of these tips:

- *Establish a regular relaxing bedtime routine.* A regular nightly routine helps the body recognize that it is bedtime. This could include taking a warm shower or bath, reading a book, or doing light stretches. When possible, try to avoid emotionally upsetting conversations and activities before attempting to sleep. Don't create to-do lists, do homework, or think of other stressors right before bedtime. Make sure to unplug from electronics at least 30 minutes before bedtime!

- *Avoid typical stressors an hour before bedtime.* Doing homework, writing a to-do list, or having talks about stressful things that came up during the day (or upcoming events) can lead to restless sleep. Cut off homework and worry talk 1 hour before bedtime.

- *Make sure that the sleep environment is pleasant.* Mattress and pillows should be comfortable. The bedroom should be cool, and lights from lamps, phones, and screens should be dimmed or shut off. Consider using blackout curtains, eyeshades, ear plugs, "white noise" machines, humidifiers, fans, and other devices that can make the bedroom more relaxing.

- *Make sure to establish a consistent wake time.* Having a consistent sleep and waking time helps regulate the body to know when it's time to get up and when it's time to go to sleep. Pushing oneself to wake up, even when tired, will help set the tone for a ready bedtime the following night.

- *Limit daytime naps to 30 minutes.* Napping does not make up for inadequate nighttime sleep. However, a short nap of 20–30 minutes can help to improve mood, alertness, and performance.

- *Avoid caffeine and other activating foods close to bedtime.* Drinking caffeinated drinks like energy drinks or coffee close to bedtime make it more difficult to fall asleep and can lead to waking up throughout the night. It might also be wise to avoid heavy or rich foods that have upset your stomach in the past a couple of hours before bedtime.

(continued)

- *Exercise to promote good-quality sleep.* As little as 10 minutes of aerobic exercise, such as walking or biking, can drastically improve nighttime sleep quality. Most people should avoid strenuous workouts close to bedtime, but it's best to find out works best for you.

- *Ensure adequate exposure to natural light.* Getting enough daylight is important to keeping a healthy sleep–wake cycle. This is particularly important for youth who may not venture outside frequently.

- *Reset your sleep–wake cycle.* For those who have already fallen into an unhealthy sleep–wake cycle (staying awake through most of the night only to sleep through most of the day), sometimes it can be helpful to try an experiment. *Force yourself to stay awake* as long as you can. Even when tired, do not let yourself fall asleep at any point during the night. When daylight comes, keep yourself awake. Eventually, your body's natural fatigue will take over, and it will welcome sleep in the next evening or two.

- *Do supplements help?* Some people find natural supplements (e.g., melatonin) helpful in creating a sense of drowsiness that puts them in the right mindset for sleep. If you would like to try such supplements, consult with your family doctor or psychiatrist to assess appropriateness and dosage.

HANDOUT 5. Myths and Facts about Medication

Are medications for anxiety or depression addictive? Will my child ever be able to stop taking them?

Most children and adults taking psychiatric medications for mood and anxiety symptoms eventually stop taking the medications and do so successfully. In fact, a discussion about stopping the meds should take place with your prescriber before any are prescribed. Most approved pediatric medications do not cause tolerance, which is the hallmark of an addictive substance (needing more of a substance to experience the same effect).

Will taking medications affect my child's growth and development?

Side effect profiles vary between different medications and should be considered on a case-by-case basis. Discuss this with your physician or prescriber.

Will these medications have dangerous side effects, like weight gain or suicidal thoughts?

As noted above, side effects may occur and are a reason to change the course of treatment if they are not tolerated. Bring up any concerning side effects to your prescriber. Ask your prescriber about the possibility of suicidal thoughts that might result from the use of antidepressants. The data suggest the benefits far outweigh the risks, but each case is individual.

Will it change my child's personality?

Psychiatric medication should make someone feel more like themself, not less so. A medication that changes a child's personality is a reason for a prescribing physician to stop the medication.

Does taking medications mean there is something wrong with my child? Does it mean they are "abnormal" or disabled?

Think of taking medication for anxiety and mood symptoms as taking medication for a medical condition, like diabetes. Taking the appropriate medication helps your child be healthy and reach their potential, even in the face of medical and psychological conditions.

We're worried the medications are not organic. We don't like to make use of artificial compounds.

Some organic substances may be highly addictive and toxic to our body, and some nonorganic substances may be life-saving. Each situation should be considered case by case, weighing the risks and benefits.

HANDOUT 6. Understanding Anxiety in Your Child or Teen

ANXIETY IS NATURAL

Anxiety is a natural emotion that can be helpful in some circumstances. It can help motivate when needed or keep one from truly threatening situations (e.g., a dark alley at night). However, it leads to trouble when it interferes with a youth's ability to handle a situation (e.g., anxiety distracts them on a test).

AVOIDANCE HURTS MORE THAN IT HELPS

Behavioral avoidance, like procrastination, withdrawal, and escape, also seems natural, but it can be problematic when the youth turns down opportunities because they misinterpret or exaggerate problems in the situation (e.g., turning down a party invitation because they assume they won't know anyone there). Approaching challenging situations can be scary, but repeated exposure to challenges helps build confidence and skills.

LEARNING COPING SKILLS HELPS

While intense feelings are natural, youth can learn how to manage their anxiety or sad feelings. Your therapist will help your child identify the triggers (e.g., situations, people, thoughts) that prompt anxiety and teach them coping skills (active problem solving, brave approach behaviors, activity scheduling, and coping thoughts) that will help youth push through their distressing feelings and reach for desired goals.

PARENTS CAN HELP

Anxious youth bring their own anxiety to the table. It's not something you "did" to them. BUT there are ways you can react to your child that help them build their coping behaviors. This includes active listening, empathizing with their feelings, and encouraging them to focus on active goals.

COGNITIVE-BEHAVIORAL THERAPY CAN HELP

A substantial evidence base has demonstrated that psychological interventions can help reduce anxiety symptoms and improve youth functioning in school, family, and social domains. Strategies that focus on increasing behavioral engagement and more realistic, positive thinking are particularly helpful. In some cases, medication treatment may also provide benefit in combination with behavioral therapies.

HANDOUT 7. Understanding Depression in Your Child or Teen

DISTINGUISH SADNESS FROM DEPRESSION

Sadness is a natural feeling that all of us feel when hard things happen (e.g., a friend moves away, the loss of a loved one, arguments with friends) or when situations do not go our way (e.g., receiving a poor grade on a test, not getting selected for the school play or team, having a privilege restricted). Sadness should draw adult attention when it begins to interfere with a youth's typical functioning (sleeping, eating, socializing) or stops them from pursuing goals and activities they care about because of isolation, withdrawal, and inactivity.

AVOIDANCE HURTS MORE THAN IT HELPS

Behavioral avoidance can seem like a natural response to sad feelings. When a teen is feeling sad or lethargic, it might seem natural for them to withdraw to their room, ignore texts or calls from friends, not go to school or participate in activities. However, repeated avoidance creates a hard habit to break. It deprives the teen of opportunities (every missed soccer practice puts the child further behind) and chances to cope (to see that they can handle the challenge if confronted). Avoidance is also different from self-care or nurturance (e.g., being realistic about demands, taking planful breaks) that is restorative and promotes continued action.

LEARNING COPING SKILLS HELPS

Depression can feel intense (painful sadness, irritable anger) or deflating (low energy, weight on shoulders). Therapy helps the youth learn the skills to manage intense pain with emotion regulation skills and evaluation of negative self-critical thoughts. Decreased activities can also be countered with the scheduling of pleasant activities, active problem solving, and approach behaviors. Together, the youth will be taught to push through the temporary sadness that defines depression.

PARENTS CAN HELP

It is natural for caregivers to feel frustrated or scared by their own child's inactivity. They don't know how to help, motivate, or encourage their child. Therapy helps caregivers understand that a youth's depression is temporary and not necessarily a reflection of the child's innate personality or of the family. In these times, the youth needs a parent's active listening and support to encourage active approach behaviors.

(continued)

COGNITIVE-BEHAVIORAL THERAPY CAN HELP

A substantial evidence base has demonstrated that psychological interventions can help reduce depressive symptoms and improve youth functioning in school, family, and social domains. Strategies that focus on increasing behavioral engagement and more realistic, positive thinking are particularly helpful. In some cases, medication treatment may also provide benefit in combination with behavioral therapies.

HANDOUT 8. The Accommodation Spiral

Look at the example below to see how accommodation and indirect encouragement can send mixed messages:

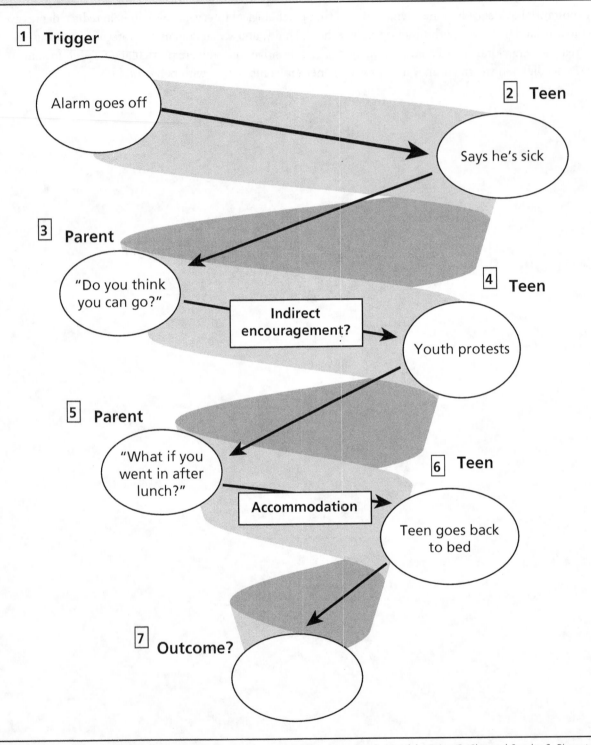

1 Trigger — Alarm goes off

2 Teen — Says he's sick

3 Parent — "Do you think you can go?"

Indirect encouragement?

4 Teen — Youth protests

5 Parent — "What if you went in after lunch?"

Accommodation

6 Teen — Teen goes back to bed

7 Outcome?

HANDOUT 9. The Passivity–Discouragement Spiral

Look at the example below to see how accommodation and passivity can reinforce discouragement:

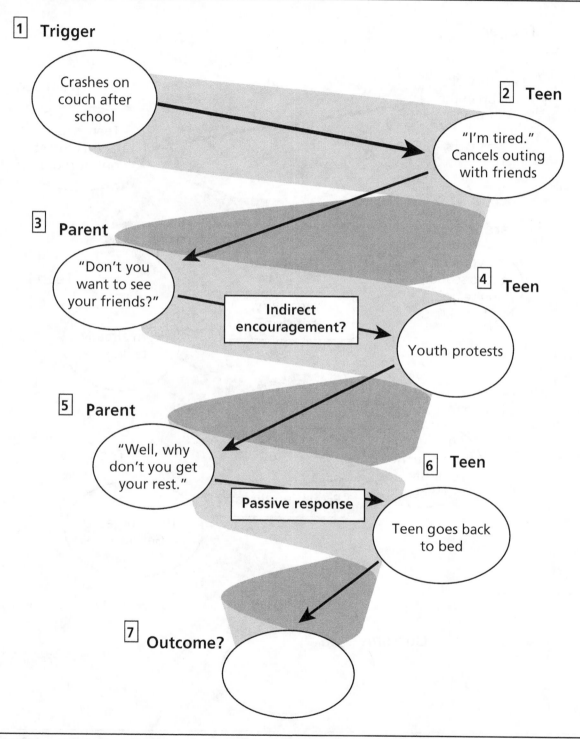

1 **Trigger**
Crashes on couch after school

2 **Teen**
"I'm tired." Cancels outing with friends

3 **Parent**
"Don't you want to see your friends?"

Indirect encouragement?

4 **Teen**
Youth protests

5 **Parent**
"Well, why don't you get your rest."

Passive response

6 **Teen**
Teen goes back to bed

7 **Outcome?**

HANDOUT 10. The Aggressive–Coercive Spiral

Look at the example below to see how negativity and criticism can escalate aggression and resistance:

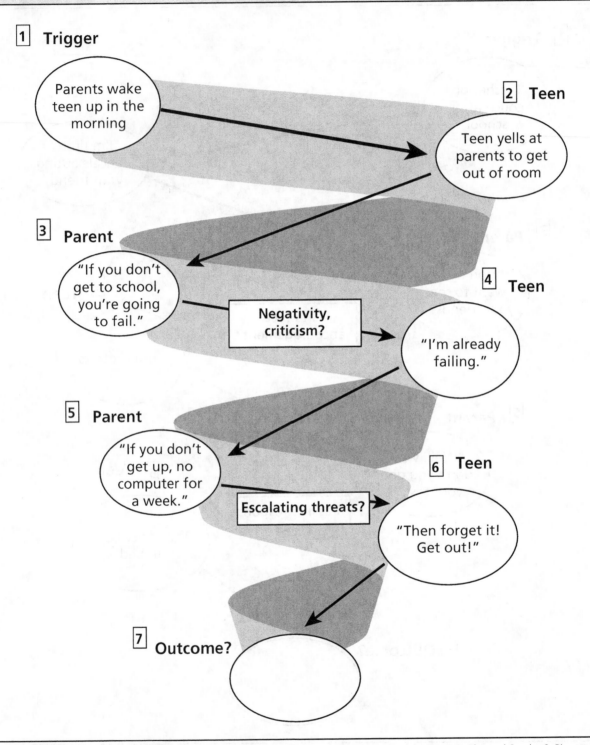

1 **Trigger**

Parents wake teen up in the morning

2 **Teen**

Teen yells at parents to get out of room

3 **Parent**

"If you don't get to school, you're going to fail."

Negativity, criticism?

4 **Teen**

"I'm already failing."

5 **Parent**

"If you don't get up, no computer for a week."

Escalating threats?

6 **Teen**

"Then forget it! Get out!"

7 **Outcome?**

HANDOUT 11. Common Parenting Traps and Helpful Solutions

COMMON PARENTING TRAPS

The Accommodation Spiral

Watching your child become upset is difficult. It's a natural instinct to try and soothe them. Some of the ways parents do that is by solving the child's problems for them or rescuing the child. Examples include ordering food for a child in a restaurant or writing a teacher for help when the child will not do so. These actions solve the problem in the short term but keep the child from learning how to do it themself.

The Passivity–Discouragement Spiral

When a child seems down, tired, or unmotivated, sometimes our instinct is to give into their mood: "They seem so tired; maybe it's just better they don't go to soccer practice." This approach might feel compassionate in the moment, but repeated permissions to withdraw and isolate reinforce the idea that withdrawal is the best solution to down moods.

The Aggressive–Coercive Spiral

Caregivers could be forgiven if long-standing anxiety or depression leads to frustration. This can lead to using anger or criticism to try and motivate kids and teens. However, shame and criticism (even if unintentional or well-meaning) make it less likely the youth will comply or feel motivated to problem-solve on their own.

COACH AND APPROACH TIPS THAT CAN HELP

Labeled Praise: Catch Them Being Good

Children and teens are keenly sensitive to caregiver signals and social attention. The best way to motivate change is to show your kids that you are noticing. Make sure you focus on the positive behaviors you want to reinforce because "negative" attention is just as potent as positive attention.

Empathize and Encourage

Caregivers can hone their motivational behaviors by focusing on two key concepts:

- **Empathize:** Make active listening a habit by practicing reflecting and amplifying what your child is saying. For example, "I know getting to school in the morning is really difficult for you."
- **Encourage:** Provide calm encouragement to move forward, emphasizing your child's ability to cope. For example, "And I know you can push yourself over this hump."

Remember to *STOP* after **three** empathize and encouragement statements to prevent falling into any of the parenting traps.

HANDOUT 12. Cognitive–Behavioral Model of Depression

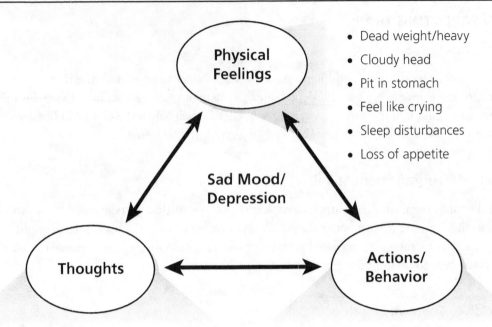

- Dead weight/heavy
- Cloudy head
- Pit in stomach
- Feel like crying
- Sleep disturbances
- Loss of appetite

Sad Mood/ Depression

Thoughts

- "I mess up everything."
- "Math is for losers."
- "Nothing will work out."
- "People don't ever help out."
- Unrealistically negative, pessimistic, self-critical, critical of others

Actions/ Behavior

- Withdrawal, isolation, pushing others away, avoidance of stressors, inability to get going
- Crying, sleeping, eating changes
- Attention and reassurance seeking, neediness
- Irritability, snapping, using sarcasm
- Rumination

HANDOUT 13. Facts about Depression

WHAT IS DEPRESSION?

Depression is a common psychological disorder that can impact a youth's social, emotional, academic, and family functioning. Identifying depression early is key to successful treatment, which can include psychological and medical interventions.

- Sadness is a familiar experience for all of us, but prolonged periods of depressed mood, sadness, and tearfulness might be the sign of more significant problems. In children and teens, sadness can mask itself as irritability and negativity.

- Loss of interest in things the youth used to care about is an important change in functioning that should be noticed.

- Sleep disruption, fatigue, change in eating habits, physical symptoms (e.g., headaches, stomachaches, muscle pain), and cognitive changes (poor concentration, slow thinking) are all common.

- Thoughts about suicide should not be dismissed as temporary or attention seeking. Any indication of suicidal ideation deserves further evaluation and potential safety planning.

- Common impairment includes significant impact on the youth's functioning in academics, friendships, and family. Self-care (e.g., maintaining sleeping, eating, and hygiene routines) often suffers as a result of depression.

- The youth does not suffer alone. Depression also impacts family and friends since the affected youth often manifests irritability, anger, and other negative/critical behaviors.

- Psychological interventions have been found to help. Cognitive-behavioral therapy (CBT) and interpersonal therapy have been found useful in individual and group formats.

- Medications can also help. Effective medical interventions, including selective serotonin reuptake inhibitors (SSRIs) such as fluoxetine and sertraline, have been found to be effective in treating depression alone and in combination with CBT.

HANDOUT 14. Habituation Curve

This handout illustrates the effect of rescue/escape on learning in the case of depression. Procrastination and escape are negatively reinforced by the tension that is created by breaking inertia and the frustration caused by the call for sustained effort. Escape prevents the youth from experiencing natural habituation to distress or learning they can tolerate the frustration.

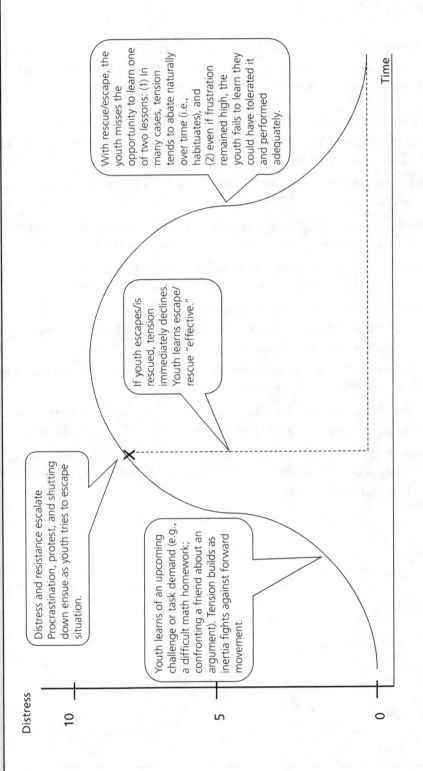

HANDOUT 15. Facts about Suicide and Self–Injurious Thoughts and Behaviors

WHAT ARE SUICIDE AND NONSUICIDAL SELF-INJURY?

Each year about 18% of teens in the United States seriously consider suicide and 9% attempt to kill themselves. Nonsuicidal self-injury, in which one causes bodily harm to themself without an explicit wish to die, has been reported in from 13–45% of teens.

- **Suicidal ideation (SI)** refers to thoughts about killing oneself. Suicidal ideation is characterized by negative, hopeless, and self-critical thinking and can include methods and plans for harming oneself.

- **Suicidal behaviors (suicide attempts, SA)** are actions a youth takes to harm themself that can lead to an injury whereby the youth wants to die. Common methods that teens use in a suicide attempt include prescription and nonprescription drug overdose, firearms, and suffocation/hanging.

- **Nonsuicidal self-injuries (NSSIs)** are self-inflicted injuries caused by a youth when there is no expressed wish to die. These include cuts, scratches, burns, and banging/hitting oneself. A youth might engage in nonsuicidal self-injuries to make themself feel better or stop feeling sadness, anxiety, or anger.

- **Who is at risk for suicide?** More girls attempt suicide, but more boys complete suicide. A prior suicide attempt increases the chances of ultimately completing suicide. Family history of suicide, drug or alcohol abuse, and access to firearms are key risk factors. Sexual minority youth are a particularly vulnerable group, with teens identifying as lesbian, gay, or bisexual reaching 3 times the risk for suicidality; nearly half of trans men and women report a prior attempt.

- **It is OK to ask questions about suicide?** Asking about suicide and self-harm does not increase the chances a youth will make a suicide attempt or experience intense SI. Thus, open communication and education are critical. However, evidence does show that graphic/visual depictions of suicide in the media or recent attempts in the youth's social network can trigger intensified SI. Caregivers should monitor vulnerable youth when such events occur.

- **Warning signs.** Please be alert if a youth shows any of the following signs of increased SI: statements about death or the desire to die; increased and sudden social isolation; giving away personal possessions; intensification of depressed mood, hopelessness, and apathy. Thoughts about suicide should not be dismissed as temporary or attention seeking. Any indication of suicidal ideation deserves further evaluation and potential safety planning.

- **How should we respond?** While suicidal ideation can be severe and frightening, it can also be fleeting. One of the most effective strategies to manage ideation and prevent suicide attempts is to enact short-term *safety planning* that includes: (1) recognizing the signs of SI, (2) accessing internal coping skills and interpersonal supports, and (3) securing the home by cutting off methods that could be used for harm (e.g., medications, firearms, rope, sharps).

- **Cognitive-behavioral therapy (CBT) can help.** Suicidal and nonsuicidal self-injury commonly co-occur in the context of depression and anxiety disorders. The coping skills a therapist teaches can help a youth learn how to manage intense emotions and make effective change in their life for long-term prevention.

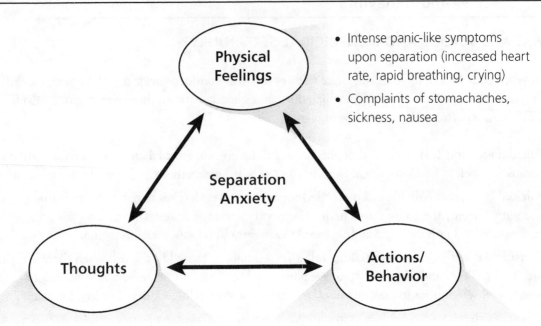

Physical Feelings

- Intense panic-like symptoms upon separation (increased heart rate, rapid breathing, crying)
- Complaints of stomachaches, sickness, nausea

Separation Anxiety

Thoughts

Actions/ Behavior

- "My parents will get into an accident."
- "A robber will break in and steal me."
- "I *can't* sleep on my own."
- Worry about harm to self or parent upon separation, or being able to handle self or problems when separated.

- Clinging behavior, reassurance, and attention seeking
- Protests, arguments, complaints, oppositionality
- Refusal to separate at home, school, or elsewhere

HANDOUT 17. Habituation Curve

This handout illustrates the effect of rescue/escape on learning in the case of a separation anxious youth. Rescue/escape is negatively reinforced by its immediate impact on distress reduction. The youth fails to experience natural habituation of distress and fails to learn distress tolerance.

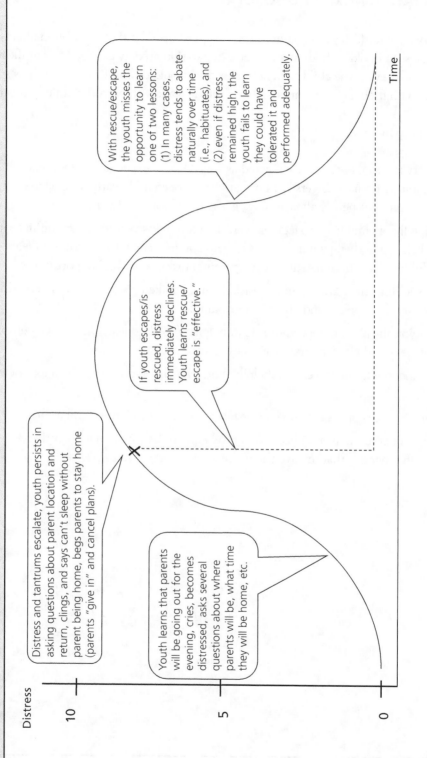

HANDOUT 18. Facts about Separation Anxiety

WHAT IS SEPARATION ANXIETY DISORDER?

Separation anxiety disorder (SEP) is a common psychological disorder that most often affects younger children but can be seen in older children and teens. Separation anxiety can lead to significant conflict within the family and prevent the child from activities they would ordinarily enjoy, such as sports, clubs, and spending time with friends. Interventions often include work with both the child and caregivers.

Other features to keep in mind:

- Some anxiety is normal and to be expected as a child faces expectations for greater independence. Fear of separating from caregivers is a normative part of a child's early development and may come about due to transient new challenges (e.g., going to school or being in a new setting)

- Treatment will not eliminate anxiety, or even the natural instinct to prefer familiar settings. Cognitive-behavioral therapy (CBT) aims to help children cope with separation fears so they do not hold the children back from meeting developmental tasks, goals, and opportunities.

- Characteristic thoughts, actions, and physical feelings make up separation anxiety. Knowing these helps demystify the problem and offers goals to aim for.

- Caregivers typically play an important role in helping the child learn new brave behaviors, including the development of their own anxiety management skills.

- Practice is essential for improvement: helping both the child and caregivers adopt new thinking and action patterns.

- Rewarding efforts to cope is essential, as new behaviors will feel unnatural at first.

- Psychological interventions have been found to help. Studies show that cognitive-behavioral therapy, particularly in programs that involve the parents and caregivers, is useful.

HANDOUT 19. Cognitive–Behavioral Model of Social Anxiety

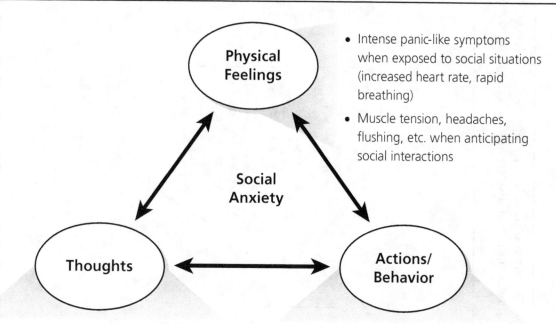

- "I'm going to mess up."
- "Everyone will see how bad I am."
- "I'll always be known as a loser."
- Fear of evaluation, embarrassment, and the consequences of poor performance

- Intense panic-like symptoms when exposed to social situations (increased heart rate, rapid breathing)
- Muscle tension, headaches, flushing, etc. when anticipating social interactions

- Avoidance/refusal/escape of social activities (parties, get-togethers) or demands (classwork, extracurriculars)
- Disruption in performance (self-presentation, awkward social skills)

HANDOUT 20. Habituation Curve

This handout illustrates the effect of escape on learning in the case of a socially anxious youth. Escape is negatively reinforced by its immediate impact on distress reduction. The youth fails to experience natural habituation of distress and fails to learn distress tolerance.

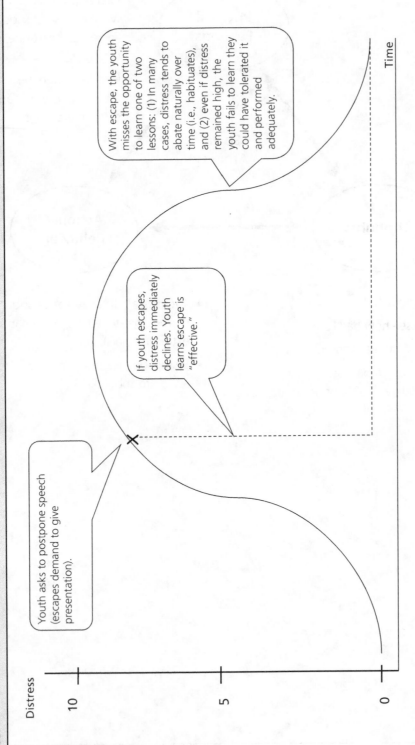

HANDOUT 21. Facts about Social Anxiety

WHAT IS SOCIAL ANXIETY DISORDER?

Social anxiety disorder (SAD) is a common psychological disorder most often identified in youth between the ages of 10 and 13 years. It is marked by intense fear and anxiety in social situations where the youth fears evaluation from, or embarrassment in front of, others. Some anxiety is normal and expected in novel social or performance situations; social anxiety disorder reflects greater difficulty than would be expected for a youth of the same age.

Other features include:

- Shyness is not problematic, but it may become so if it inhibits a youth from engaging in developmental tasks.

- Youth will vary in socialization goals and interests. Some youth will need fewer friends and activities than others and goals can be made around finding key social connections and participation opportunities.

- Treatment will not change anyone's basic personality or temperament. If the youth is naturally more introverted, it is likely they will retain elements of that.

- Cognitive-behavioral therapy (CBT) aims to help such teens manage anxiety so as to not hold themselves back from desired goals, values, experiences, and opportunities.

- Characteristic thoughts (e.g., mind reading, worrying about being evaluated), actions (e.g., avoiding social situations), and physical feelings (e.g., heart racing, blushing) make up social anxiety. Knowing these helps demystify the problem and highlight areas of intervention goals to practice.

- Practice is essential for improvement, both for making new social skills more natural, but also to gather evidence that contradicts fearful assumptions and predictions.

- Caregivers can play an important role in reinforcing skills by arranging plenty of opportunities for practice, and by taking an "empathize and encourage" stance.

- Rewarding efforts to cope is essential, as new behaviors will feel unnatural at first.

HANDOUT 22. Cognitive–Behavioral Model of Generalized Anxiety Disorder

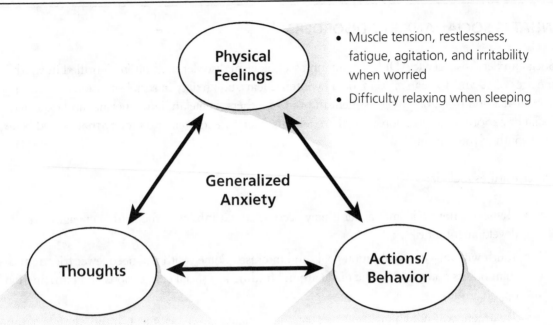

- Muscle tension, restlessness, fatigue, agitation, and irritability when worried
- Difficulty relaxing when sleeping

- Persistent "what if's . . . "
- "Will I be prepared? Safe?"
- "What happens if things go wrong?"
- "I won't be able to recover..."
- Self-imposed perfectionism, rigid sets of rules, worries about self, family, school, health, etc.

- Worry, rumination
- Avoidance, procrastination in managing demands, hassles, or addressing stressors
- Perfectionism, rigidity
- Attention and reassurance seeking, neediness

HANDOUT 23. Habituation Curve

This handout illustrates the effect of escape on learning in the case of GAD in youth. Escape is negatively reinforced by its immediate impact on distress reduction. The youth fails to experience natural habituation of distress and fails to learn distress tolerance.

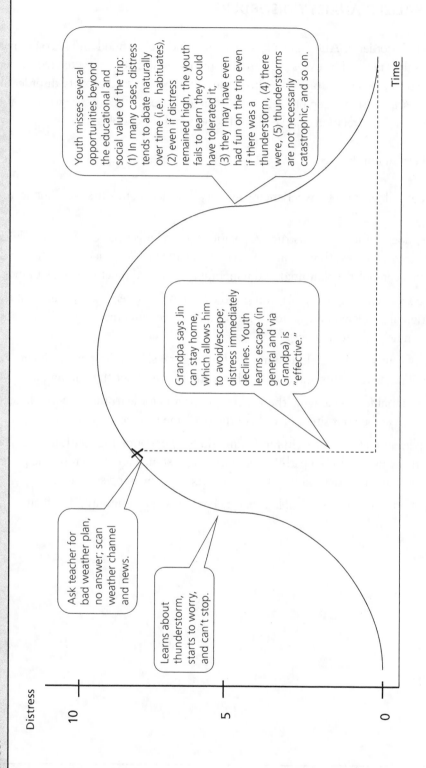

Youth misses several opportunities beyond the educational and social value of the trip: (1) In many cases, distress tends to abate naturally over time (i.e., habituates), (2) even if distress remained high, the youth fails to learn they could have tolerated it, (3) they may have even had fun on the trip even if there was a thunderstorm, (4) there were, (5) thunderstorms are not necessarily catastrophic, and so on.

Grandpa says Jin can stay home, which allows him to avoid/escape; distress immediately declines. Youth learns escape (in general and via Grandpa) is "effective."

Ask teacher for bad weather plan, no answer; scan weather channel and news.

Learns about thunderstorm, starts to worry, and can't stop.

Distress

10

5

0

Time

HANDOUT 24. Facts about Worriers

WHAT IS GENERALIZED ANXIETY DISORDER?

Generalized Anxiety Disorder (GAD) begins to surface in middle childhood and becomes more prominent in the teenage years. It is marked by excessive and uncontrollable worries characterized by numerous "what if" statements and continuous reassurance seeking. Youth with generalized anxiety disorder also tend to report significant muscle tension, sleep problems, and overall distress. The intense worry can interfere with academic performance, social relations, and completing personal or school goals.

Other features to keep in mind:

- Worry is a natural reaction to experiencing anxiety. It reflects one's first attempt at "solving" a problem.
- When worry does not lead to constructive solutions, it no longer serves problem-solving functions. Rather, it reflects a process that is aimed at seeking artificial safety via superstitious beliefs (e.g., perfectionistic, compulsive planning) and temporary emotional relief (e.g., reassurance seeking).
- Reassurance seeking, compulsive planning, and escape provide temporary relief, but they do not solve the original problem and lead to longer-term negative outcomes (e.g., failure to build skills, missing out on helpful experiences).
- The nature of youth worries reflects multiple thinking traps, including overestimates of the occurrence of negative events and catastrophic assumptions about the outcomes.
- Practice is essential for challenging these assumptions and for learning how to tolerate the anxiety that comes with ambiguous situations where the outcome is uncertain.
- Caregivers play an important role in reinforcing skills by encouraging youth to face challenges independently by taking an "empathize and encourage" stance and "catching the positive" when they effectively cope and approach, rather than avoid anxiety-provoking situations.
- Rewarding efforts to cope is essential, as new behaviors will feel unnatural at first.

HANDOUT 25. Facts about School Refusal in Children and Teens

WHAT IS SCHOOL REFUSAL?

A substantial number of middle schoolers (14%) and high schoolers (21%) miss 10% of school days a year or more, qualifying for chronic absenteeism, according to the U.S. Department of Education. School refusal (SR) refers to absenteeism that stems from youth anxiety, depression, and emotion dysregulation. Caregivers are generally aware of the student's absenteeism and the youth shows little evidence of other behavioral problems (such as serious rule breaking, physical altercations at school). School refusal tends to intensify during transitions to new schools, new school years, and after breaks.

What does school refusal look like? It includes any school routine disruption, including:

- Initial tardiness at beginning of day.
- Partial or full absences from school day.
- Frequent trips to school nurse or counselor offices.
- School attendance, but youth exhibits significant dread and distress in school.
- Family fights and arguments centering around school issues.

Why does my child have trouble going to school?

Attendance problems are related to what we call "negative affect," an overall, diffuse feeling of dread, sadness, or anxiety that surfaces when the youth approaches or thinks about going to school. It feels unexplainable to the child or teen. Other ways to describe this are:

- Anxiety, school performance, social anxiety
- Panic/dread when arriving at school, separation from home or loved ones
- Depressed mood, dysphoria, hopelessness about school situation

What is not school refusal?

Poor school attendance can occur due to the following issues, but these are <u>NOT</u> considered school refusal:

- Absences where teen is engaging in illegal or delinquent behaviors
- School suspension for conduct, aggression, or bullying other peers
- Absences are primarily linked to academic problems or school grades

(continued)

Cognitive-behavioral therapy (CBT) can help.

Your cognitive-behavioral therapist is teaching your child coping skills that can help them learn how to manage intense emotions and make effective change in their life for long-term prevention. Skills like problem solving, developing coping thoughts, behavioral activation, and distress tolerance can help your youth manage the intense negative affect underlying school refusal.

Parents play an important role.

- Parents do not "cause" school refusal. But there are certain messages that we subtly send that can either minimize attendance problems or discourage the youth from trying. Your therapist will help you identify some of those patterns.
- Cognitive-behavioral therapy will help parents gain confidence in structuring a school reentry plan by teaching skills like "empathize and encourage," and building meaningful reward plans.

HANDOUT 26. Cognitive–Behavioral Model of School Refusal Behavior

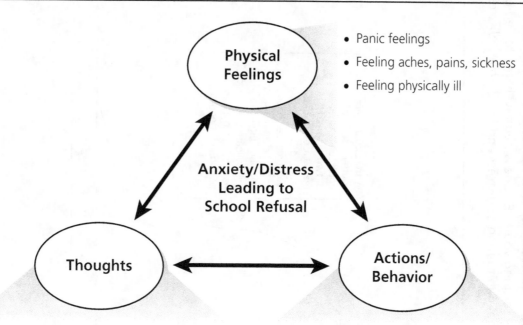

- Panic feelings
- Feeling aches, pains, sickness
- Feeling physically ill

Physical Feelings

Anxiety/Distress Leading to School Refusal

Thoughts

Actions/ Behavior

- "School's too hard."
- "The kids and teachers are mean to me."
- "I can't handle it."
- "What will happen at home if I leave?"
- "Why bother—no one cares."

- Resisting, delaying, protesting
- Avoiding, escaping
- Arguing, fighting
- Begging, reassurance seeking

HANDOUT 27. Habituation Curve

This handout illustrates the effect of escape on learning in the case of a school refusing youth. Escape is negatively reinforced by its immediate impact on distress reduction. The youth fails to experience natural habituation of distress and fails to learn distress tolerance.

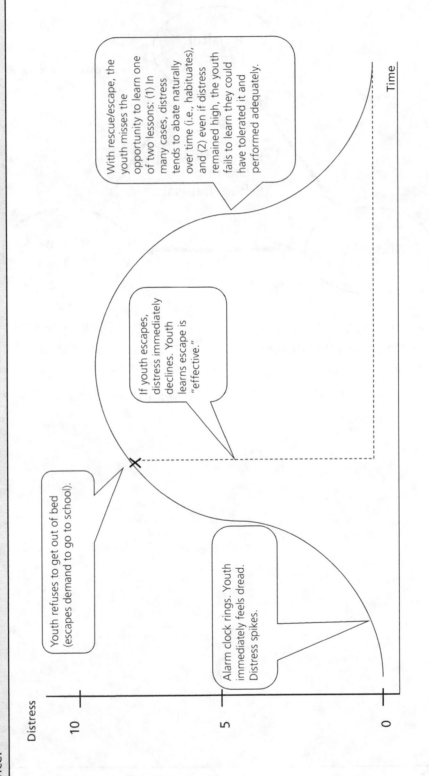

WORKSHEET 1. Trigger and Response

Tell us about your triggers and how you reacted. Describe your feelings, what you did (action), what happened right away (immediate outcome), and then what happened later (long-term outcome).

```
┌─────────────┐      ┌──────────────────┐      ┌──────────────┐
│ Antecedent  │ ───▶ │   Behavioral and │ ───▶ │ Consequences │
│             │      │ Emotional Response│      │              │
└─────────────┘      └──────────────────┘      └──────────────┘
```

Trigger	Feeling (emotional response)	Action (behavioral response)	Immediate Results (What keeps it going?)	Long-Term Results (What gets you in trouble?)
Example: I had to give a speech in class.	Fear, panic	Asked my teacher if I could go to nurse's office—feeling sick.	Teacher said "yes." Huge relief!	Now I have to do the speech another time. Teacher was annoyed.

WORKSHEET 2. Thoughts, Feelings, and Actions Tracker

What kind of thoughts do you have when feeling sad, anxious, or distressed? How do you act when thinking that way? What happens (outcome) from thinking that way?

Trigger	Feeling	Thought	Action	Outcome?
Example: My parents fought about my bad grades.	Sadness	"I'm causing my parents to fight with each other."	Go to my room, put in my earbuds.	Feeling lonely, isolated. Avoid my parents.

WORKSHEET 3. Change Plan

> The therapist and youth can fill this out together (use help from parents as needed) to discuss what they would like to get out of their collaborative work. Using this worksheet, try to identify the youth's goals, and the challenges and supports that are needed to reach those goals.

1) The changes I want to make are:

> (e.g., decrease anxiety/sad mood, improve grades, make more friends, do more fun activities)

2) The most important reasons I want to make these changes are:

> (e.g., my happiness, my family, my social life, my grades)

3) The steps I plan to take in changing are:

> (e.g., come to sessions, try skills at home, practice)

Things that could interfere with the change plan:

4) How much trouble do you think you'll have getting to session each week (e.g., scheduling)?

	0	1	2	3	4
	Not at all				Very Much

> To overcome this, I will: (e.g., talk to my teacher)

(continued)

5) How much do you think things will get in the way of you practicing the skills we go over here at home?

0	1	2	3	4
Not at all				Very Much

To overcome this, I will: (e.g., use reminders to self to practice each day)

6) How much do you feel as if coming to session each week might be too much work?

0	1	2	3	4
Not at all				Very Much

To overcome this, I will: (e.g., talk to my group leaders, make a deal with myself to work hard now for a better future)

7) How much do you feel as if using these skills at home will be too much work?

0	1	2	3	4
Not at all				Very Much

To overcome this, I will: (e.g., ask parents for help, make a deal with myself to work hard now for a better future)

8) How much do you feel that a lack of support from others will be a problem for you in using the skills we practice here at home?

0	1	2	3	4
Not at all				Very Much

Person: (e.g., parents, friends, group leaders)

Possible ways to help: (e.g., share work, ask group leaders, parents, or friends for more support)

(continued)

9) How much do you feel as if these skills will work at home?

0   1   2   3   4

Not at all   Very Much

To overcome this, I will: (e.g., remember it takes time and practice, talk to my group leaders)

10) Overall, how comfortable do you think you'll feel practicing these skills with us in session?

0   1   2   3   4

Not at all   Very Much

To overcome this, I will: (e.g., practice until I feel more comfortable)

11) How comfortable do you think you'll feel practicing these skills at home?

0   1   2   3   4

Not at all   Very Much

To overcome this, I will: (e.g., practice until I feel more comfortable)

12) How likely do you think it is that you will continue for the entire treatment?

0   1   2   3   4

Not at all   Very Much

To overcome this, I will: (e.g., remember initial treatment goal and make sure I meet it)

WORKSHEET 4. Feelings Thermometer

Pick a feeling to describe (e.g., sadness, nervousness, anger). Then try to think about that feeling on a 0–10 scale. What words would you use to describe each rating? Can you remember a time when you've felt that way?

What feeling you are rating:

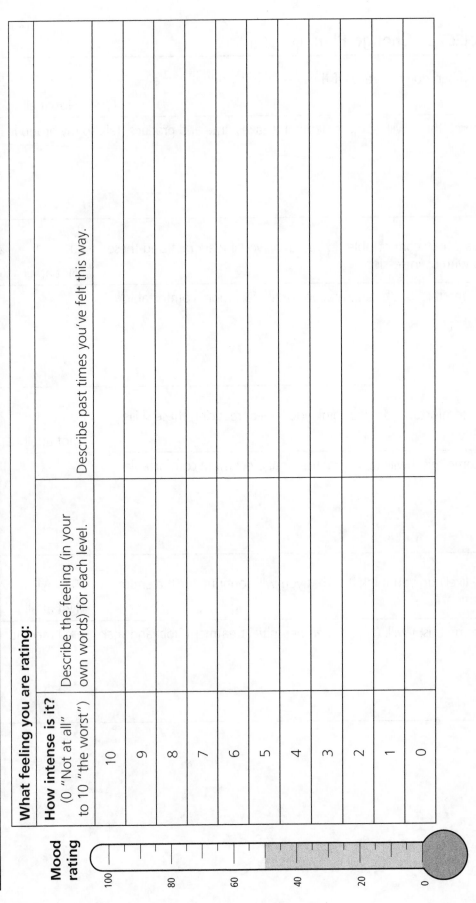

Mood rating	How intense is it? (0 "Not at all" to 10 "the worst")	Describe the feeling (in your own words) for each level.	Describe past times you've felt this way.
100	10		
80	9		
	8		
60	7		
	6		
	5		
40	4		
	3		
20	2		
	1		
0	0		

378

WORKSHEET 5. Thinking Traps Tracker

What thinking traps do you fall into when feeling sad, anxious, or distressed? For each situation, describe and rate how you feel. Describe your automatic thought (the first thought that comes into your head). What thinking trap might you be falling into? How does that make you feel (the result)?

Trigger	Feeling (rate 0–10: "not at all" to "excruciating")	Thought	Thinking Trap	Result?
Example: I hear the alarm go off on the day of a big test.	Fear, panic (7)	"I'm not ready for the test!" "This will kill my grade!"	Fortune-telling, catastrophizing	Felt worse (9)

379

WORKSHEET 6. *In Vivo* Exposure/Behavioral Experiment

Complete this worksheet with the youth as you are preparing for a behavioral experiment.

1. Situation (What's the situation?):

2. Feelings: **Distress Rating:** _____

3. Anxious/Negative Thoughts: **Thinking Traps (See list below.)**

Thinking Traps: mind reading, fortune-telling, catastrophizing, jumping to conclusions, what if's, discounting the positives, looking for the negatives, overgeneralizing, all-or-nothing thinking, should statements, taking things too personally, blaming.

4. Coping Thoughts (How do you respond to your anxious thoughts?):

Challenge Questions: Do I know for certain that _____? Am I 100% sure that _____? What evidence do I have that _____? What is the worst that could happen? How bad is that? Do I have a crystal ball?

5. Achievable Behavioral Goals (What do you want to accomplish?):

Goal	Accomplished?
a.	
b.	
c.	

6. Rewards:

Reward	Earned?
a.	
b.	
c.	

WORKSHEET 7. Coping Reminders Success Summary

You have learned a lot of great skills during our work together. Take a moment to think through the strategies that work best for you.

Key Negative Thoughts to Watch For:

1.

2.

3.

My Thinking Traps:

1.

2.

3.

My Key Coping Thoughts:

1.

2.

3.

People Who Can Help Me:

1.

2.

3.

Actions and Behaviors That Help Me:

1.

2.

3.

I Remember When I Struggled with _____.

What Helped Me Most Was:

What I Need to Keep Practicing:

My Therapy Take-Home Message:

What Is a Sign That I May Want to Check In:

WORKSHEET 8. Coordination Checklist: Consulting with a Prescribing Physician

Pre-referral	
About Physician	
	Full name (and how the providers would like to be addressed)
	Years of practice (with kids)?
	Subspecialty in psychiatry or otherwise (addiction, forensics, etc.)?
	Is referral for psychopharmacology alone or in conjunction with psychotherapy? You want to be clear that the referral is for psychopharmacological evaluation.
	Office location
	Time/day availability
	Pricing for intake and follow-up sessions
	Any commercial or other health insurance that is accepted
	Types of cases with whom they will not work (eating disorder, suicidal, self-harm, etc.)
	Preferred method of communication
	Offer to present the patient (briefly) and see if the provider thinks they may be a good fit.
	Be prepared to answer any of the above questions about yourself.
About Patient	
	Consent/release of information signed by caregiver?
	General patient information and family demographics
	Chief complaint
	History of presenting disorder
	Course/progression of symptoms
	Pertinent past history; developmental, family, and social history; notable medical history
	Assessment: highlights and diagnosis, main areas of impairment
	Cognitive-behavioral case formulation
	Course of current psychotherapeutic treatment
	Reason for psychopharmacological consultation at this time
	Expectation from the consultation
	Notable patient and family concerns communicated to therapist

(continued)

Post-referral	
	Ask for provider's formulation.
	Obtain specific recommendations.
	Understand potential side effects and benefits of offered treatment (or lack of).
	Further medical work up recommended?
	Other diagnostic consideration that may require additional evaluations
	In case of medication recommendation, ask for titration schedule and end goals.
	Collaboration schedule: When would the therapist like to be contacted (increased risk, change in medications, etc.)?
	When would the prescribing psychiatrist like to be contacted?

WORKSHEET 9. Parent–Child Chain Analysis

Can you identify any parenting traps? What alternatives could you try?

	Action/Response	Parenting Trap	Potential Solution or Skills to Use?
Prompting Event			
Child Action			
Parent Response			
Child Reaction			
Parent Response			
Conflict/Problem Behavior			
Outcome 1 (What happened?)			
Outcome 2			
Outcome 3			

WORKSHEET 10. Daily Renewable Rewards Chart

Brainstorm step-by-step goals and rewards to go with each level. Then track success!

Theme:

Goals (incremental levels)	Reward (incremental levels)	Sun	Mon	Tue	Wed	Thu	Fri	Sat	# of Days Achieved

WORKSHEET 11. Goals Tracker

Work with your therapist to brainstorm possible specific, meaningful, and achievable goals. Think through what outcomes you expect to see. And then, keep track of how your child does each week.

Parent Goals	Desired Outcomes	Week 1	Week 2	Week 3	Week 4	Week 5
Example: Improve sad mood; enjoy life more.	Rate sad mood (0–10). Rate weekly enjoyment (0–10).	Sad: 9 Joy: 0				

Youth Goals	Desired Outcomes	Week 1	Week 2	Week 3	Week 4	Week 5
Example: Looked after my little sister.						

WORKSHEET 12. Activity Tracker

Sometimes we don't even know when we're getting stuck. Over the next week, track your activities, mood, and important events that happen each day! Then rate your mood from 0 to 10:

0 = "The worst mood I've ever felt." **5** = "I'm feeling OK but not great." **10** = "The best I've ever felt."

Example:

Looked after my little sister.
7

	Monday	Tuesday	Wednesday	Thursday	Friday	Saturday	Sunday
Morning							
Lunch							
Afternoon							
After school/late afternoon							
Evening							

Week of: _____

387

WORKSHEET 13. Getting Active and Building Mastery

We all feel down and get stuck sometimes. When you feel stuck, bored, disengaged, or depressed, think up active, pleasant, or mastery activities to get un-stuck:

- Physical activation: Try physical or mental exercise or exertion.
- Pleasant activities: Try anything that you find fun and pleasant.
- Mastery exercises: Try something that helps you build a skill.
- Problem-solve: Brainstorm solutions to solve the problem, using problem-solving STEPS.

List Situations That Get You Stuck (lead to avoidance, withdrawal, procrastination, quitting, isolation)	Proactive Pleasant, Mastery, or Problem-Solving Options

WORKSHEET 14. Goals and Rewards Chart

Whenever we're trying new skills, we should reward ourselves for making the effort. First, brainstorm achievable, meaningful goals. Then decide how you would reward yourself for each accomplishment.

Goals I Can Match Myself

	Reward	M	T	W	TR	F	Sat	Sun	# of Days Achieved

Goals I Need Others' Help for

	Reward	M	T	W	TR	F	Sat	Sun	# of Days Achieved

389

WORKSHEET 15. Problem–Solving STEPS

To solve problems, take these steps: say what the problem is, think of solutions, examine each solution, pick one solution and try it, and see if it worked!

Say What the Problem Is:

| Think of Solutions | Examine Each Solution | | Rank |
	Pros	Cons	
1.			
2.			
3.			
4.			
5.			
6.			
7.			
8.			
9.			
10.			

Pick One Solution and Try It:

WORKSHEET 16. Coping Thoughts Tracker

Brainstorm coping thoughts that could respond to your thinking trap! Try and come up with coping statements that are more realistic and ask, "How am I not seeing the whole picture?"

Trigger	Thought	Thinking Trap	Coping Thought	Result?

WORKSHEET 17. Suicidal Risk Heuristic: Severity, History, Intent, Plan (SHIP)

Client Name:	Date:

Severity	
Frequency and duration	
Intensity	

History	
Chronicity and history of SI	
NSSI history	
SA history	
Impulsive/risk behaviors	
Chronic stressors/ risk factors	

(continued)

Intent	
Stated or inferred intent	
Preparatory acts	

Plan	
Planned methods	
Access to methods	

WORKSHEET 18. Acute Suicide Risk Algorithm

Circle any endorsed risk indicators to determine level of acute risk.

☐ Low: Youth may not need a safety plan.

☐ Moderate and High Risk: Youth will routinely require some elements of safety planning.

☐ Severe Risk and some High Risk: Therapist should be prepared to alert mobile response or direct youth to emergency room.

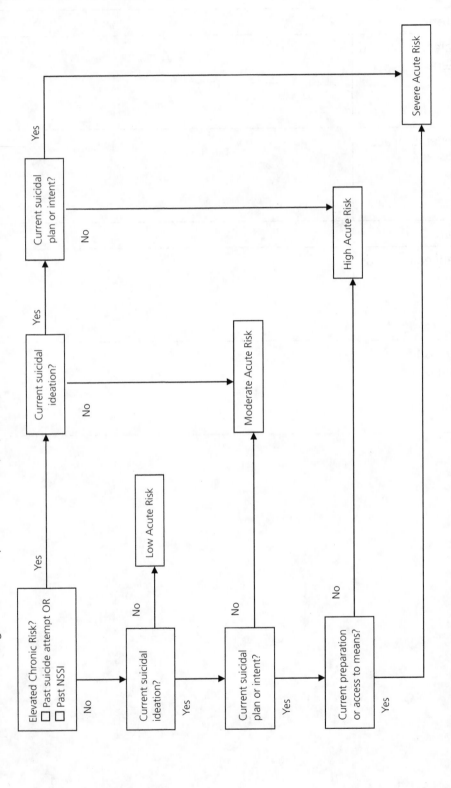

WORKSHEET 19. Assessment of Chronic Risk in Youth (ACRY)

Patient Name: _____   Date Completed: _____

Primary Therapist: _____   Date Reviewed: _____

Psychiatrist (Y/N): _____

Other Team Provider(s): _____

☐ Baseline (past 6 months)

☐ Follow-up (past 3 months)

RISK FACTOR	Current		Lifetime		COMMENTS
	YES	NO	YES	NO	
Suicide Attempt *If yes in past 2 years →* **HIGH**	Date(s): # attempts: Med attn:		Date(s): # attempts: Med attn:		
Assaultive/Violent Behavior *If yes past 2 months and caused bodily harm and led to arrest/ hospitalization → HIGH*					
Suicidal Ideation	Passive/Active Intent/Plan		Passive/Active Intent/Plan		
Suicidal Behaviors					
Homicidal Ideation	Passive/Active Intent/Plan		Passive/Active Intent/Plan		
Psychiatric Hospitalizations	#:		#:		
Psychiatric Emergency Room Visits	#:		#:		
Nonsuicidal Self-Injurious Behaviors	Med attn?		Med attn?		
High-Risk Behaviors					

(continued)

From Dackis, Eisenberg, Mowrey, and Pimentel (2021). For permission to reproduce this worksheet, contact Taylor & Francis.

RISK FACTOR	Current		Lifetime		COMMENTS
	YES	NO	YES	NO	
Substance/Alcohol Use					
Treatment Noncompliance					
Medical Condition/ Complications					
Perceived Burden to Others					
Child Maltreatment/ Trauma					
Impulsivity	Low/Mod/High		Low/Mod/High		
Other					

PROTECTIVE FACTORS

☐ Family cohesion, connectedness
☐ Perceived parental involvement
☐ Involvement of other caring adult/teacher
☐ School connectedness, positive feelings toward
☐ School safety
☐ Academic achievement
☐ Social support/positive friendships

☐ Verbal, cooperative/engaged in treatment
☐ Attendance/engagement in sports/religion
☐ Reasons for living
☐ Restricted access to means
☐ Self-esteem

DESIGNATE OVERALL RISK

Low Risk	Moderate Risk	High Risk

(continued)

Instructions/Glossary

- <u>Date Reviewed</u> = Baseline refers to the first time completing based on past 6 months; follow-up every 3 months.

- <u>Suicide Attempt</u> = Nonfatal self-directed potentially injurious behavior with any intent to die. State number of attempts, dates, whether medical attention needed. **If SA over the past 2 years** → <u>designate "high risk"</u>

- <u>Assaultive/Violent Behavior</u> = Any act of inflicting physical harm (intentional or reckless) toward another; **If caused bodily harm to another in past 2 months AND resulted in patient arrest/hospitalization** → **designate "high risk"**

- <u>Suicidal Ideation</u> = Thoughts or images related to killing oneself; circle if SI was passive, active, included intent/plan

- Intent: evidence that the individual intended to kill oneself, that death was likely outcome

- Plan: thought specifically or behaviorally made plans for how to kill oneself

- <u>Suicidal Behaviors</u> = Any communication of suicide to others, behaviors leading others to believe suicide may occur, preparatory behaviors (e.g., collecting pills, writing notes stating suicidal thoughts)

- <u>Homicidal Ideation</u> = Any thoughts or images related to killing oneself; circle whether HI was passive and/or active, and/or included intent and/or plan (see above for definitions)

- <u>Psychiatric Hospitalizations</u> = Psychiatric inpatient hospitalizations OR medical inpatient hospitalizations occurring due to psychiatric presenting concerns (e.g., medical stabilization for eating disorder, after SA); mark number

- <u>Psychiatric ER Visits</u> = Emergency room/observation visits (only for psychiatric reasons), mark number

- <u>NSSI Behaviors</u> = Intentional self-directed harm to the surface of one's body that results in injury or potential for injury to oneself, with no conscious intention to die. Note whether medical attention was needed

- <u>High-Risk Behaviors</u> = Health risk behaviors including eating disorder behaviors (restriction, purging, binging), risky sexual behaviors (prostitution, unprotected sex), truancy, running away, weapon carrying, specify behavior type

- <u>Substance/Alcohol Use</u> = Any use of substances that are not prescribed; consider and document frequency of use, which substances under comments

- <u>Treatment Noncompliance</u> = Inconsistent or nonattendance of therapy, group, and/or psychiatry appointments, inappropriate/inconsistent pager use, medication noncompliance, refusal to complete UTox

- <u>Medical Condition</u> = Any diagnosis/exacerbation that would contribute to risk; consider the following categories as increasing risk: cardiovascular, allergy/asthma, headaches, back/neck pain, dermatological conditions

- <u>Perceived Burden</u> = Patient has endorsed feeling like a burden to others verbally or on self-report measures

- <u>Child Maltreatment/Trauma</u> = **Physical neglect** refers to failure to provide for the child's basic physical needs and also includes lack of supervision, moral–legal neglect, and educational neglect; **Emotional maltreatment** involves extreme thwarting of children's basic emotional needs for psychological safety and security; **Physical abuse** involves nonaccidental physical injury to the child resulting in bruises, welts, burns, choking, and broken bones. **Sexual abuse** involves attempted or actual sexual contact between the child and caregiver/adult for purposes of the caregiver/adult's sexual satisfaction or financial benefit. Also include other reported traumas unrelated to maltreatment.

- <u>Impulsivity</u> = Choose from following anchors: **Low:** patient frequently exhibits effective behavioral control; **Moderate:** occasionally exhibits effective behavioral control; **High:** infrequently exhibits effective behavioral control

- <u>Other</u> = Consider other factors (e.g., family history of suicide/violence, gang membership, bullying, minority status, significant COVID-related stress, etc.)

- Check off any protective factors; **Designate overall chronic risk by circling either low, moderate, or high risk.**

WORKSHEET 20. Safety Plan

> Therapist and client (and caregiver when appropriate) work together to clarify warning signs that the youth might experience elevated self-harm thoughts; then, they brainstorm coping strategies to help manage thoughts and feelings and prevent harm.

Step 1: Warning signs
1.
2.
3.

Step 2: Internal coping strategies: things I can do to distract myself without contacting anyone
1.
2.
3.

Step 3: Social situations and people who can help to distract me
1.
2.
3.

Step 4: People whom I can ask for help
1.
2.
3.

Step 5: Professionals or agencies I can contact during a crisis
1.
2.
3.
4.

Step 6: Making the environment safe
1.
2.
3.

Step 7: Regular check-in's
1.
2.

Adapted from Stanley and Brown (2012). For permission to reproduce this worksheet, contact Elsevier.

WORKSHEET 21. Suicidal Ideation Intensity Thermometer

When it comes to thoughts about harming ourselves, it is important that we can describe the feeling and intensity to others. Try to rate the intensity of your suicidal thoughts and feelings on a 0 to 10 scale. What words would you use to describe each rating? Can you remember a time when you've felt that way?

Suicidal Thoughts/ Feeling Intensity	What feeling you are rating:	
	How intense is it? (0 "Not at all" to 10 "the worst")	Describe the feeling (in your own words) for each level.	Describe past times you've felt this way.
	10		
	9		
	8		
	7		
	6		
	5		
	4		
	3		
	2		
	1		
	0		

399

WORKSHEET 22. Chain Analysis of Suicidal Ideation and Self-Harm

The goal of chain analysis is to become more aware of the thoughts, emotions, and actions that spiral out of control when you fall into an emotional spiral. Work with your therapist to spell out your emotional spiral and the events that trigger them.

Name:	Date:	
Vulnerabilty Factors:		
Prompting Event:		
	Action/ Emotion/ Thought	
	What did you do?	Potential solution or skills to use?
Link 1		
Link 2		
Link 3		
Link 4		
What problems does this lead to (e.g., self-harm, SI, risk taking)?		
What happened afterward?		
Short-term outcome		
Long-term outcome		

400

WORKSHEET 23. Social Skills Checklist

Use behavioral observation and report from the youth, family, and other reporters to assess social skills strengths and concerns.

	Notable Strength	Never a Problem	Sometimes a Problem	Always a Problem	Comment
Nonverbals, Cues, and Posture					
Eye contact					
Expressing interest Smiling, nodding					
Shrinking and hiding					
Hiding behind clothes Hiding behind smartphones, headphones, books, electronics					
Standing in the periphery					
Handshakes					
Spoken Conversations: Starting, Joining, Maintaining					
The conversation volley: responding, reciprocity					
Volume and tone					
Expressing interest					
Written "Conversations": Texting and Social Media Communication					
The conversation volley					
Group chatting					
Social media To like or not to like					
Social media comments					
Writing an email					
Other Target?					

WORKSHEET 24. Weekly Parent–Child Interaction Patterns

Track your interactions with your child over the week and try to identify any parenting traps you fall into. What happened right away (immediate outcome) and then what happened later (long-term outcome)?

Day	Event	Child's Action	Parent's Response	Parent Pattern?	Immediate Result? Did behavior get better or worse right away?	Long-term Result? What happened over the next couple of days?
Example: Monday	Math tutor scheduled for next day.	Upset—Rick says he's overwhelmed.	Talked with him; canceled math tutor.	Accommodation	It stopped the complaining.	He continued protesting the next couple of days.

WORKSHEET 25. School–Family Coordination Plan: Role Assignments

Brainstorm with student, parents, teachers, and school liaisons what each person can do to help accomplish the goals of the school reentry plan.

Situation	Child Role	Parent Role	School Role
1. Morning routine	a. b. c.	a. b. c.	
2. School arrival	a. b. c.	a. b. c.	
3. During school day	a. b. c.	a. b. c.	
4. Departure/ after school	a. b. c.	a. b. c.	

Resources for Therapists and Families

ORGANIZATIONS AND WEBSITES

Association for Behavioral and Cognitive Therapies

www.abct.org/Home

Fact sheets can be found at *www.abct.org/docs/factsheets/adolesc_suicide.pdf.*

Society of Clinical Child and Adolescent Psychology

https://effectivechildtherapy.org

Fact sheets can be found at *https://effectivechildtherapy.org/concerns-symptoms-disorders/disorders/self-injurious-thoughts-and-behaviors.*

Anxiety and Depression Association of America

https://adaa.org

American Academy of Child and Adolescent Psychiatry

www.aacap.org/AACAP/Families_and_Youth/Youth_Resources/Home.aspx

American Foundation for Suicide Prevention

https://afsp.org

JED Foundation (a nonprofit that protects emotional health and prevents suicide for youth and young adults)

www.jedfoundation.org

Anxiety Canada Youth

https://youth.anxietycanada.com

Society for Adolescent Health and Medicine

www.adolescenthealth.org/Home.aspx

988 Suicide & Crisis Lifeline

www.988lifeline.org/chat

National Suicide Prevention Lifeline

https://suicidepreventionlifeline.org

Substance Abuse and Mental Health Services Administration (SAMHSA)

https://findtreatment.samhsa.gov

CBT-BASED SELF-HELP BOOKS FOR KIDS AND TEENS

The reader can also find a comprehensive list of self-help books for adults and teens at the Association for Behavioral and Cognitive Therapies, Self-Help Book Recommendations:

Mary Alvord and Anne McGrath, *Conquer Negative Thinking for Teens: A Workbook to Break the Nine Thought Habits That Are Holding You Back*

Regine Galanti, *Anxiety Relief for Teens: Essential CBT Skills and Mindfulness Practices to Overcome Anxiety and Stress*

Regine Galanti, *When Harley Has Anxiety: A Fun CBT Skills Activity Book to Help Manage Worries and Fears*

Muniya Khanna and Deborah Roth Ledley, *The Worry Workbook for Kids: Helping Children to Overcome Anxiety and the Fear of Uncertainty (An Instant Help Book for Parents and Kids)*

John March and Christine Benton, *Talking Back to OCD: The Program That Helps Kids and Teens Say "No Way"—and Parents Say "Way to Go"*

Anthony Puliafico and Joanna Robin, *The OCD Workbook for Kids: Skills to Help Children Manage Obsessive Thoughts and Compulsive Behaviors (An Instant Help Book for Parents and Kids)*

Michael Tompkins and Katherine Martinez, *My Anxious Mind*

CBT-BASED SELF-HELP BOOKS FOR PARENTS

Anne Marie Albano, *You and Your Anxious Child: Free Your Child from Fears and Worries and Create a Joyful Family Life*

Tamar Chansky, *Freeing Your Child from Anxiety: Practical Strategies to Overcome Fears, Worries, and Phobias and Be Prepared for Life—from Toddlers to Teens*

Ilyse Dobrow DiMarco, *Mom Brain: Proven Strategies to Fight the Anxiety, Guilt, and Overwhelming Emotions of Motherhood—and Relax into Your New Self*

Mary Fristad and Jill Goldberg Arnold, *Raising a Moody Child: How to Cope with Depression and Bipolar Disorder*

Donna Pincus, *Growing Up Brave: Expert Strategies for Helping Your Child Overcome Fear, Stress, and Anxiety*

Ronald Rapee, Ann Wignall, Susan H. Spence, Vanessa Cobham, and Heidi Lyneham, *Helping Your Anxious Child: A Step-by-Step Guide for Parents*

References

Abrutyn, S., & Mueller, A. S. (2014). Are suicidal behaviors contagious in adolescence? Using longitudinal data to examine suicide suggestion. *American Sociological Review, 79*(2), 211–227.

Albano, A. M. (1995). Treatment of social anxiety in adolescents. *Cognitive and Behavioral Practice, 2*(2), 271–298.

Albano, A. M., & DiBartolo, P. M. (2007). *Cognitive-behavioral therapy for social phobia in adolescents: Stand up, speak out, therapist guide.* New York: Oxford University Press.

Aldao, A., & Nolen-Hoeksema, S. (2010). Specificity of cognitive emotion regulation strategies: A transdiagnostic examination. *Behaviour Research and Therapy, 48*(10), 974–983.

Alden, L. E., & Taylor, C. T. (2004). Interpersonal processes in social phobia. *Clinical Psychology Review, 24*(7), 857–882.

Alfano, C. A. (2012). Are children with "pure" generalized anxiety disorder impaired? A comparison with comorbid and healthy children. *Journal of Clinical Child & Adolescent Psychology, 41*(6), 739–745.

Allen, C. H., Kluger, B. M., & Buard, I. (2017). Safety of transcranial magnetic stimulation in children: A systematic review of the literature. *Pediatric Neurology, 68,* 3–17.

Allen, J. L., Lavallee, K. L., Herren, C., Ruhe, K., & Schneider, S. (2010). DSM-IV criteria for childhood separation anxiety disorder: Informant, age, and sex differences. *Journal of Anxiety Disorders, 24*(8), 946–952.

American Psychiatric Association. (2013). *Diagnostic and statistical manual of mental disorders* (5th ed., DSM-5). Washington, DC: Author.

APA Presidential Task Force on Evidence-Based Practice. (2006). Evidence-based practice in psychology. *The American Psychologist, 61*(4), 271–285.

Asarnow, J. R., Porta, G., Spirito, A., Emslie, G., Clarke, G., Wagner, K. D., . . . Brent, D. A. (2011). Suicide attempts and nonsuicidal self-injury in the treatment of resistant depression in adolescents: Findings from the TORDIA study. *Journal of the American Academy of Child & Adolescent Psychiatry, 50*(8), 772–781.

Aschenbrand, S. G., Kendall, P. C., Webb, A., Safford, S. M., & Flannery-Schroeder, E. (2003). Is childhood separation anxiety disorder a predictor of adult panic disorder and agoraphobia? A seven-year longitudinal study. *Journal of the American Academy of Child & Adolescent Psychiatry, 42*(12), 1478–1485.

Auerbach, R. P., Stewart, J. G., & Johnson, S. L. (2016). Impulsivity and suicidality in adolescent inpatients. *Journal of Abnormal Child Psychology, 45*(1), 91–103.

Avenevoli, S., Swendsen, J., He, J. P., Burstein, M., & Merikangas, K. R. (2015). Major depression in the National Comorbidity Survey–Adolescent Supplement: Prevalence, correlates, and treatment. *Journal of the American Academy of Child & Adolescent Psychiatry, 54*(1), 37–44.

Bacow, T. L., Pincus, D. B., Ehrenreich, J. T., & Brody, L. R. (2009). The metacognitions questionnaire for children: Development and validation in a clinical sample of children and adolescents with anxiety disorders. *Journal of Anxiety Disorders, 23*(6), 727–736.

Badin, E., Alvarez, E., & Chu, B. C. (2020). Cognitive behavioral therapy for child and adolescent anxiety: CBT in a nutshell. In R. D. Friedberg & B. J. Nakamura (Eds.), *Cognitive behavioral therapy in youth: Tradition and innovation* (pp. 41–71). New York: Humana (Springer).

Baller, R. D., & Richardson, K. K. (2002). Social integration, imitation, and the geographic patterning of suicide. *American Sociological Review, 67*(6), 873–888.

Baly, M. W., Cornell, D. G., & Lovegrove, P. (2014). A longitudinal investigation of self- and peer reports of bullying victimization across middle school. *Psychology in the Schools, 51*(3), 217–240.

Barlow, D. H. (1988). *Anxiety and its disorders: The nature and treatment of anxiety and panic.* New York: Guilford Press.

Barlow, D. H., Allen, L. B., & Choate, M. L. (2004). Toward a unified treatment for emotional disorders. *Behavior Therapy, 35*(2), 205–230.

Barmish, A. J., & Kendall, P. C. (2005). Should parents be co-clients in cognitive-behavioral therapy for anxious youth? *Journal of Clinical Child & Adolescent Psychology, 34*(3), 569–581.

Batejan, K. L., Jarvi, S. M., & Swenson, L. P. (2015). Sexual orientation and non-suicidal self-injury: A meta-analytic review. *Archives of Suicide Research, 19*(2), 131–150.

Battaglia, M., Touchette, É., Garon-Carrier, G., Dionne, G., Côté, S. M., Vitaro, F., . . . Boivin, M. (2016). Distinct trajectories of separation anxiety in the preschool years: Persistence at school entry and early-life associated factors. *Journal of Child Psychology and Psychiatry, 57*(1), 39–46.

Beck, A. T., Steer, R. A., & Brown, G. K. (1996). *Manual for the Beck Depression Inventory-II.* San Antonio, TX: Psychological Corporation.

Becker-Haimes, E. M., Tabachnick, A. R., Last, B. S., Stewart, R. E., Hasan-Granier, A., & Beidas, R. S. (2020). Evidence base update for brief, free, and accessible youth mental health measures. *Journal of Clinical Child & Adolescent Psychology, 49*(1), 1–17.

Beesdo, K., Bittner, A., Pine, D. S., Stein, M. B., Höfler, M., Lieb, R., & Wittchen, H. U. (2007). Incidence of social anxiety disorder and the consistent risk for secondary depression in the first three decades of life. *Archives of General Psychiatry, 64*(8), 903–912.

Beidas, R. S., Stewart, R. E., Walsh, L., Lucas, S., Downey, M. M., Jackson, K., . . . Mandell, D. S. (2015). Free, brief, and validated: Standardized instruments for low-resource mental health settings. *Cognitive and Behavioral Practice, 22*(1), 5–19.

Beidel, D. C., & Turner, S. M. (1998). *Shy children, phobic adults: Nature and treatment of social phobia.* Washington, DC: American Psychological Association.

Beidel, D. C., Turner, S. M., & Morris, T. L. (2000). Behavioral treatment of childhood social phobia. *Journal of Consulting and Clinical Psychology, 68*(6), 1072–1080.

Bell-Dolan, D. J., Last, C. G., & Strauss, C. C. (1990). Symptoms of anxiety disorders in normal children. *Journal of the American Academy of Child & Adolescent Psychiatry, 29*(5), 759–765.

Berg, I. (2002). School avoidance, school phobia, and truancy. In M. Lewis (Ed.), *Child and adolescent psychiatry: A comprehensive textbook* (3rd ed., pp. 1260–1266). Sydney, Australia: Lippincott Williams & Wilkins.

Bernstein, G. A., Borchardt, C. M., Perwien, A. R., Crosby, R. D., Kushner, M. G., Thuras, P. D., & Last, C. G. (2000). Imipramine plus cognitive-behavioral therapy in the treatment of school refusal. *Journal of the American Academy of Child & Adolescent Psychiatry, 39*(3), 276–283.

Bernstein, G. A., Garfinkel, B. D., & Borchardt, C. M. (1990). Comparative studies of pharmacotherapy for school refusal. *Journal of the American Academy of Child & Adolescent Psychiatry, 29*(5), 773–781.

Bickman, L. (2008). A measurement feedback system (MFS) is necessary to improve mental health outcomes. *Journal of the American Academy of Child & Adolescent Psychiatry, 47*(10), 1114–1119.

Bickman, L., Kelley, S. D., Breda, C., de Andrade, A. R., & Riemer, M. (2011). Effects of routine feedback to clinicians on mental health outcomes of youths: Results of a randomized trial. *Psychiatric Services, 62*(12), 1423–1429.

Biederman, J., Hirshfeld-Becker, D. R., Rosenbaum, J. F., Hérot, C., Friedman, D., Snidman, N., . . . Faraone, S. V. (2001). Further evidence of association between behavioral inhibition and social anxiety in children. *American Journal of Psychiatry, 158*(10), 1673–1679.

Birmaher, B., Brent, D., & AACAP Work Group on Quality Issues. (2007). Practice parameter for the assessment and treatment of children and adolescents with depressive disorders. *Journal of the American Academy of Child & Adolescent Psychiatry, 46*(11), 1503–1526.

Blöte, A. W., Miers, A. C., Heyne, D. A., & Westenberg, P. M. (2015). Social anxiety and the school environment of adolescents. In K. Ranta, A. La Greca, L. J. Garcia-Lopez, & M. Marttunen (Eds.), *Social anxiety and phobia in adolescents* (pp. 151–181). Cham, Switzerland: Springer.

Bögels, S. M., & Mansell, W. (2004). Attention processes in the maintenance and treatment of social phobia: Hypervigilance, avoidance and self-focused attention. *Clinical Psychology Review, 24*(7), 827–856.

Borkovec, T. D., Shadick, R. N., & Hopkins, M. (1991). The nature of normal and pathological worry. In R. M. Rapee & D. H. Barlow (Eds.), *Chronic anxiety: Generalized anxiety disorder and mixed anxiety-depression* (pp. 29–51). New York: Guilford Press.

Brand, S., Hatzinger, M., Beck, J., & Holsboer-Trachsler, E. (2009). Perceived parenting styles, personality traits and sleep patterns in adolescents. *Journal of Adolescence, 32*(5), 1189–1207.

Brausch, A. M., & Girresch, S. K. (2012). A review of empirical treatment studies for adolescent nonsuicidal self-injury. *Journal of Cognitive Psychotherapy, 26*(1), 3.

Brent, D., Emslie, G., Clarke, G., Wagner, K. D., Asarnow, J. R., Keller, M., . . . Birmaher, B. (2008). Switching to another SSRI or to venlafaxine with or without cognitive behavioral therapy for adolescents with SSRI-resistant depression: The TORDIA randomized controlled trial. *JAMA, 299*(8), 901–913.

Brent, D., Greenhill, L., Compton, S., Emslie, G., Wells, K., Walkup, J. T., . . . Turner, J. B. (2009). The treatment of Adolescent Suicide Attempters Study (TASA): Predictors of suicidal events in an open treatment trial. *Journal of the American Academy of Child and Adolescent Psychiatry, 48*(10), 987–996.

Brent, D. A., Kerr, M. M., Goldstein, C., Bozigar, J., Wartella, M., & Allan, M. J. (1989). An outbreak of suicide and suicidal behavior in a high school. *Journal of the American Academy of Child & Adolescent Psychiatry, 28*(6), 918–924.

Bridge, J. A., Iyengar, S., Salary, C. B., Barbe, R. P., Birmaher, B., Pincus, H. A., . . . Brent, D. A. (2007). Clinical response and risk for reported suicidal ideation and suicide attempts in pediatric antidepressant treatment: A meta-analysis of randomized controlled trials. *JAMA, 297*(15), 1683–1696.

Brinkmeyer, M. Y., & Eyberg, S. M. (2003). Parent–child interaction therapy for oppositional children. In A. E. Kazdin & J. R. Weisz (Eds.), *Evidence-based psychotherapies for children and adolescents* (pp. 204–223). New York: Guilford Press.

Brookmeyer, K. A., Fanti, K. A., & Henrich, C. C. (2006). Schools, parents, and youth violence: A multilevel, ecological analysis. *Journal of Clinical Child & Adolescent Psychology, 35*(4), 504–514.

Brown, A. M., & Whiteside, S. P. (2008). Relations among perceived parental rearing behaviors, attachment style, and worry in anxious children. *Journal of Anxiety Disorders, 22*(2), 263–272.

Brown, G. W., & Harris, T. O. (2008). Depression and the serotonin transporter 5-HTTLPR polymorphism: A review and a hypothesis concerning gene–environment interaction. *Journal of Affective Disorders, 111*(1), 1–12.

Brückl, T. M., Wittchen, H. U., Höfler, M., Pfister, H., Schneider, S., & Lieb, R. (2007). Childhood separation anxiety and the risk of subsequent psychopathology: Results from a community study. *Psychotherapy and Psychosomatics, 76*(1), 47–56.

Bukowski, W. M., Laursen, B., & Hoza, B. (2010). The snowball effect: Friendship moderates escalations in depressed affect among avoidant and excluded children. *Development and Psychopathology, 22*(4), 749–757.

Cartwright-Hatton, S., Mather, A., Illingworth, V., Brocki, J., Harrington, R., & Wells, A. (2004). Development and preliminary validation of the Meta-Cognitions Questionnaire—Adolescent Version. *Journal of Anxiety Disorders, 18*(3), 411–422.

Cartwright-Hatton, S., McNicol, K., & Doubleday, E. (2006). Anxiety in a neglected population: Prevalence of anxiety disorders in pre-adolescent children. *Clinical Psychology Review, 26*(7), 817–833.

Centers for Disease Control and Prevention. (2022). Suicide rising across the US: Vital signs. Retrieved from *www.cdc.gov/vitalsigns/suicide.*

Cha, C. B., Augenstein, T. M., Frost, K. H., Gallagher, K., D'Angelo, E. J., & Nock, M. K. (2016). Using implicit and explicit measures to predict nonsuicidal self-injury among adolescent inpatients. *Journal of the*

American Academy of Child & Adolescent Psychiatry, 55(1), 62–68.

Chorpita, B. F., Albano, A. M., & Barlow, D. H. (1996). Cognitive processing in children: Relation to anxiety and family influences. *Journal of Clinical Child Psychology, 25*(2), 170–176.

Chorpita, B. F., & Daleiden, E. L. (2009). Mapping evidence-based treatments for children and adolescents: Application of the distillation and matching model to 615 treatments from 322 randomized trials. *Journal of Consulting and Clinical Psychology, 77*(3), 566–579.

Chorpita, B. F., Daleiden, E. L., Ebesutani, C., Young, J., Becker, K. D., Nakamura, B. J., . . . Smith, R. L. (2011). Evidence-based treatments for children and adolescents: An updated review of indicators of efficacy and effectiveness. *Clinical Psychology: Science and Practice, 18*(2), 154–172.

Chorpita, B. F., Moffitt, C. E., & Gray, J. (2005). Psychometric properties of the Revised Child Anxiety and Depression Scale in a clinical sample. *Behaviour Research and Therapy, 43*(3), 309–322.

Chorpita, B. F., & Weisz, J. R. (2009). *Modular approach to therapy for children with anxiety, depression, trauma, or conduct problems (MATCH-ADTC).* Satellite Beach, FL: PracticeWise.

Chorpita, B. F., Yim, L., Moffitt, C., Umemoto, L. A., & Francis, S. E. (2000). Assessment of symptoms of DSM-IV anxiety and depression in children: A revised child anxiety and depression scale. *Behaviour Research and Therapy, 38*(8), 835–855.

Choudhury, M. S., Pimentel, S. S., & Kendall, P. C. (2003). Childhood anxiety disorders: Parent–child (dis)agreement using a structured interview for the DSM-IV. *Journal of the American Academy of Child & Adolescent Psychiatry, 42*(8), 957–964.

Christon, L. M., McLeod, B. D., & Jensen-Doss, A. (2015). Evidence-based assessment meets evidence-based treatment: An approach to science-informed case conceptualization. *Cognitive and Behavioral Practice, 22*(1), 36–48.

Chu, B. C. (2019). Evidence-based therapist flexibility: Making treatments work for clients. In M. J. Prinstein, E. A. Youngstrom, E. J. Mash, & R. A. Barkley (Eds.), *Treatment of disorders in childhood and adolescence* (4th ed., pp. 27–46). New York: Guilford Press.

Chu, B. C., Chen, J., Mele, C., Temkin, A., & Xue, J. (2017). Transdiagnostic approaches to emotion regulation: Basic mechanisms and treatment research. In C. A. Essau, S. Leblanc, & T. H. Ollendick (Eds.), *Emotion regulation and psychopathology in children and adolescents* (pp. 419–452). Oxford, UK: Oxford University Press.

Chu, B. C., Crocco, S. T., Esseling, P., Areizaga, M. J., Lindner, A. M., & Skriner, L. C. (2016). Transdiagnostic group behavioral activation and exposure therapy for youth anxiety and depression: Initial randomized controlled trial. *Behaviour Research and Therapy,* *76,* 65–75.

Chu, B. C., Guarino, D., Mele, C., O'Connell, J., & Coto, P. (2019). Developing an online early detection system for school attendance problems: Results from a research-community partnership. *Cognitive and Behavioral Practice, 26*(1), 35–45.

Chu, B. C., Skriner, L. C., & Staples, A. M. (2014). Behavioral avoidance across child and adolescent psychopathology. In J. Ehrenreich-May & B. C. Chu (Eds.), *Transdiagnostic treatments for children and adolescents: Principles and practice* (pp. 84–110). New York: Guilford Press.

Clarke, G. N., Rohde, P., Lewinsohn, P. M., Hops, H., & Seeley, J. R. (1999). Cognitive-behavioral treatment of adolescent depression: Efficacy of acute group treatment and booster sessions. *Journal of the American Academy of Child & Adolescent Psychiatry, 38*(3), 272–279.

Cohen, P., Cohen, J., Kasen, S., Velez, C. N., Hartmark, C., Johnson, J., . . . Streuning, E. L. (1993). An epidemiological study of disorders in late childhood and adolescence—I. Age-and gender-specific prevalence. *Journal of Child Psychology and Psychiatry, 34*(6), 851–867.

Comer, J. S., Kendall, P. C., Franklin, M. E., Hudson, J. L., & Pimentel, S. S. (2004). Obsessing/worrying about the overlap between obsessive–compulsive disorder and generalized anxiety disorder in youth. *Clinical Psychology Review, 24*(6), 663–683.

Connolly, S. D., & Bernstein, G. A. (2007). Practice parameter for the assessment and treatment of children and adolescents with anxiety disorders. *Journal of the American Academy of Child & Adolescent Psychiatry, 46*(2), 267–283.

Corville-Smith, J., Ryan, B. A., Adams, G. R., & Dalicandro, T. (1998). Distinguishing absentee students from regular attenders: The combined influence of personal, family, and school factors. *Journal of Youth and Adolescence, 27*(5), 629–640.

Costello, E. J., Copeland, W., & Angold, A. (2011). Trends in psychopathology across the adolescent years: What changes when children become adolescents, and when adolescents become adults? *Journal of Child Psychology and Psychiatry, 52*(10), 1015–1025.

Costello, E. J., Erkanli, A., & Angold, A. (2006). Is there an epidemic of child or adolescent depression? *Journal of Child Psychology and Psychiatry, 47*(12), 1263–1271.

Costello, E. J., Mustillo, S., Erkanli, A., Keeler, G., & Angold, A. (2003). Prevalence and development of psychiatric disorders in childhood and adolescence. *Archives of General Psychiatry, 60*(8), 837–844.

Côté, S. M., Boivin, M., Liu, X., Nagin, D. S., Zoccolillo, M., & Tremblay, R. E. (2009). Depression and anxiety symptoms: Onset, developmental course and risk factors during early childhood. *Journal of Child Psychology and Psychiatry, 50*(10), 1201–1208.

Craske, M. G., Kircanski, K., Zelikowsky, M., Mystkowski, J., Chowdhury, N., & Baker, A. (2008). Optimizing inhibitory learning during exposure therapy. *Behaviour Research and Therapy, 46*(1), 5–27.

Craske, M. G., Treanor, M., Conway, C. C., Zbozinek, T., & Vervliet, B. (2014). Maximizing exposure therapy: An inhibitory learning approach. *Behaviour Research and Therapy, 58,* 10–23.

Cuffe, S. P. (2007). Suicide and SSRI medications in children and adolescents: An update. *American Journal of Child and Adolescent Psychiatry.* Retrieved from *www.aacap.org/AACAP/Medical_Students_and_Residents/Mentorship_Matters/DevelopMentor/Suicide_and_SSRI_Medications_in_Children_and_Adolescents_An_Update.aspx*

Cuijpers, P., Van Straten, A., & Warmerdam, L. (2007). Behavioral activation treatments of depression: A meta-analysis. *Clinical Psychology Review, 27*(3), 318–326.

Cullen, K. R., Amatya, P., Roback, M. G., Albott, C. S., Westlund Schreiner, M., Ren, Y., . . . Reigstad, K. (2018). Intravenous ketamine for adolescents with treatment-resistant depression: An open-label study. *Journal of Child and Adolescent Psychopharmacology, 28*(7), 437–444.

Cummings, C. M., Caporino, N. E., & Kendall, P. C. (2014). Comorbidity of anxiety and depression in children and adolescents: 20 years after. *Psychological Bulletin, 140*(3), 816–845.

Dackis, M. N., Eisenberg, R., Mowrey, W. B., & Pimentel, S. S (2021). The Assessment of Chronic Risk in Youth (ACRY): Development and initial validation in a clinical sample. *Evidence-Based Practice in Child and Adolescent Mental Health, 6,* 65–82.

de Lijster, J. M., Dierckx, B., Utens, E. M., Verhulst, F. C., Zieldorff, C., Dieleman, G. C., & Legerstee, J. S. (2016). The age of onset of anxiety disorders: A meta-analysis. *Canadian Journal of Psychiatry, 62*(4), 237–246.

De Los Reyes, A., & Kazdin, A. E. (2005). Informant discrepancies in the assessment of childhood psychopathology: A critical review, theoretical framework, and recommendations for further study. *Psychological Bulletin, 131*(4), 483–509.

Degnan, K. A., Almas, A. N., & Fox, N. A. (2010). Temperament and the environment in the etiology of childhood anxiety. *Journal of Child Psychology and Psychiatry, 51*(4), 497–517.

Deno, S. L., Reschly, A. L., Lembke, E. S., Magnusson, D., Callender, S. A., Windram, H., & Stachel, N. (2009). Developing a school-wide progress-monitoring system. *Psychology in the Schools, 46*(1), 44–55.

Dexter-Mazza, E. T., & Freeman, K. A. (2003). Graduate training and the treatment of suicidal clients: The students' perspective. *Suicide and Life-Threatening Behavior, 33*(2), 211–218.

DiBartolo, P. M., & Helt, M. (2007). Theoretical models of affectionate versus affectionless control in anxious families: A critical examination based on observations of parent–child interactions. *Clinical Child and Family Psychology Review, 10*(3), 253–274.

Dickson, J. M., & MacLeod, A. K. (2004). Approach and avoidance goals and plans: Their relationship to anxiety and depression. *Cognitive Therapy and Research, 28*(3), 415–432.

DiCorcia, D. J., Arango, A., Horwitz, A. G., & King, C. A. (2017). Methods and functions of non-suicidal self-injury among adolescents seeking emergency psychiatric services. *Journal of Psychopathology and Behavioral Assessment, 39*(4), 693–704.

Dimidjian, S., Barrera Jr., M., Martell, C., Muñoz, R. F., & Lewinsohn, P. M. (2011). The origins and current status of behavioral activation treatments for depression. *Annual Review of Clinical Psychology, 7,* 1–38.

Donovan, M. R., Glue, P., Kolluri, S., & Emir, B. (2010). Comparative efficacy of antidepressants in preventing relapse in anxiety disorders—A meta-analysis. *Journal of Affective Disorders, 123*(1–3), 9–16.

Dummit, E. S., III, Klein, R. G., Tancer, N. K., Asche, B., Martin, J., & Fairbanks, J. A. (1997). Systematic assessment of 50 children with selective mutism. *Journal of the American Academy of Child & Adolescent Psychiatry, 36*(5), 653–660.

Egger, H. L., Costello, J. E., & Angold, A. (2003). School refusal and psychiatric disorders: A community study. *Journal of the American Academy of Child & Adolescent Psychiatry, 42*(7), 797–807.

Fan, F., Su, L., & Su, Y. (2008). Anxiety structure by gender and age groups in a Chinese children sample of 12 cities. *Chinese Mental Health Journal, 22*(4), 241–245.

Feldman, B. N., & Freedenthal, S. (2006). Social work education in suicide intervention and prevention: An unmet need? *Suicide and Life-Threatening Behavior, 36*(4), 467–480.

Ferster, C. B. (1973). A functional analysis of depression. *American Psychologist, 28*(10), 857–870.

Festa, C. C., & Ginsburg, G. S. (2011). Parental and peer predictors of social anxiety in youth. *Child Psychiatry & Human Development, 42*(3), 291–306.

Fisak, B., & Grills-Taquechel, A. E. (2007). Parental modeling, reinforcement, and information transfer: Risk factors in the development of child anxiety? *Clinical Child and Family Psychology Review, 10*(3), 213–231.

Foa, E. B., Huppert, J. D., & Cahill, S. P. (2006). Emotional processing theory: An update. In B. O. Rothbaum (Ed.), *Pathological anxiety: Emotional processing in etiology and treatment* (pp. 3–24). New York: Guilford Press.

Foxx, R. M. (2013). The maintenance of behavioral change: The case for long-term follow-ups. *American Psychologist, 68*(8), 728–736.

Friedman, R. (2014). Antidepressants' black box warning—10 years later. *New England Journal of Medicine, 371,* 66–68.

Garber, J., & Weersing, V. R. (2010). Comorbidity of anxiety and depression in youth: Implications for treatment and prevention. *Clinical Psychology: Science and Practice, 17*(4), 293–306.

Gariepy, G., Honkaniemi, H., & Quesnel-Vallee, A. (2016). Social support and protection from depression: Systematic review of current findings in Western countries. *British Journal of Psychiatry, 209*(4), 284–293.

Gazelle, H., & Ladd, G. W. (2003). Anxious solitude and peer exclusion: A diathesis–stress model of internalizing trajectories in childhood. *Child Development, 74*(1), 257–278.

Gearing, R. E., Schwalbe, C. S., Lee, R., & Hoagwood, K. E. (2013). The effectiveness of booster sessions in CBT treatment for child and adolescent mood and anxiety disorders. *Depression and Anxiety, 30*(9), 800–808.

Ginsburg, G. S., Becker-Haimes, E. M., Keeton, C., Kendall, P. C., Iyengar, S., Sakolsky, D., . . . Piacentini, J. (2018). Results from the child/adolescent anxiety multimodal extended long-term study (CAMELS): Primary anxiety outcomes. *Journal of the American Academy of Child & Adolescent Psychiatry, 57*(7), 471–480.

Ginsburg, G. S., Drake, K. L., Tein, J. Y., Teetsel, R., & Riddle, M. A. (2015). Preventing onset of anxiety disorders in offspring of anxious parents: A randomized controlled trial of a family-based intervention. *American Journal of Psychiatry, 172*(12), 1207–1214.

Glew, G. M., Fan, M. Y., Katon, W., Rivara, F. P., & Kernic, M. A. (2005). Bullying, psychosocial adjustment, and academic performance in elementary school. *Archives of Pediatrics & Adolescent Medicine, 159*(11), 1026–1031.

Goldston, D. B., & Compton, J. S. (2007). Adolescent suicidal and nonsuicidal self-harm behaviors and risks. In E. J. Mash & R. A. Barkley (Eds.), *Assessment of childhood disorders* (pp. 305–343). New York: Guilford Press.

Gosselin, P., Langlois, F., Freeston, M. H., Ladouceur, R., Laberge, M., & Lemay, D. (2007). Cognitive variables related to worry among adolescents: Avoidance strategies and faulty beliefs about worry. *Behaviour Research and Therapy, 45*(2), 225–233.

Gould, M. S., & Kramer, R. A. (2001). Youth suicide prevention. *Suicide and Life-Threatening Behavior, 31*(Suppl. 1), 6–31.

Gould, M. S., Kleinman, M. H., Lake, A. M., Forman, J., & Midle, J. B. (2014). Newspaper coverage of suicide and initiation of suicide clusters in teenagers in the USA, 1988–96: A retrospective, population-based, case-control study. *The Lancet Psychiatry, 1*(1), 34–43.

Gould, M. S., Marrocco, F. A., Kleinman, M., Thomas,

J. G., Mostkoff, K., Cote, J., & Davies, M. (2005). Evaluating iatrogenic risk of youth suicide screening programs. *JAMA, 293*(13), 1635–1643.

Gould, M. S., Wallenstein, S., Kleinman, M. H., O'Carroll, P., & Mercy, J. (1990). Suicide clusters: An examination of age-specific effects. *American Journal of Public Health, 80*(2), 211–212.

Grant, K. E., Compas, B. E., Thurm, A. E., McMahon, S. D., Gipson, P. Y., Campbell, A. J., . . . Westerholm, R. I. (2006). Stressors and child and adolescent psychopathology: Evidence of moderating and mediating effects. *Clinical Psychology Review, 26*(3), 257–283.

Greco, L. A., Baer, R. A., & Smith, G. T. (2011). Assessing mindfulness in children and adolescents: development and validation of the Child and Adolescent Mindfulness Measure (CAMM). *Psychological Assessment, 23*(3), 606–614.

Greco, L. A., Blackledge, J. T., Coyne, L. W., & Ehrenreich, J. (2005). Integrating acceptance and mindfulness into treatments for child and adolescent anxiety disorders. In S. M. Orsillo & L. Roemer (Eds.), *Acceptance and mindfulness-based approaches to anxiety: Conceptualization and treatment* (pp. 301–322). Boston: Springer.

Haas, A. P., Rodgers, P. L., & Herman, J. L. (2014). *Suicide attempts among transgender and gender nonconforming adults.* New York: American Foundation for Suicide Prevention. Retrieved from *https://queeramnesty.ch/docs/AFSP-Williams-Suicide-Report-Final.pdf.*

Halldorsson, B., & Creswell, C. (2017). Social anxiety in pre-adolescent children: What do we know about maintenance? *Behaviour Research and Therapy, 99*(1), 19–36.

Hamilton, B. E., Minino, A. M., Martin, J. A., Kochanek, K. D., Strobino, D. M., & Guyer, B. (2007). Annual summary of vital statistics: 2005. *Pediatrics, 119*(2), 345–360.

Hammen, C. (2009). Adolescent depression: Stressful interpersonal contexts and risk for recurrence. *Current Directions in Psychological Science, 18*(4), 200–204.

Hamza, C. A., Stewart, S. L., & Willoughby, T. (2012). Examining the link between non-suicidal self-injury and suicidal behavior: A review of the literature and an integrated model. *Clinical Psychology Review, 32*(6), 482–495.

Hankin, B. L., & Abramson, L. Y. (2001). Development of gender differences in depression: An elaborated cognitive vulnerability–transactional stress theory. *Psychological Bulletin, 127*(6), 773–796.

Harvey, A. G., Watkins, E., Mansell, W., & Shafran, R. (2004). *Cognitive behavioural processes across psychological disorders: A transdiagnostic approach to research and treatment.* Oxford, UK: Oxford University Press.

Hatzenbuehler, M. L., & Keyes, K. M. (2013). Inclusive anti-bullying policies and reduced risk of suicide attempts in lesbian and gay youth. *Journal of Adolescent Health, 53*(1), S21–S26.

Havik, T., Bru, E., & Ertesvåg, S. K. (2015). School factors associated with school refusal-and truancy-related reasons for school non-attendance. *Social Psychology of Education, 18*(2), 221–240.

Hawkins, S. M., & Heflin, L. J. (2011). Increasing secondary teachers' behavior-specific praise using a video self-modeling and visual performance feedback intervention. *Journal of Positive Behavior Interventions, 13*(2), 97–108.

Hayward, C., Killen, J. D., Kraemer, H. C., & Taylor, C. B. (1998). Linking self-reported childhood behavioral inhibition to adolescent social phobia. *Journal of the American Academy of Child & Adolescent Psychiatry, 37*(12), 1308–1316.

Heffer, T., Good, M., Daly, O., MacDonell, E., & Willoughby, T. (2019). The longitudinal association between social-media use and depressive symptoms among adolescents and young adults: An empirical reply to Twenge et al. (2018). *Clinical Psychological Science, 7*(3), 462–470.

Hendron, M., & Kearney, C. A. (2016). School climate and student absenteeism and internalizing and externalizing behavioral problems. *Children & Schools, 38*(2), 109–116.

Heyne, D., Gren-Landell, M., Melvin, G., & Gentle-Genitty, C. (2019). Differentiation between school attendance problems: Why and how? *Cognitive and Behavioral Practice, 26*(1), 8–34.

Heyne, D., King, N. J., Tonge, B. J., Rollings, S., Young, D., Pritchard, M., & Ollendick, T. H. (2002). Evaluation of child therapy and caregiver training in the treatment of school refusal. *Journal of the American Academy of Child & Adolescent Psychiatry, 41*(6), 687–695.

Higa-McMillan, C. K., Francis, S. E., Rith-Najarian, L., & Chorpita, B. F. (2016). Evidence base update: 50 years of research on treatment for child and adolescent anxiety. *Journal of Clinical Child & Adolescent Psychology, 45*(2), 91–113.

Hirshfeld, D. R., Rosenbaum, J. F., Biederman, J., Bolduc, E. A., Faraone, S. V., Snidman, N., . . . Kagan, J. (1992). Stable behavioral inhibition and its association with anxiety disorder. *Journal of the American Academy of Child & Adolescent Psychiatry, 31*(1), 103–111.

Hirshfeld-Becker, D. R., Micco, J., Henin, A., Bloomfield, A., Biederman, J., & Rosenbaum, J. (2008). Behavioral inhibition. *Depression and Anxiety, 25*(4), 357–367.

Hock, E., McBride, S., & Gnezda, M. T. (1989). Maternal separation anxiety: Mother–infant separation from the maternal perspective. *Child Development, 60*(4), 793–802.

Hodges, J., & Oei, T. P. (2007). Would Confucius benefit from psychotherapy? The compatibility of cognitive behaviour therapy and Chinese values. *Behaviour Research and Therapy, 45*(5), 901–914.

Hoffman, L. J., & Chu, B. C. (2019). When is seeking safety functional? Taking a pragmatic approach to distinguishing coping from safety. *Cognitive and Behavioral Practice, 26*(1), 176–185.

Hopko, D. R., Armento, M. E., Cantu, M. S., Chambers, L. L., & Lejuez, C. W. (2003). The use of daily diaries to assess the relations among mood state, overt behavior, and reward value of activities. *Behaviour Research and Therapy, 41*(10), 1137–1148.

Hopko, D. R., Robertson, S., & Lejuez, C. W. (2006). Behavioral activation for anxiety disorders. *The Behavior Analyst Today, 7*(2), 212.

Horwitz, A. G., Czyz, E. K., Berona, J., & King, C. A. (2018). Rumination, brooding, and reflection: Prospective associations with suicide ideation and suicide attempts. *Suicide and Life-Threatening Behavior, 49*(4), 1085–1093.

Hughes, E. K., Gullone, E., Dudley, A., & Tonge, B. (2010). A case-control study of emotion regulation and school refusal in children and adolescents. *Journal of Early Adolescence, 30*(5), 691–706.

Hunnicutt Hollenbaugh, K. M., & Lenz, A. S. (2018). Preliminary evidence for the effectiveness of dialectical behavior therapy for adolescents. *Journal of Counseling & Development, 96*(2), 119–131.

Hwang, W. C., Wood, J. J., Lin, K. M., & Cheung, F. (2006). Cognitive-behavioral therapy with Chinese Americans: Research, theory, and clinical practice. *Cognitive and Behavioral Practice, 13*(4), 293–303.

Inderbitzen-Nolan, H. M., Anderson, E. R., & Johnson, H. S. (2007). Subjective versus objective behavioral ratings following two analogue tasks: A comparison of socially phobic and non-anxious adolescents. *Journal of Anxiety Disorders, 21*(1), 76–90.

Jack, S. P., Petrosky, E., Lyons, B. H., Blair, J. M., Ertl, A. M., Sheats, K. J., & Betz, C. J. (2018). Surveillance for violent deaths—National violent death reporting system, 27 states, 2015. *MMWR Surveillance Summaries, 67*(11), 1–32. Retrieved from *www.cdc.gov/mmwr/volumes/67/ss/ss6711a1.htm.*

Jacobson, N. S., Martell, C. R., & Dimidjian, S. (2001). Behavioral activation treatment for depression: Returning to contextual roots. *Clinical Psychology: Science and Practice, 8*(3), 255–270.

Jensen-Doss, A., & Weisz, J. R. (2008). Diagnostic agreement predicts treatment process and outcomes in youth mental health clinics. *Journal of Consulting and Clinical Psychology, 76*(5), 711–722.

Joiner, T. E. Jr. (2000). Depression's vicious scree: Self-propagating and erosive processes in depression chronicity. *Clinical Psychology: Science and Practice, 7*(2), 203–218.

Kagan, J. (1994). *Galen's prophecy.* New York: Basic Books.

Kagan, J., Reznick, J. S., & Snidman, N. (1988). Biological bases of childhood shyness. *Science, 240*(4849), 167–171.

Kallapiran, K., Koo, S., Kirubakaran, R., & Hancock, K. (2015). Effectiveness of mindfulness in improving

mental health symptoms of children and adolescents: A meta-analysis. *Child and Adolescent Mental Health, 20*(4), 182–194.

Kann, L., McManus, T., Harris, W. A., Shanklin, S. L., Flint, K. H., Hawkins, J., . . . Whittle, L. (2016). Youth risk behavior surveillance—United States, 2015. *Morbidity and Mortality Weekly Report: Surveillance Summaries, 65*(6), 1–174. Retrieved from *www.cdc.gov/healthyyouth/data/yrbs/pdf/2015/ss6506_updated.pdf.*

Kaufman, J., Birmaher, B., Axelson, D., Perepletchikova, F., Brent, D., & Ryan, N. (2016). Kiddie Schedule for Affective Disorders and Schizophrenia. Retrieved from *www.kennedykrieger.org/sites/default/files/library/documents/faculty/ksads-dsm-5-screener.pdf.*

Kazdin, A. E. (2001). *Behavior modification in applied settings.* New York: Wadsworth.

Kearney, C. (2007). *Getting your child to say "yes" to school: A guide for parents of youth with school refusal behavior.* New York: Oxford University Press.

Kearney, C. A. (2002). Identifying the function of school refusal behavior: A revision of the School Refusal Assessment Scale. *Journal of Psychopathology and Behavioral Assessment, 24*(4), 235–245.

Kearney, C. A. (2008). School absenteeism and school refusal behavior in youth: A contemporary review. *Clinical Psychology Review, 28*(3), 451–471.

Kearney, C. A., & Albano, A. M. (2007). *When children refuse school: A cognitive-behavioral therapy approach* (2nd ed.). Oxford, UK. Oxford University Press.

Kearney, C. A., & Graczyk, P. (2014). A response to intervention model to promote school attendance and decrease school absenteeism. *Child Youth Care Forum, 43*(1), 1–25.

Kearney, C. A., & Silverman, W. K. (1990). A preliminary analysis of a functional model of assessment and treatment for school refusal behavior. *Behavior Modification, 14*(3), 340–366.

Kearney, C. A., & Silverman, W. K. (1999). Functionally based prescriptive and nonprescriptive treatment for children and adolescents with school refusal behavior. *Behavior Therapy, 30*(4), 673–695.

Kelly, K. T. (2000). Are no-suicide contracts effective in preventing suicide in suicidal patients seen by primary care physicians? *Archives of Family Medicine, 9*(10), 1119–1121.

Kelly, K. T., & Knudson, M. P. (2000). Are no-suicide contracts effective in preventing suicide in suicidal patients seen by primary care physicians? *Archives of Family Medicine, 9*(10), 1119–1121.

Kendall, P. C., Compton, S. N., Walkup, J. T., Birmaher, B., Albano, A. M., Sherrill, J., . . . Keeton, C. (2010). Clinical characteristics of anxiety disordered youth. *Journal of Anxiety Disorders, 24*(3), 360–365.

Kendall, P. C., & Hedtke, K. A. (2006). *Cognitive-behavioral therapy for anxious children: Therapist manual.* New York: Workbook.

Kendall, P. C., & Pimentel, S. S. (2003). On the physiological symptom constellation in youth with generalized anxiety disorder (GAD). *Journal of Anxiety Disorders, 17*(2), 211–221.

Kennard, B. D., Clarke, G. N., Weersing, V. R., Asarnow, J. R., Shamseddeen, W., Porta, G., . . . Keller, M. B. (2009). Effective components of TORDIA cognitive–behavioral therapy for adolescent depression: Preliminary findings. *Journal of Consulting and Clinical Psychology, 77*(6), 1033.

Kertz, S. J., Petersen, D. R., & Stevens, K. T. (2019). Cognitive and attentional vulnerability to depression in youth: A review. *Clinical Psychology Review, 71*, 63–77.

Kessler, R. C., Avenevoli, S., Costello, E. J., Georgiades, K., Green, J. G., Gruber, M. J., . . . Sampson, N. A. (2012). Prevalence, persistence, and sociodemographic correlates of DSM-IV disorders in the National Comorbidity Survey Replication Adolescent Supplement. *Archives of General Psychiatry, 69*(4), 372–380.

Kessler, R. C., Berglund, P., Demler, O., Jin, R., Merikangas, K. R., & Walters, E. E. (2005). Lifetime prevalence and age-of-onset distributions of DSM-IV disorders in the National Comorbidity Survey Replication. *Archives of General Psychiatry, 62*(6), 593–602.

Kessler, R. C., Chiu, W. T., Demler, O., Merikangas, K. R., & Walters, E. E. (2005). Prevalence, severity, and comorbidity of 12-month DSM-IV disorders in the National Comorbidity Survey Replication. *Archives of General Psychiatry, 62*(6), 617–627.

Kessler, R. C., Petukhova, M., Sampson, N. A., Zaslavsky, A. M., & Wittcehn, H. (2012). Twelve-month and lifetime prevalence and lifetime morbid risk of anxiety and mood disorders in the United States, *International Journal of Methods in Psychiatric Research, 21*(3), 169–184.

Kiekens, G., Hasking, P., Bruffaerts, R., Claes, L., Baetens, I., Boyes, M., . . . Whitlock, J. (2017). What predicts ongoing nonsuicidal self-injury? *Journal of Nervous and Mental Disease, 205*(10), 762–770.

King, C. A., & Merchant, C. R. (2008). Social and interpersonal factors relating to adolescent suicidality: A review of the literature. *Archives of Suicide Research, 12*(3), 181–196.

King, N. J., & Bernstein, G. A. (2001). School refusal in children and adolescents: A review of the past 10 years. *Journal of the American Academy of Child & Adolescent Psychiatry, 40*(2), 197–205.

King, N., Tonge, B. J., Heyne, D., & Ollendick, T. H. (2000). Research on the cognitive-behavioral treatment of school refusal: A review and recommendations. *Clinical Psychology Review, 20*(4), 495–507.

King, N. J., Tonge, B. J., Heyne, D., Pritchard, M., Rollings, S., Young, D., . . . Ollendick, T. H. (1998). Cognitive-behavioral treatment of school-refusing children: A controlled evaluation. *Journal of the American Academy of Child & Adolescent Psychiatry, 37*(4), 395–403.

Klein, D. F. (1964). Delineation of two drug-responsive anxiety syndromes. *Psychopharmacologia, 5*(6), 397–408.

Kley, H., Tuschen-Caffier, B., & Heinrichs, N. (2012). Safety behaviors, self-focused attention and negative thinking in children with social anxiety disorder, socially anxious and non-anxious children. *Journal of Behavior Therapy and Experimental Psychiatry, 43*(1), 548–555.

Kõlves, K., & De Leo, D. (2017). Suicide methods in children and adolescents. *European Child & Adolescent Psychiatry, 26*(2), 155–164.

Kossowsky, J., Pfaltz, M. C., Schneider, S., Taeymans, J., Locher, C., & Gaab, J. (2013). The separation anxiety hypothesis of panic disorder revisited: A meta-analysis. *American Journal of Psychiatry, 170*(7), 768–781.

Lakdawalla, Z., Hankin, B. L., & Mermelstein, R. (2007). Cognitive theories of depression in children and adolescents: A conceptual and quantitative review. *Clinical Child and Family Psychology Review, 10*(1), 1–24.

Lambert, M. J., Harmon, C., Slade, K., Whipple, J. L., & Hawkins, E. J. (2005). Providing feedback to psychotherapists on their patients' progress: Clinical results and practice suggestions. *Journal of Clinical Psychology, 61*(2), 165–174.

Lambert, M. J., Whipple, J. L., Hawkins, E. J., Vermeersch, D. A., Nielsen, S. L., & Smart, D. W. (2003). Is it time for clinicians to routinely track patient outcome? A meta-analysis. *Clinical Psychology: Science and Practice, 10*(3), 288–301.

Langer, D. A., & Jensen-Doss, A. (2018). Shared decision-making in youth mental health care: Using the evidence to plan treatments collaboratively. *Journal of Clinical Child & Adolescent Psychology, 47*(5), 821–831.

Last, C. G., Hansen, C., & Franco, N. (1998). Cognitive-behavioral treatment of school phobia. *Journal of the American Academy of Child & Adolescent Psychiatry, 37*(4), 404–411.

Last, C. G., & Strauss, C. C. (1990). School refusal in anxiety-disordered children and adolescents. *Journal of the American Academy of Child & Adolescent Psychiatry, 29*(1), 31–35.

Lavallee, K., Herren, C., Blatter-Meunier, J., Adornetto, C., In-Albon, T., & Schneider, S. (2011). Early predictors of separation anxiety disorder: Early stranger anxiety, parental pathology and prenatal factors. *Psychopathology, 44*(6), 354–361.

Legerstee, J. S., Garnefski, N., Jellesma, F. C., Verhulst, F. C., & Utens, E. M. (2010). Cognitive coping and childhood anxiety disorders. *European Child & Adolescent Psychiatry, 19*(2), 143–150.

Legerstee, J. S., Tulen, J. H., Dierckx, B., Treffers, P. D., Verhulst, F. C., & Utens, E. M. (2010). CBT for childhood anxiety disorders: Differential changes in selective attention between treatment responders and non-responders. *Journal of Child Psychology and Psychiatry, 51*(2), 162–172.

Levinson, D. F. (2006). The genetics of depression: A review. *Biological Psychiatry, 60*(2), 84–92.

Lewinsohn, P. M., & Graf, M. (1973). Pleasant activities and depression. *Journal of Consulting and Clinical Psychology, 41*(2), 261–268.

Lewinsohn, P. M., Holm-Denoma, J. M., Small, J. W., Seeley, J. R., & Joiner, T. E., Jr. (2008). Separation anxiety disorder in childhood as a risk factor for future mental illness. *Journal of the American Academy of Child & Adolescent Psychiatry, 47*(5), 548–555.

Lewinsohn, P. M., & Libet, J. (1972). Pleasant events, activity schedules, and depressions. *Journal of Abnormal Psychology, 79*(3), 291–295.

Lewinsohn, P. M., Rohde, P., & Seeley, J. R. (1996). Adolescent suicidal ideation and attempts: Prevalence, risk factors, and clinical implications. *Clinical Psychology: Science and Practice, 3*(1), 25–46.

Lewis-Morrarty, E., Degnan, K. A., Chronis-Tuscano, A., Rubin, K. H., Cheah, C. S., Pine, D. S., . . . Fox, N. A. (2012). Maternal over-control moderates the association between early childhood behavioral inhibition and adolescent social anxiety symptoms. *Journal of Abnormal Child Psychology, 40*(8), 1363–1373.

Leyfer, O., Gallo, K. P., Cooper-Vince, C., & Pincus, D. B. (2013). Patterns and predictors of comorbidity of DSM-IV anxiety disorders in a clinical sample of children and adolescents. *Journal of Anxiety Disorders, 27*(3), 306–311.

Lighthouse Project the Columbia Lighthouse Project. (2016). Retrieved from *https://cssrs.columbia.edu*.

Linehan, M. M. (1993). *Diagnosis and treatment of mental disorders: Cognitive-behavioral treatment of borderline personality disorder.* New York: Guilford Press.

Liu, M., Wu, L., & Yao, S. (2016). Dose–response association of screen time-based sedentary behaviour in children and adolescents and depression: A meta-analysis of observational studies. *British Journal of Sports Medicine, 50*(20), 1252–1258.

Liu, R. T., & Mustanski, B. (2012). Suicidal ideation and self-harm in lesbian, gay, bisexual, and transgender youth. *American Journal of Preventive Medicine, 42*(3), 221–228.

Lloyd-Richardson, E. E., Perrine, N., Dierker, L., & Kelley, M. L. (2007). Characteristics and functions of non-suicidal self-injury in a community sample of adolescents. *Psychological Medicine, 37*(8), 1183–1192.

Manicavasagar, V., Silove, D., Curtis, J., & Wagner, R. (2000). Continuities of separation anxiety from early life into adulthood. *Journal of Anxiety Disorders, 14*(1), 1–18.

Manos, R. C., Kanter, J. W., & Busch, A. M. (2010). A critical review of assessment strategies to measure the behavioral activation model of depression. *Clinical Psychology Review, 30*(5), 547–561.

March, J., Silva, S., Petrycki, S., Curry, J., Wells, K., Fairbank, J., . . . Severe, J. (2004). Fluoxetine, cognitive-behavioral therapy, and their combination for adolescents with depression: Treatment for Adolescents with Depression Study (TADS) randomized controlled trial. *JAMA, 292*(7), 807–820.

Marshal, M. P., Dietz, L. J., Friedman, M. S., Stall, R., Smith, H. A., McGinley, J., . . . Brent, D. A. (2011). Suicidality and depression disparities between sexual minority and heterosexual youth: A meta-analytic review. *Journal of Adolescent Health, 49*(2), 115–123.

Martin, C., Cabrol, S., Bouvard, M. P., Lepine, J. P., & Mouren-Simeoni, M. C. (1999). Anxiety and depressive disorders in fathers and mothers of anxious school-refusing children. *Journal of the American Academy of Child & Adolescent Psychiatry, 38*(7), 916–922.

Mash, E. J., & Hunsley, J. (2005). Evidence-based assessment of child and adolescent disorders: Issues and challenges. *Journal of Clinical Child and Adolescent Psychology, 34*(3), 362–379.

Masi, G., Mucci, M., & Millepiedi, S. (2001). Separation anxiety disorder in children and adolescents. *CNS Drugs, 15*(2), 93–104.

Maynard, B. R., Brendel, K. E., Bulanda, J. J., Heyne, D., Thompson, A. M., & Pigott, T. D. (2015). Psychosocial interventions for school refusal with primary and secondary school students: A systematic review. *Campbell Systematic Reviews, 11*(1), 1–76.

Maynard, B. R., Brendel, K. E., Bulanda, J. J., & Pigott, T. (2013). Protocol: Psychosocial interventions for school refusal behavior with elementary and secondary school students. *Campbell Systematic Reviews, 9*(1), 1–33.

Maynard, B. R., Heyne, D., Brendel, K. E., Bulanda, J. J., Thompson, A. M., & Pigott, T. D. (2018). Treatment for school refusal among children and adolescents: A systematic review and meta-analysis. *Research on Social Work Practice, 28*(1), 56–67.

Maynard, B. R., McCrea, K. T., Pigott, T. D., & Kelly, M. S. (2012). Indicated truancy interventions: Effects on school attendance among chronic truant students. *Campbell Systematic Reviews, 8*(1), 1–84.

Maynard, B. R., Salas-Wright, C. P., Vaughn, M. G., & Peters, K. E. (2012). Who are truant youth? Examining distinctive profiles of truant youth using latent profile analysis. *Journal of Youth and Adolescence, 41*(12), 1671–1684.

McLeod, B. D., Weisz, J. R., & Wood, J. J. (2007). Examining the association between parenting and childhood depression: A meta-analysis. *Clinical Psychology Review, 27*(8), 986–1003.

McLeod, B. D., Wood, J. J., & Weisz, J. R. (2007). Examining the association between parenting and childhood anxiety: A meta-analysis. *Clinical Psychology Review, 27*(2), 155–172.

McShane, G., Walter, G., & Rey, J. M. (2001). Characteristics of adolescents with school refusal. *Australian & New Zealand Journal of Psychiatry, 35*(6), 822–826.

Melvin, G. A., Dudley, A. L., Gordon, M. S., Klimkeit, E., Gullone, E., Taffe, J., & Tonge, B. J. (2017). Augmenting cognitive behavior therapy for school refusal with fluoxetine: A randomized controlled trial. *Child Psychiatry & Human Development, 48*(3), 485–497.

Melvin, G. A., & Gordon, M. S. (2019). Antidepressant medication: Is it a viable and valuable adjunct to cognitive-behavioral therapy for school refusal? *Cognitive and Behavioral Practice, 26*(1), 107–118.

Merikangas, K. R., He, J. P., Burstein, M., Swanson, S. A., Avenevoli, S., Cui, L., . . . Swendsen, J. (2010). Lifetime prevalence of mental disorders in U.S. adolescents: Results from the National Comorbidity Survey Replication–Adolescent Supplement (NCS-A). *Journal of the American Academy of Child & Adolescent Psychiatry, 49*(10), 980–989.

Merikangas, K. R., Stevens, D. E., Fenton, B., Stolar, M., O'Malley, S., Woods, S. W., & Risch, N. (1998). Co-morbidity and familial aggregation of alcoholism and anxiety disorders. *Psychological Medicine, 28*(4), 773–788.

Miers, A. C., Blöte, A. W., Bokhorst,C. L., & Westenberg, P. M. (2009). Negative self-evaluations and the relation to performance level in socially anxious children and adolescents. *Behavior Research and Therapy, 47*(12), 1043–1049.

Miers, A. C., Blöte, A. W., de Rooij, M., Bokhorst, C. L., & Westenberg, P. M. (2012). Trajectories of social anxiety during adolescence and relations with cognition, social competence, and temperament. *Journal of Abnormal Child Psychology, 41*(1), 97–110.

Miers, A. C., Blöte, A. W., & Westenberg, P. M. (2011). Negative social cognitions in socially anxious youth: Distorted reality or a kernel of truth? *Journal of Child and Family Studies, 20*(2), 214–223.

Miller, W. R., & Rollnick, S. (2012). *Motivational interviewing: Helping people change.* New York: Guilford Press.

Moore, P. S., Whaley, S. E., & Sigman, M. (2004). Interactions between mothers and children: Impacts of maternal and child anxiety. *Journal of Abnormal Psychology, 113*(3), 471–476.

Moses, T. (2018). Suicide attempts among adolescents with self-reported disabilities. *Child Psychiatry & Human Development, 49*(3), 420–433.

Mueller, A. S., James, W., Abrutyn, S., & Levin, M. L. (2015). Suicide ideation and bullying among US adolescents: Examining the intersections of sexual orientation, gender, and race/ethnicity. *American Journal of Public Health, 105*(5), 980–985.

Muris, P. (2011). Further insights in the etiology of fear, anxiety and their disorders in children and adolescents: The partial fulfillment of a prophecy. *Journal of Child and Family Studies, 20*(2), 133–134.

Muris, P., Meesters, C., Merckelbach, H., & Hülsenbeck, P. (2000). Worry in children is related to perceived parental rearing and attachment. *Behaviour Research and Therapy, 38*(5), 487–497.

Muris, P., Meesters, C., Merckelbach, H., Sermon, A.,

& Zwakhalen, S. (1998). Worry in children. *Journal of the American Academy of Child and Adolescent Psychiatry, 37*(7), 703–710.

Nadeem, E., Cappella, E., Holland, S., Coccaro, C., & Crisonino, G. (2016). Development and piloting of a classroom-focused measurement feedback system. *Administration and Policy in Mental Health and Mental Health Services Research, 43*(3), 379–393.

Nestor, B. A., Cheek, S. M., & Liu, R. T. (2016). Ethnic and racial differences in mental health service utilization for suicidal ideation and behavior in a nationally representative sample of adolescents. *Journal of Affective Disorders, 202*(15), 197–202.

Nischal, A., Tripathi, A., Nischal, A., & Trivedi, J. K. (2012). Suicide and antidepressants: What current evidence indicates. *Mens Sana Monographs, 10*(1), 33–44.

Nock, M. K. (2010). Self-injury. *Annual Review of Clinical Psychology, 6*(1), 339–363.

Nock, M. K., Borges, G., Bromet, E. J., Cha, C. B., Kessler, R. C., & Lee, S. (2008). Suicide and suicidal behavior. *Epidemiologic Reviews, 30*(1), 133–154.

Nock, M. K., Green, J. G., Hwang, I., McLaughlin, K. A., Sampson, N. A., Zaslavsky, A. M., & Kessler, R. C. (2013). Prevalence, correlates, and treatment of lifetime suicidal behavior among adolescents: Results from the National Comorbidity Survey replication adolescent supplement. *JAMA Psychiatry, 70*(3), 300–310.

Nock, M. K., Holmberg, E. B., Photos, V. I., & Michel, B. D. (2007). Self-injurious thoughts and behaviors interview: Development, reliability, and validity in an adolescent sample. *Psychological Assessment, 19*(3), 309–317.

Nock, M. K., Joiner, T. E., Jr., Gordon, K. H., Lloyd-Richardson, E., & Prinstein, M. J. (2006). Non-suicidal self-injury among adolescents: Diagnostic correlates and relation to suicide attempts. *Psychiatry Research, 144*(1), 65–72.

Nock, M. K., & Kazdin, A. E. (2001). Parent expectancies for child therapy: Assessment and relation to participation in treatment. *Journal of Child and Family Studies, 10*(2), 155–180.

Nock, M. K., & Kazdin, A. E. (2005). Randomized controlled trial of a brief intervention for increasing participation in parent management training. *Journal of Consulting and Clinical Psychology, 73*(5), 872–879.

Nock, M. K., & Prinstein, M. J. (2004). A functional approach to the assessment of self-mutilative behavior. *Journal of Consulting and Clinical Psychology, 72*(5), 885–890.

Nock, M. K., & Prinstein, M. J. (2005). Contextual features and behavioral functions of self-mutilation among adolescents. *Journal of Abnormal Psychology, 114*(1), 140–146.

Nock, M. K., Prinstein, M. J., & Sterba, S. K. (2009). Revealing the form and function of self-injurious thoughts and behaviors: A real-time ecological assessment study among adolescents and young adults. *Journal of Abnormal Psychology, 118*(4), 816–827.

Okuyama, M., Okada, M., Kuribayashi, M., & Kaneko, S. (1999). Factors responsible for the prolongation of school refusal. *Psychiatry and Clinical Neurosciences, 53*(4), 461–469.

Ollendick, T. H., Benoit, K., & Grills-Taquechel, A. E. (2014). Social anxiety in children and adolescents. In J. Weeks (Ed.), *The Wiley–Blackwell handbook of social anxiety* (pp. 181–200). Chichester, UK: John Wiley & Sons.

Ollendick, T. H., & Hirshfeld-Becker, D. R. (2002). The developmental psychopathology of social anxiety disorder. *Biological Psychiatry, 51*(1), 44–58.

Ollendick, T. H., Jarrett, M. A., Grills-Taquechel, A. E., Hovey, L. D., & Wolff, J. C. (2008). Comorbidity as a predictor and moderator of treatment outcome in youth with anxiety, affective, attention deficit/hyperactivity disorder, and oppositional/conduct disorders. *Clinical Psychology Review, 28*(8), 1447–1471.

Osher, Y., & Belmaker, R. H. (2009). Omega-3 fatty acids in depression: A review of three studies. *CNS Neuroscience & Therapeutics, 15*(2), 128–133.

Oud, M., De Winter, L., Vermeulen-Smit, E., Bodden, D., Nauta, M., Stone, L., . . . Engels, R. (2019). Effectiveness of CBT for children and adolescents with depression: A systematic review and meta-regression analysis. *European Psychiatry, 57,* 33–45.

Pandey, G. N. (1997). Altered serotonin function in suicide: Evidence from platelet and neuroendocrine studies. *Annals of the New York Academy of Sciences, 836*(1), 182–201.

Paschall, M. J., & Bersamin, M. (2018). School-based health centers, depression, and suicide risk among adolescents. *American Journal of Preventive Medicine, 54*(1), 44–50.

Paulhus, D. L., & Morgan, K. L. (1997). Perceptions of intelligence in leaderless groups: The dynamic effects of shyness and acquaintance. *Journal of Personality and Social Psychology, 72*(3), 581–591.

Pediatric OCD Treatment Study Team (2004). Cognitive-behavior therapy, sertraline, and their combination for children and adolescents with obsessive–compulsive disorder: The Pediatric OCD Treatment Study (POTS) randomized controlled trial. *JAMA, 292*(16), 1969–1976.

Peris, T. S., Compton, S. N., Kendall, P. C., Birmaher, B., Sherrill, J., March, J., . . . Piacentini, J. (2015). Trajectories of change in youth anxiety during cognitive-behavior therapy. *Journal of Consulting and Clinical Psychology, 83*(2), 239–252.

Persons, J. B. (2006). Case formulation-driven psychotherapy. *Clinical Psychology: Science and Practice, 13*(2), 167–170.

Pettit, J. W., Buitron, V., & Green, K. L. (2018). Assessment and management of suicide risk in children and adolescents. *Cognitive and Behavioral Practice, 25*(4), 460–472.

Pettit, J. W., Temple, S. R., Norton, P. J., Yaroslavsky, I., Grover, K. E., Morgan, S. T., & Schatte, D. J. (2009). Thought suppression and suicidal ideation: Preliminary evidence in support of a robust association. *Depression and Anxiety, 26*(8), 758–763.

Phillips, D. P. (1974). The influence of suggestion on suicide: Substantive and theoretical implications of the Werther effect. *American Sociological Review, 39*(3), 340–354.

Piacentini, J., Bennett, S., Compton, S. N., Kendall, P. C., Birmaher, B., Albano, A. M., . . . Rynn, M. (2014). 24-and 36-week outcomes for the Child/Adolescent Anxiety Multimodal Study (CAMS). *Journal of the American Academy of Child & Adolescent Psychiatry, 53*(3), 297–310.

Platt, B., Kadosh, K. C., & Lau, J. Y. (2013). The role of peer rejection in adolescent depression. *Depression and Anxiety, 30*(9), 809–821.

Plener, P. L., Schumacher, T. S., Munz, L. M., & Groschwitz, R. C. (2015). The longitudinal course of nonsuicidal self-injury and deliberate self-harm: A systematic review of the literature. *Borderline Personality Disorder and Emotion Dysregulation, 2*(1), 1–11.

Raifman, J., Moscoe, E., Austin, S. B., & McConnell, M. (2017). Difference-in-differences analysis of the association between state same-sex marriage policies and adolescent suicide attempts. *JAMA Pediatrics, 171*(4), 350–356.

Rao, P. A., Beidel, D. C., Turner, S. M., Ammerman, R. T., Crosby, L. E., & Sallee, F. R. (2007). Social anxiety disorder in childhood and adolescence: Descriptive psychopathology. *Behaviour Research and Therapy, 45*(6), 1181–1191.

Rao, U., Hammen, C. L., & Poland, R. E. (2009). Risk markers for depression in adolescents: Sleep and HPA measures. *Neuropsychopharmacology, 34*(8), 1936–1945.

Rapee, R. M. (1997). Potential role of childrearing practices in the development of anxiety and depression. *Clinical Psychology Review, 17*(1), 47–67.

Rapee, R. M. (2014). Preschool environment and temperament as predictors of social and nonsocial anxiety disorders in middle adolescence. *Journal of the American Academy of Child & Adolescent Psychiatry, 53*(3), 320–328.

Rapee, R. M., & Spence, S. H. (2004). The etiology of social phobia: Empirical evidence and an initial model. *Clinical Psychology Review, 24*(7), 737–767.

Reid, K. (2005). The causes, views and traits of school absenteeism and truancy: An analytical review. *Research in Education, 74*(1), 59–82.

Reid, W. H. (1998). Promises, promises: Don't rely on patients' no-suicide/no-violence "contracts." *Journal of Practical Psychiatry and Behavioral Health, 4*(3), 316–318.

Reinke, W. M., Lewis-Palmer, T., & Martin, E. (2007). The effect of visual performance feedback on teacher use of behavior-specific praise. *Behavior Modification, 31*(3), 247–263.

Renaud, J., Brent, D. A., Baugher, M., Birmaher, B., Kolko, D. J., & Bridge, J. (1998). Rapid response to psychosocial treatment for adolescent depression: A two-year follow-up. *Journal of the American Academy of Child & Adolescent Psychiatry, 37*(11), 1184–1190.

Rice, F., Harold, G., & Thapar, A. (2002). The genetic aetiology of childhood depression: A review. *Journal of Child Psychology and Psychiatry, 43*(1), 65–79.

Rizvi, S. L., & Ritschel, L. A. (2014). Mastering the art of chain analysis in dialectical behavior therapy. *Cognitive and Behavioral Practice, 21*(3), 335–349.

Robinson, J. L., Kagan, J., Reznick, J. S., & Corley, R. (1992). The heritability of inhibited and uninhibited behavior: A twin study. *Developmental Psychology, 28*(6), 1030–1037.

Roemer, L., & Borkovec, T. D. (1993). Worry: Unwanted cognitive activity that controls unwanted somatic experience. In D. M. Wegner & J. W. Pennebaker (Eds.), *Handbook of mental control* (pp. 220–238). Century Psychology Series. Upper Saddle River, NJ: Prentice Hall.

Rood, L., Roelofs, J., Bögels, S. M., Nolen-Hoeksema, S., & Schouten, E. (2009). The influence of emotion-focused rumination and distraction on depressive symptoms in non-clinical youth: A meta-analytic review. *Clinical Psychology Review, 29*(7), 607–616.

Ross, S., & Heath, N. (2002). A study of the frequency of self-mutilation in a community sample of adolescents. *Journal of Youth and Adolescence, 31*(1), 67–77.

Rubin, K. H., Burgess, K. B., & Hastings, P. D. (2002). Stability and social–behavioral consequences of toddlers' inhibited temperament and parenting behaviors. *Child Development, 73*(2), 483–495.

Rudolph, K. D., Flynn, M., & Abaied, J. L. (2008). A developmental perspective on interpersonal theories of youth depression. In J. R. Z. Abela & B. L. Hankin (Eds.), *Handbook of depression in children and adolescents* (pp. 79–102). New York: Guilford Press.

Rudolph, K. D., & Hammen, C. (1999). Age and gender as determinants of stress exposure, generation, and reactions in youngsters: A transactional perspective. *Child Development, 70*(3), 660–677.

Rudolph, K. D., Hammen, C., Burge, D., Lindberg, N., Herzberg, D., & Daley, S. E. (2000). Toward an interpersonal life-stress model of depression: The developmental context of stress generation. *Development and Psychopathology, 12*(2), 215–234.

Rueger, S. Y., Malecki, C. K., Pyun, Y., Aycock, C., & Coyle, S. (2016). A meta-analytic review of the association between perceived social support and depression in childhood and adolescence. *Psychological Bulletin, 142*(10), 1017–1067.

Ruscio, A. M., Brown, T. A., Chiu, W. T., Sareen, J.,

Stein, M. B., & Kessler, R. C. (2007). Social fears and social phobia in the USA: Results from the National Comorbidity Survey Replication. *Psychological Medicine, 38*(1), 15–28.

Salkovskis, P. M. (1991). The importance of behaviour in the maintenance of anxiety and panic: A cognitive account. *Behavioural and Cognitive Psychotherapy, 19*(1), 6–19.

Sander, J. B., & McCarty, C. A. (2005). Youth depression in the family context: Familial risk factors and models of treatment. *Clinical Child and Family Psychology Review, 8*(3), 203–219.

Scaini, S., Ogliari, A., Eley, T. C., Zavos, H. M., & Battaglia, M. (2012). Genetic and environmental contributions to separation anxiety: A meta-analytic approach to twin data. *Depression and Anxiety, 29*(9), 754–761.

Segrin, C. (2000). Social skills deficits associated with depression. *Clinical Psychology Review, 20*(3), 379–403.

Selby, E. A., Anestis, M. D., & Joiner, T. E. (2008). Understanding the relationship between emotional and behavioral dysregulation: Emotional cascades. *Behaviour Research and Therapy, 46*(5), 593–611.

Shaffer, D., & Pfeffer, C. R. (2001). Practice parameter for the assessment and treatment of children and adolescents with suicidal behavior. *Journal of the American Academy of Child & Adolescent Psychiatry, 40*(7), 24S–51S.

Shear, K., Jin, R., Ruscio, A. M., Walters, E. E., & Kessler, R. C. (2006). Prevalence and correlates of estimated DSM-IV child and adult separation anxiety disorder in the National Comorbidity Survey Replication. *American Journal of Psychiatry, 163*(6), 1074–1083.

Sheeber, L., & Sorensen, E. (1998). Family relationships of depressed adolescents: A multimethod assessment. *Journal of Clinical Child Psychology, 27*(3), 268–277.

Shirk, S. R., Crisostomo, P. S., Jungbluth, N., & Gudmundsen, G. R. (2013). Cognitive mechanisms of change in CBT for adolescent depression: Associations among client involvement, cognitive distortions, and treatment outcome. *International Journal of Cognitive Therapy, 6*(4), 311–324.

Silove, D., Harris, M., Morgan, A., Boyce, P., Manicavasagar, V., Hadzi-Pavlovic, D., & Wilhelm, K. (1995). Is early separation anxiety a specific precursor of panic disorder–agoraphobia? A community study. *Psychological Medicine, 25*(2), 405–411.

Silverman, W. K., La Greca, A. M., & Wasserstein, S. (1995). What do children worry about? Worries and their relation to anxiety. *Child Development, 66*(3), 671–686.

Simon, G. E., Savarino, J., Operskalski, B., & Wang, P. S. (2006). Suicide risk during antidepressant treatment. *American Journal of Psychiatry, 163*(1), 41–47.

Songco, A., Hudson, J. L., & Fox, E. (2020). A cognitive model of pathological worry in children and adolescents: A systematic review. *Clinical Child and Family Psychology Review, 23*(2), 229–249.

Sornberger, M. J., Heath, N. L., Toste, J. R., & McLouth, R. (2012). Nonsuicidal self-injury and gender: Patterns of prevalence, methods, and locations among adolescents. *Suicide and Life-Threatening Behavior, 42*(3), 266–278.

Spence, S. H., & Rapee, R. M. (2016). The etiology of social anxiety disorder: An evidence-based model. *Behaviour Research and Therapy, 86*(1), 50–67.

Stack, S. (1987). The sociological study of suicide: Methodological issues. *Suicide and Life-Threatening Behavior, 17*(2), 133–150.

Stack, S. (2003). Media coverage as a risk factor in suicide. *Journal of Epidemiology & Community Health, 57*(4), 238–240.

Stack, S. (2005). Suicide in the media: A quantitative review of studies based on nonfictional stories. *Suicide and Life-Threatening Behavior, 35*(2), 121–133.

Stack, S. (2009). Copycat effects of fictional suicide: A meta-analysis. In S. Stack & D. Lester (Eds.), *Suicide and the creative arts* (pp. 231–243). New York: Nova Science.

Stahl, S. M. (1998). Basic psychopharmacology of antidepressants: Part 1. Antidepressants have seven distinct mechanisms of action. *Journal of Clinical Psychiatry, 59*(Suppl. 4), 5–14.

Stanley, B., & Brown, G. K. (2012). Safety planning intervention: A brief intervention to mitigate suicide risk. *Cognitive and Behavioral Practice, 19*(2), 256–264.

Stanley, B., Brown, G., Brent, D. A., Wells, K., Poling, K., Curry, J., . . . Hughes, J. (2009). Cognitive-behavioral therapy for suicide prevention (CBT-SP): Treatment model, feasibility, and acceptability. *Journal of the American Academy of Child & Adolescent Psychiatry, 48*(10), 1005–1013.

Stone, D. M., Simon, T. R., Fowler, K. A., Kegler, S. R., Yuan, K., Holland, K. M., . . . Crosby, A. E. (2018). Vital signs: Trends in state suicide rates—United States, 1999–2016 and circumstances contributing to suicide—27 states, 2015. *Morbidity and Mortality Weekly Report, 67*(22), 617–624.

Suarez, L., & Bell-Dolan, D. (2001). The relationship of child worry to cognitive biases: Threat interpretation and likelihood of event occurrence. *Behavior Therapy, 32*(3), 425–442.

Sullivan, E. M., Annest, J. L., Simon, T. R., Luo, F., & Dahlberg, L. L. (2015). Suicide trends among persons aged 10–24 years—United States, 1994–2012. *Morbidity and Mortality Weekly Report, 64*(8), 201.

Sullivan, P. F., Neale, M. C., & Kendler, K. S. (2000). Genetic epidemiology of major depression: Review and meta-analysis. *American Journal of Psychiatry, 157*(10), 1552–1562.

Sumter, S. R., Bokhorst, C. L., Miers, A. C., Van Pelt, J., & Westenberg, P. M. (2010). Age and puberty differences in stress responses during a public speaking task:

Do adolescents grow more sensitive to social evaluation? *Psychoneuroendocrinology, 35*(10), 1510–1516.

Sutphen, R. D., Ford, J. P., & Flaherty, C. (2010). Truancy interventions: A review of the research literature. *Research on Social Work Practice, 20*(2), 161–171.

Tang, T. Z., & DeRubeis, R. J. (1999). Reconsidering rapid early response in cognitive behavioral therapy for depression. *Clinical Psychology: Science and Practice, 6*(3), 283–288.

Tiwari, S., Podell, J. C., Martin, E. D., Mychailyszyn, M. P., Furr, J. M., & Kendall, P. C. (2008). Experiential avoidance in the parenting of anxious youth: Theory, research, and future directions. *Cognition and Emotion, 22*(3), 480–496.

Treatment for Adolescents with Depression Study Team. (2009). The Treatment for Adolescents with Depression Study (TADS): Outcomes over 1 year of naturalistic follow-up. *American Journal of Psychiatry, 166*(10), 1141–1149.

Twenge, J. M., Joiner, T. E., Rogers, M. L., & Martin, G. N. (2018). Increases in depressive symptoms, suicide-related outcomes, and suicide rates among U.S. adolescents after 2010 and links to increased new media screen time. *Clinical Psychological Science, 6*(1), 3–17.

Underwood, M. D., Kassir, S. A., Bakalian, M. J., Galfalvy, H., Dwork, A. J., Mann, J. J., & Arango, V. (2018). Serotonin receptors and suicide, major depression, alcohol use disorder and reported early life adversity. *Translational Psychiatry 8*(1), 279–294.

U. S. Department of Education. (2001). The Elementary and Secondary Education Act (The No Child Left Behind Act of 2001). Retrieved July 25, 2003, from *www2.ed.gov/nclb/overview/intro/execsumm.html*

U. S. Department of Education (2019). Chronic absenteeism in the nation's schools: A hidden educational crisis. Retrieved from *www2.ed.gov/datastory/chronicabsenteeism.html#:~:text=Students%20who%20are%20chronically%20absent,of%20falling%20behind%20in%20school.*

Verduin, T. L., & Kendall, P. C. (2003). Differential occurrence of comorbidity within childhood anxiety disorders. *Journal of Clinical Child & Adolescent Psychology, 32*(2), 290–295.

Vidair, H. B., Feyijinmi, G. O., & Feindler, E. L. (2016). Termination in cognitive-behavioral therapy with children, adolescents, and parents. *Psychotherapy, 54*(1), 15–21.

Walkup, J. T. (2017). Antidepressant efficacy for depression in children and adolescents: Industry and NIMH funded studies. *American Journal of Psychiatry, 147*(5), 430–437.

Walkup, J. T., Albano, A. M., Piacentini, J., Birmaher, B., Compton, S. N., Sherrill, J. T., . . . Iyengar, S. (2008) Cognitive behavioral therapy, sertraline, or a combination in childhood anxiety. *New England Journal of Medicine, 359*(26), 2753–2766.

Wan, L. B., Levitch, C. F., Perez, A. M., Brallier, J. W.,

Iosifescu, D. V., Chang, L. C., . . . Murrough, J. W. (2015). Ketamine safety and tolerability in clinical trials for treatment-resistant depression. *Journal of Clinical Psychiatry, 76*(3), 247–252.

Wasserman, D., Hoven, C. W., Wasserman, C., Wall, M., Eisenberg, R., Hadlaczky, G., . . . Carli, V. (2015). School-based suicide prevention programmes: The SEYLE cluster-randomised, controlled trial. *The Lancet, 385*(9977), 1536–1544.

Watson, D. (2005). Rethinking the mood and anxiety disorders: A quantitative hierarchical model for DSM-V. *Journal of Abnormal Psychology, 114*(4), 522–536.

Weems, C. F., Silverman, W. K., & La Greca, A. M. (2000). What do youth referred for anxiety problems worry about? Worry and its relation to anxiety and anxiety disorders in children and adolescents. *Journal of Abnormal Child Psychology, 28*(1), 63–72.

Weersing, V. R., Jeffreys, M., Do, M. T., Schwartz, K. T., & Bolano, C. (2017). Evidence base update of psychosocial treatments for child and adolescent depression. *Journal of Clinical Child and Adolescent Psychology, 46*(1), 11–43.

Weisz, J. R., Chorpita, B. F., Frye, A., Ng, M. Y., Lau, N., Bearman, S. K., . . . Hoagwood, K. E. (2011). Youth top problems: Using idiographic, consumer-guided assessment to identify treatment needs and to track change during psychotherapy. *Journal of Consulting and Clinical Psychology, 79*(3), 369–380.

Weisz, J. R., Thurber, C. A., Sweeney, L., Proffitt, V. D., & LeGagnoux, G. L. (1997). Brief treatment of mild-to-moderate child depression using primary and secondary control enhancement training. *Journal of Consulting and Clinical Psychology, 65*(4), 703.

Wells, A. (2006). The metacognitive model of worry and generalised anxiety disorder. In G. C. L. Davey & A. Wells (Eds.), *Worry and its psychological disorders: Theory, assessment and treatment* (pp. 179–199). New York: Wiley Publishing.

Whaley, S. E., Pinto, A., & Sigman, M. (1999). Characterizing interactions between anxious mothers and their children. *Journal of Consulting and Clinical Psychology, 67*(6), 826–836.

Wierzbicki, M., & Sayler, M. K. (1991). Depression and engagement in pleasant and unpleasant activities in normal children. *Journal of Clinical Psychology, 47*(4), 499–505.

Wilkins, J. (2008). School characteristics that influence student attendance: Experiences of students in a school avoidance program. *High School Journal, 91*(3), 12–24.

Wilson, C., Budd, B., Chernin, R., King, H., Leddy, A., Maclennan, F., & Mallandain, I. (2011). The role of meta-cognition and parenting in adolescent worry. *Journal of Anxiety Disorders, 25*(1), 71–79.

Wingate, L. R., Joiner, T. E., Jr., Walker, R. L., Rudd, M. D., & Jobes, D. A. (2004). Empirically informed approaches to topics in suicide risk assessment. *Behavioral Sciences & the Law, 22*(5), 651–665.

Wolff, J., Frazier, E., Davis, S., Freed, R. D., Esposito-Smythers, C., Liu, R., & Spirito, A. (2017). Depression and suicidality. In C. A. Flessner & J. C. Piacentini (Eds.), *Clinical handbook of psychological disorders in children and adolescents: A step by step treatment manual* (pp. 55–93). New York: Guilford Press.

Wolitzky-Taylor, K., Bobova, L., Zinbarg, R. E., Mineka, S., & Craske, M. G. (2012). Longitudinal investigation of the impact of anxiety and mood disorders in adolescence on subsequent substance use disorder onset and vice versa. *Addictive Behaviors, 37*(8), 982–985.

Wood, J. J., McLeod, B. D., Sigman, M., Hwang, W. C., & Chu, B. C. (2003). Parenting and childhood anxiety: Theory, empirical findings, and future directions. *Journal of Child Psychology and Psychiatry, 44*(1), 134–151.

World Health Organization. (2014). *Global health observatory data: World health statistics 2014.* Geneva: Author. Retrieved from *www.who.int/gho*.

Wu, X., Liu, F., Cai, H., Huang, L., Li, Y., Mo, Z., & Lin, J. (2013). Cognitive behaviour therapy combined fluoxetine treatment superior to cognitive behaviour therapy alone for school refusal. *International Journal of Pharmacology, 9*(3), 197–203.

Yap, M. B. H., Pilkington, P. D., Ryan, S. M., & Jorm, A. F. (2014). Parental factors associated with depression and anxiety in young people: A systematic review and meta-analysis. *Journal of Affective Disorders, 156*, 8–23.

Yoman, J. (2008). A primer on functional analysis. *Cognitive and Behavioral Practice, 15*(3), 325–340.

Young, J. F., Mufson, L., & Benas, J. S. (2014). Interpersonal psychotherapy for youth depression and anxiety. In J. Ehrenreich-May & B. C. Chu (Eds.), *Transdiagnostic treatments for children and adolescents: Principles and practice* (pp. 183–202). New York: Guilford Press.

Youngstrom, E. A., Choukas-Bradley, S., Calhoun, C. D., & Jensen-Doss, A. (2015). Clinical guide to the evidence-based assessment approach to diagnosis and treatment. *Cognitive and Behavioral Practice, 22*(1), 20–35.

Index

Note. f or *t* after a page number indicates a figure or a table.